AGE AND GENDER CONSIDERATIONS IN PSYCHIATRIC DIAGNOSIS

A Research Agenda for DSM-V

AGE AND GENDER CONSIDERATIONS IN PSYCHIATRIC DIAGNOSIS

Edited by

William E. Narrow, M.D., M.P.H.
Michael B. First, M.D.
Paul J. Sirovatka, M.S.
Darrel A. Regier, M.D., M.P.H.

Published by the
American Psychiatric Association
Arlington, Virginia

Note: The authors have worked to ensure that all information in this book is accurate at the time of publication and consistent with general psychiatric and medical standards, and that information concerning drug dosages, schedules, and routes of administration is accurate at the time of publication and consistent with standards set by the U.S. Food and Drug Administration and the general medical community. As medical research and practice continue to advance, however, therapeutic standards may change. Moreover, specific situations may require a specific therapeutic response not included in this book. For these reasons and because human and mechanical errors sometimes occur, we recommend that readers follow the advice of physicians directly involved in their care or the care of a member of their family.

The findings, opinions, and conclusions of this report do not necessarily represent the views of the officers, trustees, or all members of the American Psychiatric Association. The views expressed are those of the authors of the individual chapters.

Manufactured in China by Everbest Printing Company through Four Colour Imports, Ltd.
11 10 09 08 07 5 4 3 2 1
First Edition

Typeset in Adobe's Frutiger and AGaramond.

American Psychiatric Publishing, Inc.
1000 Wilson Boulevard
Arlington, VA 22209-3901
www.appi.org

Library of Congress Cataloging-in-Publication Data
Age and gender considerations in psychiatric diagnosis : a research agenda for DSM-V / edited by William E. Narrow... [et al.].—1st ed.
p. ; cm.
Includes bibliographical references and index.
ISBN 978-0-89042-295-3 (pbk. : alk. paper) 1. Mental illness—Sex factors. 2. Mental illness—Age factors. 3. Mental illness—Diagnosis. 4. Diagnostic and statistical manual of mental disorders. I. Narrow, William E., 1957–
[DNLM: 1. Diagnostic and statistical manual of mental disorders. 5th ed. 2. Diagnostic and statistical manual of mental disorders. 5th ed. 3. Mental Disorders—diagnosis. 4. Age Factors. 5. Research. 6. Sex Factors. WM 141 A265 2007]
RC455.4.S45A34 2007
616.89'075—dc22

2007018817

British Library Cataloguing in Publication Data
A CIP record is available from the British Library.

CONTENTS

CONTRIBUTORS ix
PREFACE xv
ACKNOWLEDGMENTS xix

PART I
Sex/Gender

1 INTRODUCTION 3
Katharine A. Phillips, M.D., and Michael B. First, M.D.

2 WHY GENDER MATTERS 7
Katherine L. Wisner, M.D., M.S., and Regina Dolan-Sewell, Ph.D.

3 DSM'S APPROACH TO GENDER: History and Controversies 19
Thomas A. Widiger, Ph.D.

4 GENDER AND THE PREVALENCE OF PSYCHIATRIC DISORDERS 31
Bridget F. Grant, Ph.D., Ph.D., and Myrna M. Weissman, Ph.D.

5 NEUROBIOLOGY AND SEX/GENDER 47
Margaret Altemus, M.D.

6 SOCIOCULTURAL FACTORS AND GENDER 65
Katherine Shear, M.D., Katherine A. Halmi, M.D.,
Thomas A. Widiger, Ph.D., and Cheryl Boyce, Ph.D.

7 A DEVELOPMENTAL PERSPECTIVE, WITH A FOCUS ON CHILDHOOD TRAUMA 81
Adrian Angold, M.B., MRCPsych, and
Christine Marcelle Heim, Ph.D.

8 THE LONGITUDINAL LABORATORY OF WOMEN'S REPRODUCTIVE HEALTH 101
Katherine L. Wisner, M.D., M.S.

9 CLINICAL VALIDATORS OF DIAGNOSES:
Symptom Expression, Course, and Treatment. 113
Kimberly A. Yonkers, M.D., William E. Narrow, M.D., M.P.H., and Katherine A. Halmi, M.D.

10 GENDER AND DIAGNOSTIC CRITERIA. 127
Thomas A. Widiger, Ph.D., and Michael B. First, M.D.

11 CONCLUDING THOUGHTS 139
Katharine A. Phillips, M.D., and Michael B. First, M.D.

PART II
Early Childhood

12 DIAGNOSIS OF PSYCHOPATHOLOGY IN INFANTS, TODDLERS, AND PRESCHOOL CHILDREN 145
Irene Chatoor, M.D., Daniel S. Pine, M.D., and William E. Narrow, M.D., M.P.H.

13 A RESEARCH AGENDA FOR POSTTRAUMATIC STRESS DISORDER IN INFANTS, TODDLERS, AND PRESCHOOL CHILDREN. 151
Michael S. Scheeringa, M.D., M.P.H.

14 REACTIVE ATTACHMENT DISORDER. 163
Charles H. Zeanah Jr., M.D.

15 MEASUREMENT OF PSYCHOPATHOLOGY IN CHILDREN UNDER THE AGE OF SIX. 177
Adrian Angold, M.B., MRCPsych, Helen Link Egger, M.D., and Alice Carter, Ph.D.

16 NOSOLOGY OF MOOD DISORDERS IN PRESCHOOL CHILDREN:
State of Knowledge and Future Directions. 191
Joan L. Luby, M.D.

17 DIAGNOSIS OF ANXIETY DISORDERS IN INFANTS, TODDLERS, AND PRESCHOOL CHILDREN 201
Susan L. Warren, M.D.

18 CLASSIFYING SLEEP DISORDERS IN INFANTS AND TODDLERS. 215
Thomas F. Anders, M.D., and Ronald Dahl, M.D.

19 CLASSIFYING FEEDING DISORDERS OF INFANCY AND EARLY CHILDHOOD 227
Irene Chatoor, M.D., and Massimo Ammaniti, M.D.

20 DISRUPTIVE BEHAVIOR DISORDERS AND ADHD IN PRESCHOOL CHILDREN: Characterizing Heterotypic Continuities for a Developmentally Informed Nosology for DSM-V 243
Lauren S. Wakschlag, Ph.D., Bennett L. Leventhal, M.D., Jean Thomas, M.D., and Daniel S. Pine, M.D.

21 DIAGNOSIS OF AUTISM AND RELATED DISORDERS IN INFANTS AND VERY YOUNG CHILDREN: Setting a Research Agenda for DSM-V . . . 259
Fred Volkmar, M.D., Kasia Chawarska, Ph.D., Alice Carter, Ph.D., and Catherine Lord, Ph.D.

PART III
The Elderly

22 AGING-RELATED DIAGNOSTIC VARIATIONS: Need for Diagnostic Criteria Appropriate for Elderly Psychiatric Patients 273
Dilip V. Jeste, M.D., Dan G. Blazer, M.D., M.P.H., Ph.D., and Michael B. First, M.D.

23 LATE-LIFE DEPRESSION: A Model for Medical Classification 289
George S. Alexopoulos, M.D., Susan K. Schultz, M.D., and Barry D. Lebowitz, Ph.D.

24 CHALLENGES OF DIAGNOSING PSYCHIATRIC DISORDERS IN MEDICALLY ILL PATIENTS 305
Ira Katz, M.D., Ph.D., and Linda Ganzini, M.D., M.P.H.

25 USE OF BIOMARKERS IN THE ELDERLY: Current and Future Challenges 317
Trey Sunderland, M.D., Raquel E. Gur, M.D., Ph.D., and Steven E. Arnold, M.D.

26 IMPACT OF PSYCHOSOCIAL FACTORS ON LATE-LIFE DEPRESSION 329
Patricia A. Areán, Ph.D., and Charles F. Reynolds III, M.D.

INDEX 343

CONTRIBUTORS

Margaret Altemus, M.D.
Associate Professor, Cornell University Medical Center, New York, New York

Massimo Ammaniti, MD.
Professor of Developmental Psychopathology, Department of Dynamic and Clinical Psychology, University of Rome "La Sapienza," Rome, Italy

Thomas F. Anders, M.D.
Distinguished Professor (Emeritus), Department of Psychiatry, University of California Davis Medical Center, Sacramento, California

Adrian Angold, M.B., MRCPsych
Associate Professor, Department of Psychiatry and Behavioral Sciences, Duke University, Durham, North Carolina

Patricia A. Areán, Ph.D.
Associate Professor, Department of Psychiatry University of California, San Francisco

Steven E. Arnold, M.D.
Director, Geriatric Psychiatry and Cellular and Molecular Neuropathology Programs, Center for Neurobiology and Behavior; Associate Professor of Psychiatry, Department of Psychiatry, University of Pennsylvania, Philadelphia, Pennsylvania

George S. Alexopoulos, M.D.
Professor of Psychiatry, Weill Medical College of Cornell University, White Plains, New York

Dan G. Blazer, M.D., M.P.H., Ph.D.
J.P. Gibbons Professor of Psychiatry, Department of Psychiatry and Behavioral Sciences, Duke University Medical Center, Durham, North Carolina

Cheryl Boyce, Ph.D.
National Institute of Mental Health, National Institutes of Health, Bethesda, Maryland

Alice Carter, Ph.D.
Professor of Psychology, Department of Psychology, University of Massachusetts Boston, Boston, Massachusetts

Irene Chatoor, M.D.
Professor of Psychiatry and Behavioral Sciences and of Pediatrics, The George Washington University; Director, Infant and Toddler Mental Health Program, and Vice Chair, Department of Psychiatry, Children's National Medical Center, Washington, D.C.

Kasia Chawarska, Ph.D.
Assistant Professor, Child Study Center, University of Connecticut, Storrs, Connecticut

Ronald Dahl, M.D.
Staunton Professor of Psychiatry and Pediatrics, Department of Psychiatry, Western Psychiatric Institute and Clinic, University of Pittsburgh, Pittsburgh, Pennsylvania

Regina Dolan-Sewell, Ph.D.
Chief, Mood, Anxiety, and Regulatory Disorders Program (Retired), Division of Mental Disorders, Behavioral Research and AIDS, National Institute of Mental Health, Bethesda, Maryland

Helen Link Egger, M.D.
Assistant Professor, Department of Psychiatry and Behavioral Sciences, Duke University Medical Center, Durham, North Carolina

Michael B. First, M.D.
Professor of Clinical Psychiatry, Columbia University, New York State Psychiatric Institute, New York, New York

Linda Ganzini, M.D., M.P.H.
Director, Columbia Center for the Study of Chronic, Comorbid Mental and Physical Disorders, Portland Veterans Administration Medical Center, Portland, Oregon

Bridget F. Grant, Ph.D., Ph.D.
Chief, Laboratory of Epidemiology and Biometry, Division of Intramural Clinical and Biological Research, National Institute on Alcohol Abuse and Alcoholism, National Institutes of Health, Rockville, Maryland

Raquel E. Gur, M.D., Ph.D.
Professor of Psychiatry, Department of Psychiatry, University of Pennsylvania, Philadelphia, Pennsylvania

Katherine A. Halmi, M.D.
Director, Eating Disorders Program, Cornell Medical Center, New York Hospital, White Plains, New York

Christine Marcelle Heim, Ph.D.
Assistant Professor, Department of Psychiatry and Behavioral Sciences, Emory University, Atlanta, Georgia

Dilip V. Jeste, M.D.
Estelle and Edgar Levi Chair in Aging; Director, Sam and Rose Stein Institute for Research on Aging, and Distinguished Professor of Psychiatry and Neurosciences, University of California, San Diego, San Diego, California.

Ira Katz, M.D., Ph.D.
Professor of Geriatric Psychiatry, University of Pennsylvania, Philadelphia, Pennsylvania

Barry D. Lebowitz, Ph.D.
Deputy Director, The Sam and Rose Stein Institute for Research on Aging, University of California, San Diego, School of Medicine, La Jolla, California

Bennett L. Leventhal, M.D.
Institute for Juvenile Research, Department of Psychiatry, University of Illinois at Chicago, Chicago, Illinois

Catherine Lord, Ph.D.
Director, University of Michigan Autism and Communication Disorders Center (UMACC), Professor of Psychology and Psychiatry, Research Professor, Center for Human Growth and Development (CHGD), Ann Arbor, Michigan

Joan L. Luby, M.D.
Associate Professor of Psychiatry (Child), Washington University School of Medicine, St. Louis, Missouri

William E. Narrow, M.D., M.P.H.
Deputy Director of the American Psychiatric Institute for Research and Education and the Division of Research, American Psychiatric Association, Arlington, Virginia

Katharine A. Phillips, M.D.
Professor of Psychiatry and Human Behavior, Butler Hospital and Brown University School of Medicine, Providence, Rhode Island

Daniel S. Pine, M.D.
Chief of Developmental Studies, Mood and Anxiety Disorders Program, Chief, Section on Development and Affective Neuroscience, National Institute of Mental Health, National Institutes of Health, Bethesda, Maryland

Charles F. Reynolds III, M.D.
UPMC Endowed Chair in Geriatric Psychiatry and Professor of Psychiatry, Neurology, and Neuroscience, Intervention Research Center for Late Life Mood Disorders, Western Psychiatric Institute and Clinic, University of Pittsburgh School of Medicine, Pittsburgh, Pennsylvania

Michael S. Scheeringa, M.D., M.P.H.
Professor, Department of Psychiatry and Neurology, Tulane University Medical School, New Orleans, Louisiana,

Susan K. Schultz, M.D.
Associate Professor, Department of Psychiatry, University of Iowa College of Medicine, Iowa City, Iowa

Katherine Shear, M.D.
Marion E. Kenworthy Professor of Psychiatry, Columbia University School of Social Work, Columbia College of Physicians and Surgeons, New York, New York

Trey Sunderland, M.D.
Chevy Chase, Maryland

Jean Thomas, M.D.
Co-Director, Infant and Toddler Mental Health Program, Department of Psychiatry and Behavioral Sciences, The George Washington University School of Medicine and Children's National Medical Center, Washington, DC

Fred Volkmar, M.D.
Director, Yale Child Study Center, and Irving B. Harris Professor of Child Psychiatry, Pediatrics and Psychology, Yale University School of Medicine, New Haven, Connecticut

Lauren S. Wakschlag, Ph.D.
Institute for Juvenile Research, Department of Psychiatry, University of Illinois at Chicago, Chicago, Illinois

Susan L. Warren, M.D.
Associate Professor, Department of Psychiatry, The George Washington University, Washington, DC

Myrna M. Weissman, Ph.D.
Professor of Epidemiology in Psychiatry and Chief, Division of Clinical and Genetic Epidemiology, College of Physicians and Surgeons, Columbia University, and New York State Psychiatric Institute, New York, New York

Thomas A. Widiger, Ph.D.
Professor, University of Kentucky, Department of Psychology, Lexington, Kentucky

Katherine L. Wisner, M.D., M.S.
Professor of Psychiatry, Obstetrics and Gynecology and Reproductive Sciences, and Epidemiology, and Director, Women's Behavioral HealthCARE, Western Psychiatric Institute and Clinic, University of Pittsburgh School of Medicine, Pittsburgh, Pennsylvania

Kimberly Ann Yonkers, M.D.
Associate Professor, Departments of Psychiatry and Obstetrics and Gynecology in Reproductive Sciences, Yale University, New Haven, Connecticut

Charles H. Zeanah Jr., M.D.
Sellars-Polchow Professor of Psychiatry and Professor of Clinical Pediatrics; Director of Child and Adolescent Psychiatry; Vice Chair, Department of Psychiatry and Neurology; Executive Director, Institute of Infant and Early Childhood Mental Health, Tulane University Health Sciences Center, New Orleans, Louisiana

PREFACE

Publication of *Age and Gender Considerations in Psychiatric Diagnosis: A Research Agenda for DSM-V* coincides with the early phases of work on the *Diagnostic and Statistical Manual of Mental Disorders,* 5th Edition (DSM-V), slated for completion in 2011. Rather than being part of the official DSM-V revision process, this monograph is a continuation of the most extensive state-of-the-science assessment and research planning initiative that the American Psychiatric Association (APA) has undertaken in anticipation of any edition of DSM. In the short-term future, this monograph will serve as a valuable source document for the DSM-V Task Force and its disorder-specific workgroups. Over the longer term, we anticipate that the identification of gaps in our knowledge and specific research recommendations to address those gaps will guide funding agencies and independent investigators in the support and conduct of studies that will contribute to revised psychiatric classifications farther into the future.

The approximately 17-year interval between publication of DSM-IV (American Psychiatric Association 1994) and DSM-V has been an immensely scientifically productive era in psychiatry. Numerous factors have contributed to this energy. Beginning in the 1990s, the "decade of the brain" directed public attention to the prevalence and toll of mental disorders and greatly stimulated the contributions of researchers in diverse fields of biological and behavioral science to the study of these disorders. Between 1999 and 2004, the doubling of the National Institutes of Health budget allowed the National Institute of Mental Health (NIMH), the National Institute on Drug Abuse (NIDA), and the National Institute on Alcohol Abuse and Alcoholism (NIAAA) to more effectively mine a rich array of scientific leads to better understand, treat, and prevent mental and substance use disorders. Among the scientific developments that held the potential for significant refinements in future psychiatric classification systems have been the accelerating search for biological markers of mental disorders; the availability of a completed draft of the human genome and haplotype maps; advances in behavioral phenotyping; new statistical methodologies and software that increase the feasibility of incorporating a dimensional component into psychiatric diagnoses; and appreciation of the critical importance of developmental perspectives in research on mental disorders and mental health.

With greater emphasis assigned to clinical and translational research, patient groups encouraged funding agencies to stiffen requirements for appropriate representation in clinical trials of women of childbearing age who previously often had been excluded from such studies. Insights gained from the involvement of women often raised new questions to be addressed at the preclinical level. Yet another factor contributing to productivity—and to the timeliness of this monograph—has been the increasing globalization of psychiatric research capacities and resources. In addition to expanding the critical mass of investigators in diverse scientific areas, the growing involvement of all regions and most countries of the world in mental illness research has underscored the critical role of gender in diagnosis as well as in the experience of illness, health, and aging across the life span.

Recognizing the potential of these activities to inform psychiatric classification systems, the leadership of the APA and the NIMH agreed in 1999 to support an extended effort to develop a research agenda that would address diagnostic issues. This collaboration led to the convening of six workgroups that were charged with developing white papers on the following topics: basic nomenclature issues, neuroscience, developmental considerations, personality disorders and relational disorders, mental disorders and disability, and culture and psychiatric diagnosis. In facilitating integration of findings from genetics, neuroscience, epidemiology, neuroimaging, animal studies, behavioral research, and other research areas, the papers recommended strategies for achieving key goals for the next revision of the DSM; these included a greater emphasis on validity, progress toward a classification based on pathogenesis, and a public health perspective, including focused attention on critical populations and issues. These white papers were published in *A Research Agenda for DSM-V* (Kupfer et al. 2002).

Following publication of the first research agenda volume, three critical areas were recognized by APA membership and staff as needing further examination. In response, the APA's Committee on Psychiatric Diagnosis and Assessment commissioned additional white papers to cover diagnostic issues as they related to gender and to the age groups at each end of the life span—that is, infancy/young childhood and old age. Again, three workgroups were formed to conduct more extensive literature reviews in each of these focused areas and to develop research agendas. The workgroup on gender was co-chaired by Katharine Phillips, M.D., of Brown University and Michael First, M.D., of Columbia University; the group on geriatrics was chaired by Dilip Jeste, M.D., of the University of California at San Diego; and the group on infancy/young childhood was co-chaired by Irene Chatoor, M.D., of The George Washington University, and Daniel Pine, M.D., of the NIMH. Meeting regularly through conference calls (and for the gender and infant/young child groups, a face-to-face meeting), the workgroup members developed outlines that would address a range of issues and assigned specific topics to experts in a given area. These individual sections were integrated into single drafts, which were circulated to the entire group and to consultants and reviewers outside the groups.

The three sections of this monograph represent areas of psychiatric research that have historically been neglected but have rightfully received increasing attention in recent years. Evidence from epidemiological studies has pointed to significant gender differences in prevalence, symptom profiles, and risk factors for mental and substance use disorders. Research in gender differences has progressed beyond female hormonal explanations to more sophisticated investigations that suggest neurodevelopmental, neurophysiological, and environmental factors at play for both males and females.

Not so long ago, dementia was considered to be a normal, if not desirable, consequence of senescence, and depression in the elderly was seen as a normal reaction to end-of-life issues. It is now virtually undisputed that brain development continues well beyond early adulthood, as does psychosocial development, and that mental disorders in the elderly represent disordered rather than normative states. These disorders are now seen as worthy of investigation into their clinical features, etiology, and course, which indicates great hope for improved diagnostic criteria and future prevention and treatment initiatives.

Mental disorders in childhood present one of the greatest challenges for psychiatric research. There has been widespread dissatisfaction with the DSM-IV criteria from researchers and clinicians who work with children and adolescents. For infants and young children, there is even more doubt as to whether mental disorders are adequately described, and there is probably widespread public skepticism that children in this age group can even develop mental disorders, particularly preverbal infants. This situation has led to a growing number of researchers investigating infant and young childhood disorders and developing new or modified diagnostic criteria based on clinical samples. With an increasingly recognized research base, longitudinal clinical and epidemiological research should follow.

The work of the age and gender workgroups on the development of a wide-ranging research agenda in these areas has paralleled another, more focused research planning effort led by APA in collaboration with the World Health Organization (WHO) and the National Institutes of Health. In 2003, APA's American Psychiatric Institute for Research and Education (APIRE) was awarded a cooperative research planning conference grant to drill deeper into the research agenda–setting process initiated with the white papers. With joint funding from NIMH, NIDA, and NIAAA, this 5-year project entails a series of 12 international conferences, each of which is focusing on a particular diagnosis or cluster of diagnoses that warrant closer examination due to scientific advances or dissatisfaction with current approaches. Each conference has two co-chairs, one selected from the U.S. psychiatric research community and one from another country. Scientists invited to participate in each conference represent all regions of the world; midway through the project, 47% of conference workgroup members have been from outside the United States. The emphasis on international involvement in the project reflects the mutual interests of APA and the WHO in developing optimally compatible future editions of both DSM and the *International Classification of Diseases*' "Mental and Behavioral Disorders" section. We are particularly pleased that several of the authors who have contributed papers to this monograph also have participated in one or more of the research conference workgroups, where they have been well positioned to advocate for appropriate attention to the issues identified here.

The authors and editors hope that these white papers will help to underscore the considerable gaps in our knowledge in these three areas and to stimulate the needed research to help fill these gaps. Ultimately, such research is likely to have an important impact on future diagnostic systems and, in turn, help in increasing our understanding of the causes of mental disorders and in the development of effective preventative and treatment interventions for our patients, our families, and our communities.

William E. Narrow, M.D., M.P.H.

References

American Psychiatric Association: Diagnostic and Statistical Manual of Mental Disorders, 4th Edition. Washington, DC, American Psychiatric Association, 1994

Kupfer DJ, First MB, Regier DA (eds): A Research Agenda for DSM-V. Washington, DC, American Psychiatric Association, 2002

ACKNOWLEDGMENTS

We would like to acknowledge the scientific contributions to this book made by David J. Kupfer, M.D., former chair of the American Psychiatric Association's Committee on Psychiatric Diagnosis and Assessment, and the invaluable editorial and administrative contributions made by the following staff members of the American Psychiatric Association: Jennifer Shupinka, Kristin Edwards, and Liz McCartney.

PART I

SEX/GENDER

1

INTRODUCTION

Katharine A. Phillips, M.D.
Michael B. First, M.D.

Gender is a window to understanding mental illness. In two recent, groundbreaking reports, the Institute of Medicine emphasized the importance of sex/gender in understanding disease. Gender may affect virtually all aspects of psychopathology, including the prevalence of mental disorders, how symptoms are expressed, course of illness, whether patients seek treatment, and whether patients improve with treatment. For example, women are twice as likely as men to be depressed, but they may respond better than men to certain serotonin reuptake inhibitors. Women with bipolar disorder are more likely to have a rapid-cycling pattern. Women are more likely to be exposed to some environmental "toxins" that may influence the development of illness (e.g., sexual abuse), whereas men are more likely to be exposed to others (e.g., physical abuse). Increasingly, research is elucidating intriguing neurobiological differences between men and women that likely interact in complex ways with sociocultural factors to produce mental illness.

Much more research is needed, however, to elucidate the complex relationship between gender and psychopathology. This field, as important as it is, is still surprisingly nascent. Indeed, the Institute of Medicine report called on medical researchers to incorporate sex and gender into all research at its inception. In particular, this report underscored the need to expand research on sex differences in brain organization and function, monitor sex differences and similarities for disorders that affect both sexes, conduct additional research on sex differences, and encourage and support interdisciplinary research on sex differences.

The purpose of Part I of this book is to extend the work represented in *A Research Agenda for DSM-V* (Kupfer et al. 2002), published in 2002, into the critically important domain of sex and gender. These monographs are part of the initial phase of the research planning process for the upcoming revision of DSM-V, which is slated to formally begin in 2007. *A Research Agenda for DSM-V* consisted of six white papers that focused on nomenclature, neuroscience and genetics, developmental science, gaps in DSM-IV (personality and relational disorders), disability, and culture. These publications were developed under a partnership between the American Psychiatric Association and the National Institute of Mental Health, National Institute on Alcohol Abuse and Alcoholism, and the National Institute on Drug Abuse. Their purpose was to provide direction for and to stimulate research that will provide an improved scientific basis for future diagnostic classifications.

After the initial six papers were published, three additional white papers were developed, one of which is the white paper focusing on gender issues represented by the chapters in Part I of this book. Although the initial papers included brief sections touching on gender issues, the burgeoning research base in this area justified a more extensive review and the development of a specific research agenda.

The purpose of the chapters in the present book is the same as that of previous white papers:

1. To stimulate research that could enrich the empirical database in preparation for the revision of DSM-V and ICD-11 as well as future editions of the DSM and ICD; and
2. To suggest future research directions that will improve our understanding of the role of gender in the development, course, and outcome of psychopathology.

We also reexamine some of the perspectives covered in the six published white papers to ensure that the role of gender is adequately included (e.g., neurobiological aspects of gender and their relationship to psychopathology). We wish to emphasize that the committee that produced the contributions to the present volume was not an official part of the DSM-V revision process, because it convened prior to the formal start of DSM-V. Therefore, this volume does not contain any specific recommendations about changes in the DSM-IV diagnostic criteria. Rather, our purpose is to review the existing knowledge base to identify deficiencies and to suggest research directions that will inform future editions of DSM.

This review and our research recommendations are not intended to be comprehensive because the field of gender research has blossomed, especially in recent years, and is enormous in scope. It is not possible to comprehensively address all aspects of sex and gender and their relationship to psychopathology. Nor is it possible to address gender as it specifically pertains to each of the hundreds of disorders in DSM-IV. Rather, we approach our review and recommendations from several fundamental perspectives (e.g., neurobiological, sociocultural, developmental) that cut across diagnostic categories.

In the chapters that follow we begin by addressing the critical importance of gender to illness more generally and to psychopathology in particular. We then discuss DSM's approach to gender to date, highlighting both advantages and limitations of its approach. We review some relevant research findings on gender, identify gaps in this research and in our knowledge, and propose some of the research that is needed to fill those gaps. This review and proposed research agenda is organized around the following perspectives: 1) epidemiology, 2) etiology and pathophysiology of disorders (from both neurobiological and sociocultural perspectives), and 3) gender-related expression of psychopathology. The last category includes a life span/developmental perspective, reproductive behavior and events, a clinical perspective (e.g., course of illness and treatment response), and diagnostic criteria issues that are especially pertinent to gender (such as whether DSM should include gender-specific diagnostic criteria).

As is discussed throughout this book, it is remarkable how far gender research has come. We now know so much more than we did a decade or two ago about gender and how it impacts and shapes psychopathology. At the same time, we have much to learn. Psychiatry has recently entered an exciting era of discoveries about the brain and what causes psychiatric disorders, including the critically important role that gender plays in how psychiatric illness develops and presents. Future editions of DSM are likely to reflect disorders' etiologies and pathophysiology, once these are elucidated. Such an approach will likely more usefully guide the treatment and prevention of disease than does our current descriptive syndrome-based approach. Our current diagnostic system is largely descriptive—that is, based on the way mental disorders present rather than their underlying cause. To use an analogy from medicine, knowing that shigella, rather than cancer, is causing a patient's fever enables use of a specific antibiotic to effectively treat the fever. Therefore, in anticipation of this eventual paradigm shift, several chapters of this volume focus on gender-related aspects of illness etiology and pathophysiology (neurobiological factors and sociocultural/environmental factors). We realize that some of this research may not be directly relevant to DSM-V, because many years of work will be needed to elucidate complex pathoetiologic mechanisms of illness and translate them into changes in DSM's overall structure and definitions of disorders. Nonetheless, such research will enormously increase our understanding of psychopathology and will undoubtedly lead to changes—perhaps radical changes—in DSM in the more distant future. This book also addresses topics that are more directly relevant to clinical practice today and to changes for DSM-V. For example, we include chapters on the relationship of gender to symptom expression, treatment response, and course of illness.

In a broad sense, researchers can shed light on gender-related aspects of psychopathology using approaches such as 1) conducting new gender-focused studies, 2) including a gender component in future non-gender-focused studies, and 3) doing secondary analyses of existing data sets, examining the relationship of gender to other variables.

In this volume, we have taken both a short- and a long-term perspective. It is likely that many of our research recommendations (e.g., those that involve conducting new gender-focused studies or elucidating disorders' underlying etiology) will not bear fruit until DSM-VI or later, given that studies often take years, if not decades, to go from initial conception to publication of results in peer-reviewed journals. In addition, we aim to have a broad vision for the directions that future gender research might take—a vision that anticipates future paradigm shifts in our field and is not constrained by the limitations of our current categorical descriptive diagnostic system.

We hope that the discussions in this book will fuel new ideas and fruitful discussion about the directions that future gender research might take. We also hope that they will stimulate actual research. Gender-focused research is greatly needed to shed light on the causes of mental illness and to improve the validity of future editions of DSM. This work is also critically important for increasing clinical understanding of mental illness, developing more effective treatments, and ultimately preventing these common and often disabling disorders.

Reference

Kupfer DJ, First MB, Regier DA (eds): A Research Agenda for DSM-V. Washington, DC, American Psychiatric Association, 2002

2

WHY GENDER MATTERS

Katherine L. Wisner, M.D., M.S.
Regina Dolan-Sewell, Ph.D.

Importance of Gender in Illness and Psychopathology

The query in the title of the Institute of Medicine (IOM) report *Exploring the Biological Contributions to Human Health: Does Sex Matter?* (Institute of Medicine 2001) is answered in the authors' work with a bold statement: *sex matters at the cellular level.* In this report and a thematically related report (Institute of Medicine 1998), the IOM evaluated the biology of sex and gender differences. Recommendations from the executive summary included 1) expanding research on sex differences in brain organization and function, 2) monitoring sex differences and similarities for all human diseases that affect both sexes, 3) supporting and conducting additional research on sex differences, 4) encouraging and supporting interdisciplinary research on sex differences, and 5) reducing the potential for discrimination based on identified sex differences. These recommendations reflect a challenge to all medical fields to incorporate sex and gender into all research at its inception. The understanding of sex differences in health and illness merits serious scientific inquiry in all aspects of health research.

In an IOM report on gender susceptibility to environmental exposures (Institute of Medicine 1998), the authors emphasized that exposures to toxins (which include stress as well as chemical agents) and the physiological response to toxins are related to sex. In the development of approaches to disease prevention, health promotion, behavioral and medical interventions, and research strategies, consideration must be given to health effects that are either sex specific or overrepresented in women or men. Environmental factors such as occupation, behavior, lifestyle, hobbies, reproductive status, or physical activity are affected by gender and have a major impact on health status. Women's exposures tend to differ from those of men in the home and work setting and during childbearing, childrearing, and caretaking of elders. Exposures occur across the life span, are cumulative, and are likely to affect health. As acute toxic exposures with marked effects are eliminated, chronic low-level exposures become more important in affecting health outcomes. An example that has received attention in psychiatric research is chronic stress, its physiological sequelae, and the association of stress with the development of mood and other psychiatric disorders. Sex-specific differential susceptibility to environmental factors must also be included in etiological models of psychiatric disorders.

The IOM also promoted a broad genetic–environmental model of disease development and urged researchers to use sex-focused analyses to promote hypothesis development and to establish comparative risks for diseases in men and women. Variations in disease expression between the sexes are a rich source of information about gender similarities and differences that provide critical details about physiological disease processes at the cellular level (Kupfer et al. 2002). In their chapter in *A Research Agenda for DSM-V,* Alarcón et al. (2002) recommended that investigators consider a framework for examining sex, gender, and culture in their research. Investigators must ask how knowledge about the questions they are examining can be maximized by considering these important variables. Every type of study domain (interpretive/explanatory, pathogenic/pathoplastic, diagnostic/nosologic, therapeutic/protective, and management/services) will be enriched by including such analyses (Alarcón et al. 2002). Both sexes will benefit, and our diagnostic system will improve. Every aspect of disease phenomenology in a population—including environmental toxin exposures, vulnerability to disorders, symptomatology, characteristics of symptom expression, natural history, treatment choice, treatment response, social support, and functional capacity—may be affected by sex (Alarcón et al. 2002). Examining and elucidating variables related to disease expression offers a rich opportunity for hypothesis generation, testing, and new knowledge in psychiatry. The benefits of sex-specific analyses provide immense potential for improved conceptual models and therapies across our entire field (Wisner 2004).

Are We Attending to Sex and Gender in Mental Health Research?

As psychiatrists, are we attending to sex and gender variables in our research? One measure of this is the number of scientific publications related to these domains. Table 2–1 was generated from a search of MedLine through 2003, using the terms *sex* and *gender* for the following selected topics: psychiatry, depression, bipolar disorder, schizophrenia, and anxiety. Only English documents related to human stud-

TABLE 2–1. Sex and gender in psychiatry and disorders by year

Years	Gender and psychiatry	Sex and psychiatry	Gender and depression	Sex and depression	Gender and bipolar disorder	Sex and bipolar disorder	Gender and schizophrenia	Sex and schizophrenia	Gender and anxiety	Sex and anxiety	Total for all categories
1990	9	22	65	126	11	20	35	61	27	69	445
1991	7	10	65	140	3	20	16	49	40	63	413
1992	12	15	87	121	14	20	55	60	50	68	502
1993	8	10	102	109	15	14	52	55	58	71	494
1994	13	9	117	133	10	18	54	75	59	49	537
1995	14	14	147	138	10	12	51	74	73	69	602
1996	18	10	154	162	16	23	65	55	76	109	688
1997	17	18	187	169	16	13	66	79	91	102	758
1998	15	18	184	181	25	17	67	84	108	90	789
1999	22	23	246	183	34	28	81	90	124	102	933
2000	24	27	254	202	37	22	91	92	142	147	1,038
2001	17	11	320	239	30	31	101	83	170	124	1,126
2002	15	13	323	257	35	36	92	100	152	137	1,160
2003	26	13	370	289	40	36	125	118	195	155	1,367
2004	59	90	356	568	50	63	115	186	182	352	2,021
2005	63	104	474	703	70	94	146	209	245	405	2,513
2006	58	115	510	729	50	78	130	188	281	383	2,522

ies were included in the search. Note that the first IOM report was published in 1998 and the second in 2001. The mean number of publications in the post-IOM report epoch of 1999–2003 increased by 1.7 over the 5-year pre-IOM report epoch of 1994–1998. The greatest increases in gender-related publications occurred in the years 1999 (933–789 = 144), 2003 (1367–1160 = 207), 2004 (2021–1367 = 654), and 2005 (2513–2021 = 492). Thus, there is evidence of increased interest and scientific productivity in topics related to sex and gender in psychiatry and psychiatric disorders. Because many of the disorders that we treat occur at differential rates in men and women (see Chapter 4 in this volume, "Gender and the Prevalence of Psychiatric Disorders"), this increase is appropriate, and acceleration of publication rates is commendable.

New journals that focus on sex- and gender-specific effects have emerged. The *Journal of Gender-Specific Medicine* is the first journal to focus on exploring the impact of gender on normal physiology and on the pathophysiology of disease. The editor-in-chief, Marianne J. Legato, M.D., has recently joined a working group of biomedical journal editors to promote publication of original research in which gender is an important variable. A journal on men's health, *Journal of Men's Health and Gender,* was launched in 2004. These efforts, too, are likely to greatly advance research on sex and gender as they relate to illness.

How Are Sex and Gender Defined?

The authors of the IOM reports used the term *sex* to designate classification according to reproductive organs and chromosomal complement—that is, genetic and biological phenomena linked to having the XX or XY chromosomal complement. The reproductive hormonal milieu is an example of the distinction between males and females; however, the effects of sex extend far beyond the reproductive system. *Gender* is the term used to refer to a person's self-representation as male or female, or the psychosocial expression of living as a man or a woman. Gender is a proxy term for a highly complex set of biological, psychological, and behavioral processes. Research on gender and sex differences is often conducted as though they are the same, but the distinction is important. Sex differences that are highly correlated with cultural and socioeconomic variables have little relationship to biological differences between men and women. *Gender* is the term that captures this concept. For example, the earning power of American women remains substantially lower than that of men. This may affect women's health through multiple avenues, such as health care coverage, ability to access health care, and capacity to produce co-payments for treatment services.

The occurrence of two sexes is an experiment of nature and an opportunity to understand variability in the expression of diseases (Alarcón et al. 2002). In scientific inquiry, we seek to define and understand how populations differ from one another. The identified variables become targets of etiological hypotheses. We observe associations with gender in our work daily. When a patient with an eating disorder appears on our schedule, the assumption is that the person is female. If the patient is a male, why is he more likely than a female patient to have a severe course of illness? Why do boys have a greater likelihood than girls of developing attention-deficit/hyperactivity disorder and a learning disability? If we ask the questions, we can develop research approaches to answer them (Alarcón et al. 2002).

Sexual orientation is a related concept that is inconsistently defined across studies. There is a distinction between *sexual identity* (homosexual versus heterosexual), *sexual desire* (feelings), and *sexual behavior* (actions). An individual may define herself as a heterosexual but have sexual desire for women and be involved in sexual interactions with other women. Another individual may define herself as a lesbian and have sexual desire for women but sexual interactions only with men. Many combinations of sexual identity, desire, and behavior exist among individuals and may change over time for a particular individual. It is therefore necessary to be clear in our definitions and assessments of sexual orientation (Solarz 1999). We recognize the importance of sexual orientation as an important research arena in its own right, but this is a large topic, and in this chapter we focus on gender in psychiatry. Because sociocultural variables are prominent in mental health practice and research, the term *gender* is preferentially used in this chapter.

Gender Is Important in Nonpsychiatric Illness

Historically, from a physiological perspective women have been regarded as "small men." Research from male populations has been generalized to female populations without supporting data. The IOM reports provide a platform for widespread appreciation that the study of gender differences is a new approach to advance knowledge in all domains of health research. For example, women are 2.7 times more likely than men to develop autoimmune disorders (Jacobson et al. 1997). Women's enhanced immune systems promote resistance to infection but increase susceptibility to autoimmune disease (Yovel et al. 2000). Men also have higher levels of natural killer cell activity, which is associated with reduced frequency of autoimmune disease. Systemic lupus erythematosus primarily affects women of childbearing age and often decreases after menopause (Rider et al. 1998; van Vollenhoven et al. 1998). If we can elucidate the mechanisms that produce these gender differences, we can potentially improve the detection, treatment, and prevention of such illnesses (Greenstein 2001).

Cardiovascular disease is the leading cause of death in American women (Anderson et al. 2002). Specific cardiac arrhythmias such as atrial re-entrant tachycardias, drug-induced *torsades de pointes,* and long QT syndrome occur more frequently in women than men (Malloy and Bahinski 1999). Premenopausal women with cardiovascular risk factors are more likely to have a myocardial infarction during the late luteal phase, when estrogen levels are low (Hamelin 2000). Women are more likely to have subtle symptoms of heart attack, such as nausea, vomiting, fatigue, shortness of breath, dizziness, abdominal or mid-back pain, and indigestion, in addition to—or instead of—chest pain (Kyker and Limacher 2002). Investigators are clarifying the role of gonadal steroids and their interactions with other factors with respect to immune and cardiovascular function (Epperson et al. 1999). These studies may lead to the better identification of illness and the development of treatments that improve health outcomes for both genders. When gender-related mechanisms are understood, they will become a platform for modifying the expression of disease.

Gender Is Critically Important in Psychopathology

The burden of mental illness on health and productivity has not been recognized fully. Data from the Global Burden of Disease study conducted by the World Health Organization (Murray and Lopez 1996) revealed that mental illness accounts for more than 15% of the disease burden in established market economies (such as the United States). This is more than the disease burden inflicted by all cancers, and depression was second only to ischemic heart disease (Table 2–2). Depression is the leading cause of disability for women throughout the world. The lifetime risk of major depression in America has ranged from 10% to 25% for women. Nearly twice as many women (12%) as men (6.6%) have a depressive disorder each year. In established market economies, schizophrenia and bipolar disorder are also among the top 10 causes of disability-adjusted life years (DALYs) for women. DALYs allow comparison of the burden of disease across many different disease conditions by including both death and disability; the disability component of this measure is weighted for severity. Disability caused by major depression was found to be equivalent to that of blindness or paraplegia. In women, the leading cause of disease burden by the year 2020 is projected to be major depression (Figure 2–1) (U.S. Department of Health and Human Services 1999).

Why does depression occur at such high rates, particularly in women? The search for answers lies in the complicated fabric of etiological contributors (Wisner 2004). The modern view that many factors interact to produce disease is attributed to Engel (1977), who developed the biopsychosocial model of disease. The relative contributions of biological, psychological, and social factors vary across individuals and across phases of the life cycle. For example, in some individuals, depression occurs only in response to exposure to stressful life events, whereas in others depressive episodes occur without extraordinarily stressful stimuli (Matza et al. 2003). The burden of posttraumatic stress disorder (PTSD) in America is greater in women

TABLE 2–2. Leading sources of disease burden in established market economies, 1990

	Total (millions)[a]	Percentage of total
All causes	98.7	
1. Ischemic heart disease	8.9	9.0
2. Unipolar major depression	6.7	6.8
3. Cardiovascular disease	5.0	5.0
4. Alcohol use	4.7	4.7
5. Road traffic accidents	4.3	4.4
6. Lung and upper respiratory cancers	3.0	3.0
7. Dementia and degenerative CNS	2.9	2.9
8. Osteoarthritis	2.7	2.7
9. Diabetes	2.4	2.4
10. COPD	2.3	2.3

Note. CNS = central nervous system; COPD = chronic obstructive pulmonary disease.
[a]Measured in disability adjusted life years (lost years of healthy life regardless of whether the years were lost to premature death or disability).

than in men due to the greater effect of assaultive violence on women. Although the lifetime prevalence of traumatic events is higher in men than in women, the risk for PTSD after trauma has been shown to be twice as high in women as in men (Breslau 2002). One study found that after assault, the probability of PTSD in women and men was 36% and 6%, respectively. Prior exposure to assault was associated with an increased risk of PTSD from subsequent trauma, but the gender difference in vulnerability for PTSD was not explained solely by previous exposure.

The interaction of life stress and depression in the genesis of illness is complex. Recently, Caspi et al. (2003) found that the influence of life stress on depression was moderated by a gene-by-environment interaction. The serotonergic system has been examined for candidate genes for depression because of its central role in the pharmacological treatment of this disorder. The promoter region of the serotonin transporter gene displays short- and long-form alleles. The short-form allele has lower transcriptional efficiency of the promoter compared with the long form. For carriers of the short allele, stressful life events predicted a diagnosis of major depression; this was not shown for long-allele homozygotes. Stressful life events also predicted the occurrence of suicidal ideation and suicide attempt among individuals who carried the short-form allele but not among long-form homozygotes. Caspi et al. (2003) concluded that complex disorders may result from variations in a small number of genes whose effects are conditional upon exposure to environmental risks. Such risks may vary by gender.

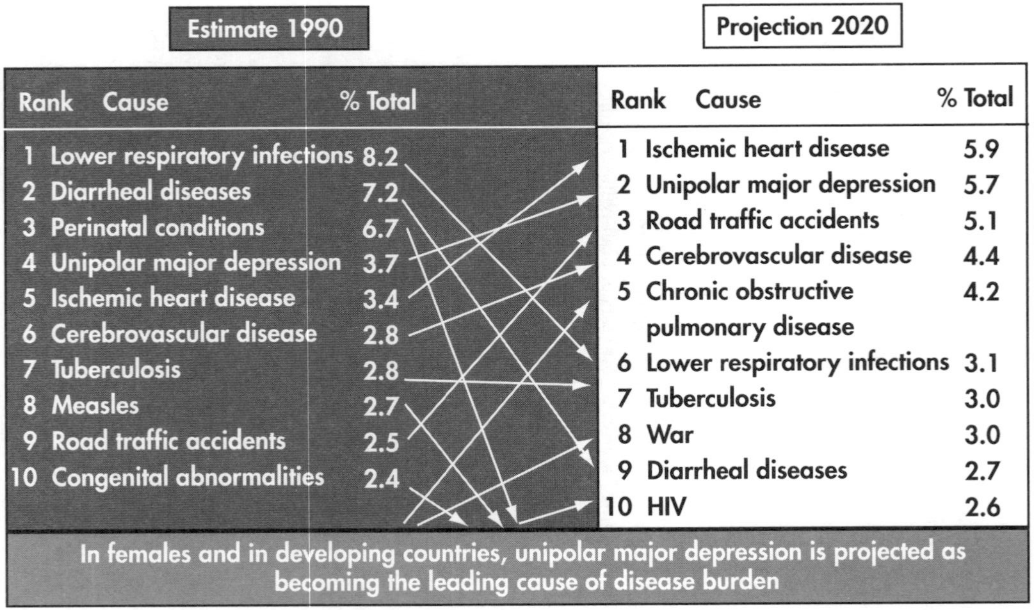

Estimate 1990
Rank Cause % Total
1 Lower respiratory infections 8.2
2 Diarrheal diseases 7.2
3 Perinatal conditions 6.7
4 Unipolar major depression 3.7
5 Ischemic heart disease 3.4
6 Cerebrovascular disease 2.8
7 Tuberculosis 2.8
8 Measles 2.7
9 Road traffic accidents 2.5
10 Congenital abnormalities 2.4
Projection 2020
Rank Cause % Total
1 Ischemic heart disease 5.9
2 Unipolar major depression 5.7
3 Road traffic accidents 5.1
4 Cerebrovascular disease 4.4
5 Chronic obstructive pulmonary disease 4.2
6 Lower respiratory infections 3.1
7 Tuberculosis 3.0
8 War 3.0
9 Diarrheal diseases 2.7
10 HIV 2.6
In females and in developing countries, unipolar major depression is projected as becoming the leading cause of disease burden

FIGURE 2–1. Disease burden measured in disability-adjusted life years (DALYs).

The Global Burden of Disease Web site is www.who.int/msa/mnh/ems/dalys/intro.htm.

Source. All material in this fact sheet is in the public domain and may be copied or reproduced without permission from the Institute. NIH Publication No. 01–4586.

A Suggested Research Approach

The life course epidemiology approach (Kuh et al. 2003) has evolved as a strategy to address the limitations of earlier etiological disease models, which focused on adult behaviors (e.g., smoking, diet) and their relationship to the onset and course of diseases (e.g., lung cancer, obesity). Biological and psychosocial factors act independently and interactively to influence health in adult life (Kuh et al. 2003). The effects of these forces are cumulative through time. A comprehensive epidemiological life course framework, as is applied to the "longitudinal laboratory of women's lives" (see Chapter 8, "The Longitudinal Laboratory of Women's Reproductive Health"), is required to meld the many etiological dimensions that interact. Time can be conceptualized as the horizontal longitudinal platform, with biopsychosocial interactions as vertical cross-sectional intersects. These processes operate across an individual's life course, or across generations, to influence health. The model promotes consideration and study of the contribution of early life factors jointly with later life influences to identify risk and protective processes across life. Factors such as genetic constitution, environmental insults, and support from individuals and institutions all need to be included to create a complex dynamic model of illness (and wellness) development. Designing studies, collecting data, and analyzing data in a way that incorporates this perspective is challenging. An example of such a study is investigating how exposures (e.g., lead, violence) during fetal life and childhood influence adult disease risk, mental health, and socioeconomic status, which in turn contribute to disparities in adult health and mortality. Such studies are enormously complex!

As a field, we have begun to appreciate and systematically assess the potential of gender-specific multimodal treatment plans for a variety of diagnoses. To use schizophrenia as an example, gender-specific treatment planning for patients with schizophrenia has been proposed convincingly (Seeman 2004) and provides a rich example of this approach. In women, symptoms more often involve depression, whereas men tend to exhibit more apathy, paucity of speech, disturbances in cognitive function, and social isolation (Usall et al. 2004). Although equal numbers of men and women develop schizophrenia, men experience symptoms earlier and have a worse prognosis than women. Such differences have implications for treatment as well as the classification and description of schizophrenia in future editions of DSM. Furthermore, the gender-specific features of schizophrenia suggest that factors that cause normal sex differences in the brain may be associated with the development of schizophrenia (Goldstein et al. 2002). For example, estrogen (17-beta-estradiol) appears to have a neuroprotective effect (Rao and Kolsch 2003), and decreases in estrogen levels at menopause may be related to the second peak of schizophrenia onset observed in women after age 50 (Seeman 2004).

Women with schizophrenia tend to respond to treatment differently than men (Seeman 2004). Because women report more mood symptoms, they often require a more complicated treatment regimen with both antidepressants and antipsychotics. Women often require lower dosages of medication and less frequent depot neuroleptic doses, develop higher prolactin levels with antipsychotic treatment, and more frequently develop obesity (Blaak 2001). The frequency of serious side effects, especially prolongation of the QT interval and the occurrence of arrhythmias, is greater. Integration of increased medical risks of both the disorder and its treatment with a care plan that includes sexuality/contraception counseling, bone density assessment, electrocardiographic monitoring, weight management, pregnancy and lactation treatment planning, childrearing, and victimization prevention (Gearon and Bellack 1999) must be achieved. Men with schizophrenia often benefit from aggressive drug regimens, treatments to reduce interpersonal violence and addiction, and behavioral programs to achieve successful integration into structured long-term settings (Tamminga 1997). If we embrace a gender-informed life-span approach to mental illness, we can devise therapies for disorders that complement the developmental capacity of each person. For example, treatment of women with schizophrenia may be improved by using different therapies during the childbearing years than in the postmenopausal years (Hallonquist et al. 1993). Testing gender-related intervention packages and their benefit on functional outcomes versus the cost of integrating and focusing such interventions is the next challenge. The process of conceptualizing gender-based medical approaches as a reorientation in medical practice is a timely challenge (James 2002).

Alarcón et al. (2002) elegantly described the advantages of including contextual variables, particularly gender and culture, in all psychiatric research. As the following chapters in this section of this volume will illustrate, critical questions about the epidemiology and pathophysiology of mental illnesses cannot be answered without considering the role of gender in mental illness across the life span. Until questions related to sex and gender are routinely investigated, and both positive and negative results are consistently reported, opportunities to more comprehensively understand the symptom expression, pathogenesis, and effective treatment of disease will surely be missed (Institute of Medicine 2001). Psychiatry has much to gain from this mandate. Let us designate a "decade of the gendered brain"!

References

Alarcón RD, Bell CC, Kirmayer LJ, et al: Beyond the funhouse mirrors: research agenda on culture and psychiatric diagnosis, in A Research Agenda for DSM-V. Edited by Kupfer DJ, First MB, Regier DA. Washington, DC, American Psychiatric Association, 2002

Anderson RN: National Vital Statistics Report, National Center for Health Statistics, Centers for Disease Control and Prevention. Washington, DC, U.S. Department of Health and Human Services, 2002

Blaak E: Gender differences in fat metabolism. Curr Opin Clin Nutr Metab Care 4:499–502, 2001

Breslau N: Gender differences in trauma and posttraumatic stress disorder. J Gend Specif Med 5:34–40, 2002

Caspi A, Sugden K, Moffitt TE, et al: Influence of life stress on depression: moderation by a polymorphism in the 5-HTT gene. Science 301:386–389, 2003

Engel GL: The need for a new medical model: a challenge for biomedicine. Science 196:129–136, 1977

Epperson CN, Wisner KL, Yamamoto B: Gonadal steroids in the treatment of mood disorders. Psychosom Med 61:676–697, 1999

Gearon JS, Bellack AS: Women with schizophrenia and co-occurring substance use disorders: an increased risk for violent victimization and HIV. Community Ment Health J 35:401–419, 1999

Goldstein JM, Seidman LJ, O'Brien LM, et al: Impact of normal sexual dimorphisms on sex differences in structural brain abnormalities in schizophrenia assessed by magnetic resonance imaging. Arch Gen Psychiatry 59:154–164, 2002

Greenstein BD: Lupus: why women? J Womens Health Gend Based Med 10:233–239, 2001

Hallonquist JD, Seeman MV, Lang M, et al: Variation in symptom severity over the menstrual cycle of schizophrenics. Biol Psychiatry 33:207–209, 1993

Hamelin B: Low estrogen linked to heart attack in premenopausal women. Presented at the American Heart Association Scientific Sessions, New Orleans, LA, November 2000

Institute of Medicine: Gender Differences in Susceptibility to Environmental Factors: A Priority Assessment. Washington, DC, National Academy Press, 1998

Institute of Medicine: Exploring the Biological Contributions to Human Health: Does Sex Matter? Washington, DC, National Academy Press, 2001

Jacobson DL, Gange SJ, Rose NR, et al: Epidemiology and estimated population burden of selected autoimmune diseases in the United States. Clin Immunol Immunopathol 84:223–243, 1997

James G: Winning In The Women's Health Care Marketplace: A Comprehensive Plan For Health Care Strategists. San Francisco, CA, Jossey-Bass, 2002

Kuh D, Ben-Shlomo Y, Lynch J, et al: Life course epidemiology. J Epidemiol Community Health 57:778–783, 2003

Kupfer DJ, First MB, Regier DA (eds): A Research Agenda for DSM-V. Washington, DC, American Psychiatric Association, 2002

Kyker KA, Limacher MC: Gender differences in the presentation and symptoms of coronary artery disease. Curr Womens Health Rep 2:115–119, 2002

Malloy KJ, Bahinski A: Cardiovascular disease and arrhythmias: unique risks in women. J Gend Specif Med 2:37–44, 1999

Matza LS, Revicki DA, Davidson JR, et al: Depression with atypical features in the National Comorbidity Survey: classification, description, and consequences. Arch Gen Psychiatry 60:817–826, 2003

Murray CJL, Lopez AD (eds): The Global Burden Of Disease and Injury Series, Vol 1: A Comprehensive Assessment of Mortality and Disability from Diseases, Injuries, and Risk Factors in 1990 and Projected to 2020. Cambridge, MA, Harvard School of Public Health on behalf of the World Health Organization and the World Bank, Harvard University Press, 1996

Rao ML, Kolsch H: Effects of estrogen on brain development and neuroprotection—implications for negative symptoms in schizophrenia. Psychoneuroendocrinology 28 (suppl 2):83–96, 2003

Rider V, Foster RT, Evans M, et al: Gender differences in autoimmune diseases: estrogen increases calcineurin expression in systemic lupus erythematosus. Clin Immunol Immunopathol 89:171–180, 1998

Seeman MV: Gender differences in the prescribing of antipsychotic drugs. Am J Psychiatry 161:1324–1333, 2004

Solarz AL (ed): Lesbian Health: Current Assessment and Directions for the Future. Washington, DC, Institute of Medicine/National Academies Press, 1999

Tamminga CA: Gender and schizophrenia. J Clin Psychiatry 58:33–37, 1997

U.S. Department of Health and Human Services: Mental Health: A Report of the Surgeon General, Executive Summary. Rockville, MD, U.S. Department of Health and Human Services, Substance Abuse and Mental Health Services Administration, Center for Mental Health Services, National Institute of Health, National Institute of Mental Health, 1999

Usall J, Araya S, Ochoa S, et al: Gender differences in a sample of schizophrenic outpatients. Compr Psychiatry 42:301–305, 2004

van Vollenhoven RF, Mortabito LM, Engleman EG, et al: Treatment of systemic lupus erythematosus with dehydroepiandrosterone: 50 patients treated up to 12 months. J Rheumatol 25:285–289, 1998

Wisner KL: Sex and psychiatry in the next 5 years (editorial). J Clin Psychiatry 65:462–463, 2004

3

DSM'S APPROACH TO GENDER

History and Controversies

Thomas A. Widiger, Ph.D.

DSM-I and DSM-II: A Minimal Focus on Gender

Gender has been approached differently in the various editions of DSM and has fueled a number of controversies. The first edition (DSM-I; American Psychiatric Association 1952) devoted an entire section to basic principles and suggested tabulations for the statistical reporting of demographic and related information, which was pertinent to the manual's purpose of facilitating the "increasing need for adequate statistical data on the mental hospital population of the country" (p. 52). Sex of the patient was included among many other items recommended for inclusion. However, no actual findings related to sex (e.g., sex ratios) were reported in the manual. DSM-I occasionally used a male pronoun when describing a few of the disorders (e.g., obsessive-compulsive reaction, depressive reaction, and emotionally unstable personality), but these likely referred to both males and females.

Unlike DSM-I, DSM-II (American Psychiatric Association 1968) did not devote a lengthy section to the statistical reporting of mental disorders, although recommendations for the tabulation of demographic and other information were again provided. However, DSM-II did include for the first time information on the gender ratio of one disorder—group delinquent reaction of childhood—stating that "the condition is more common in boys than girls" (p. 51). The authors of DSM-II went even further, commenting on gender differences in the expression of the disorder: "when group delinquency occurs with girls it usually involves sexual delinquency, although shoplifting is also common" (p. 51). Interestingly, no gender information was provided for any other diagnoses, including those that might reasonably be considered to apply only to one sex (e.g., psychosis with childbirth, and the menstrual and impotence variations of psychophysiologic genitourinary disorder). As in DSM-I, there were occasional uses of male pronouns (e.g., hysterical neurosis, paranoia, and explosive personality) that were intended to refer to both males and females. The minimal attention to gender in DSM-I and DSM-II likely reflected many factors, including a lack of research on the relationship between gender and psychopathology.

DSM-III: An Increased, Although Still Limited, Focus on Gender

DSM-III focused considerably more on gender, although gender-related information was still quite limited. DSM-III greatly expanded the text description of each disorder, which included associated features, age at onset, complications, and predisposing factors (American Psychiatric Association 1980; Spitzer et al. 1980). "The relative frequency with which the disorder is diagnosed in men and women" (American Psychiatric Association 1980, p. 32) was provided in a section devoted specifically to sex ratios. For some disorders this information was relatively specific. For example, attention-deficit disorder with hyperactivity was said to be "ten times more common in boys than in girls" (p. 42). Additional gender-specific information on the course or presentation of a disorder was also provided at times in other sections of the text. For example, a gender variation in course was noted for transsexualism (i.e., female-to-male transsexuals "are more likely to have a history of homosexuality and to have a more stable course" [p. 262]), and the text for intermittent explosive disorder stated that "the males are likely to be seen in a correctional institution and the females, in a mental health facility" (p. 296). At other times, however, information on sex/gender was less certain or specific. For example, schizophrenia was noted to be "apparently equally common in males and in females" (p. 186); for voyeurism it was stated that "although no cases of voyeurism in women have been reported in the literature, some clinicians claim to know of such cases" (p. 268); and for conversion disorder it was stated that "no definite information is available; but one particular conversion symptom, globus hystericus, the feeling of a lump in the throat that interferes with swallowing, is apparently more common in females" (p. 245). For some of the disorders it was simply acknowledged that no information was available (e.g., gender identity disorder of childhood, depersonalization disorder, psychogenic fugue, generalized anxiety disorder, posttraumatic stress disorder, and paranoid disorders). For some disorders, the sex ratio was embedded in the prevalence section (e.g., the text for somatization disorder stated that "approximately 1% of females have this disorder[, whereas] the disorder is rarely diagnosed in males" [p. 242]).

DSM-III included for the first time some different criteria sets for males and females. Different diagnostic criteria for the two sexes were provided for gender identity disorder of childhood and for inhibited sexual excitement. Different diagnostic criteria and even different code numbers were provided for inhibited orgasm in males and inhibited orgasm in females. It was also noted that premature ejaculation, "as defined, is restricted to men [and] functional vaginismus, by definition, is restricted to women" (p. 278). Some of this information could not have been provided in DSM-II because premature ejaculation, inhibited orgasm, transsexualism, and gender identity disorder of childhood were not included in that edition.

DSM-III-R and DSM-IV: Progress and Controversies

The next edition of DSM, DSM-III-R (American Psychiatric Association 1987), continued to include a section devoted specifically to sex ratio, and some of the statements concerning sex ratio were more precise than in earlier editions. For example, DSM-III-R stated that attention-deficit/hyperactivity disorder was six to nine times more common in males within clinical settings but three times more common in males in community samples. It was noted that oppositional defiant disorder was more common in males before puberty but not postpuberty. On the other hand, no reference was made to the different presentation of conduct disorder in males versus females that was noted in DSM-II and DSM-III. DSM-III-R continued to have separate male and female diagnoses for inhibited orgasm, and, in fact, this variation was expanded to include separate diagnoses for sexual arousal disorders (i.e., female sexual arousal disorder and male erectile disorder). Separate diagnostic criteria were again provided for gender identity disorder of childhood, but not for gender identity disorder of adolescence or adulthood, nontranssexual type, nor for transsexualism.

Several gender-related controversies arose during the development of DSM-III-R. The DSM-III-R revision process included an entire advisory committee devoted to examining the proposed diagnosis of late luteal phase dysphoric disorder (LLPDD); this was due in large part to concerns regarding the potential harm to women of including this diagnosis. As suggested by the chair of the Work Group to Revise DSM-III, "the inclusion of this category in the manual was perhaps the most controversial aspect of the revision of DSM-III" (Spitzer et al. 1989, p. 892). "Many nosologic issues and questions about potential harm to women emerged in the debate about the inclusion of LLPDD in DSM-III-R" (Spitzer et al. 1989, p. 894). Additional concerns were also raised with respect to the decisions to include the diagnoses of self-defeating personality disorder and sadistic personality disorder in an appendix. As stated in the DSM-III-R introduction,

> The advisory committees that had worked on the definitions of these disorders [late luteal phase dysphoric disorder, self-defeating personality disorder, and sadistic personality disorder] and the Work Group believed that there was sufficient research and clinical evidence regarding the validity of each of these categories to justify its inclusion in the revised manual. On the other hand, critics of each of these categories believed that not only was adequate evidence of the validity of these categories lacking but these categories had such a high potential for misuse, particularly against women, that they should not be included.
>
> This controversy was resolved by the inclusion of these three categories in Appendix A: Proposed Diagnostic Categories Needing Further Study. (American Psychiatric Association 1987, pp. xxv–xxvi)

Gender-related controversies continued during the development of DSM-IV (American Psychiatric Association 1994; Ross et al. 1995). Ross et al. (1995) highlighted gender-related controversies pertaining to LLPDD, personality disorders, and dissociative disorders. A work group was again devoted to an examination of LLPDD (with the name eventually changed to *premenstrual dysphoric disorder*). Self-defeating personality disorder and sadistic personality disorder, which had been approved for inclusion by the Work Group to Revise DSM-III, were deleted from the manual by the DSM-IV Task Force (Widiger 1995).

DSM-IV expanded the manual's text to include additional information on how disorders vary in their expression and course across the sexes in a section called "Specific Culture, Age, and Gender Features" (Frances et al. 1995; Ross et al. 1995). For example, it was stated that "males with a diagnosis of conduct disorder frequently exhibit fighting, stealing, vandalism, and school discipline problems [whereas] females with a conduct disorder are more likely to exhibit lying, truancy, running away, substance use, and prostitution" (American Psychiatric Association 1994, p. 88), and "women [with schizophrenia] are more likely to have later onset, more prominent mood symptoms, and a better prognosis" (p. 281).

DSM-IV-TR: A Focus on Gender Ratios

Hartung and Widiger (1998) comprehensively tabulated the sex ratio information in DSM-IV and expressed concerns over a lack of consistency in the quantity and quality of this information. They suggested that this was due not only to variation in the empirical data available to the authors of DSM-IV but also to the fact that "the information provided in the DSM-IV was prepared by different individuals, without published documentation of the bases for the conclusions" (Hartung and Widiger 1998, p. 260). This concern was addressed in part in DSM-IV-TR (American Psychiatric Association 2000), which focused on reviewing and updating the text (First and Pincus 2002). The authors of DSM-IV-TR conducted systematic literature reviews to provide written documentation for the statements made in the text, including those concerning sex ratio and gender variation in expression and course. These reviews were then critiqued by independent experts.

TABLE 3–1. Sex ratios for infancy, childhood, and adolescent disorders in DSM-IV-TR

Disorder	Sex ratio
Mental retardation	1.5M:1F
Learning disorders	
Reading disorder	3–4M:1F[a]
Mathematics disorder	—
Disorder of written expression	—
Developmental coordination disorder	—
Communication disorders	
Expressive language disorder	M>F
Mixed language disorder	M>F
Phonological disorder	M>F
Stuttering	3M:1F
Pervasive developmental disorders	
Autistic disorder	4–5M:1F
Rett's disorder	F only
Childhood disintegrative	M>F
Asperger's disorder	5M:1F
Conduct disorder	M>F
Feeding and eating disorders	
Pica	—[b]
Rumination	M>F
Feeding disorder	M=F
Tic disorders	
Tourette's disorder	2–5M:1F
Chronic motor or vocal tic	—
Transient tic disorder	—
Elimination disorders	
Encopresis	M>F
Enuresis	—
Separation anxiety disorder	M<F[c]
Selective mutism	M<F
Reactive attachment disorder	—
Stereotypic movement	—[d]
Attention-deficit/hyperactivity disorder	2–9M:1F
Oppositional defiant disorder	M>F[e]

Note. F=female; M=male; —=no information provided. Read 1.5M:1F as 1.5 males for every 1 female. [a]Equal rates might be obtained with more accurate assessments. [b]DSM-IV-TR provides no information regarding the sex ratio for pica. [c]Sex ratio tends to be equal within clinical settings. [d]Head banging occurs at a ratio of 3M:1F, whereas F>M for self-biting. [e]Sex ratio is equal for males and females after puberty.

TABLE 3–2. Sex ratios for delirium, dementia, amnestic, and substance-related disorders in DSM-IV-TR

Disorder	Sex ratio
Delirium	—[a]
Dementia	
Alzheimer's	M<F
Vascular[a]	M>F
HIV	—
Head trauma	M>F
Parkinson's disease	—
Huntington's disease	M=F
Pick's disease	—
Creutzfeldt-Jakob disease	—
Amnestic disorders	—
Substance-related disorders	
Alcohol	2–5M:1F
Amphetamine	3–4M:1F[b]
Caffeine	M>F
Cannabis	M>F
Cocaine[c]	1.5–2M:1F
Hallucinogen	3M:1F
Inhalant	3.5–4M:1F[c]
Nicotine	M>F[d]
Opioid	1.5–3M:1F
Phencyclidine	2M:1F[c]
Sedative, hypnotic, anxiolytic	M<F
Polysubstance	—

Note. F=female; M=male; — = no sex ratio information provided.
[a]Males said to be more at risk.
[b]Sex ratio more even with nonintravenous use.
[c]These ratios are in reference to emergency department visits.
[d]Smoking is decreasing more rapidly among males in the United States, and use of smokeless tobacco is much higher among males.

As a result of this systematic process, changes were made in DSM-IV-TR in the sex ratio statements for many disorders. (See Tables 3–1 through 3–4 for a comprehensive summary of the sex ratio information contained in DSM-IV-TR.) For example, whereas DSM-IV stated that factitious disorder occurs with equal frequency in males and females, DSM-IV-TR stated that it occurs more often in females. Whereas DSM-IV suggested that schizophrenia occurs with equal fre-

TABLE 3–3. Sex ratios for schizophrenic, mood, anxiety, adjustment, somatoform, dissociative, and sleep disorders in DSM-IV-TR

Disorder	Sex ratio
Schizophrenia and other psychotic disorders	
Schizophrenia	M>F
Schizophreniform disorder	—
Schizoaffective disorder	M<F
Delusional disorder	M=F[a]
Brief psychotic disorder	—
Shared psychotic disorder	M<F
Mood disorders	
Major depressive disorder	1M:2F
Dysthymic disorder	1M:2–3F[b]
Bipolar I disorder	M=F
Bipolar II disorder	M<F
Cyclothymic disorder	M=F[c]
Anxiety disorders	
Panic without agoraphobia	1M:2F
Panic with agoraphobia	1M:3F
Agoraphobia without panic	M<F
Specific phobia	1M:2F
Social phobia	M<F[d]
Obsessive-compulsive disorder	M=F
Posttraumatic stress disorder	—
Acute stress disorder	—
Generalized anxiety	1M:2F
Adjustment disorder[a]	1M:2F[b]
Somatoform disorders	
Somatization disorder	M<F
Undifferentiated somatoform disorder	M<F
Conversion disorder	1M:2–10F
Pain disorder	M<F
Hypochondriasis	M=F
Body dysmorphic disorder	M=F
Factitious disorder	M<F[e]
Dissociative disorders	
Dissociative amnesia	—
Dissociative fugue	—
Dissociative identity disorder	1M:3–9F
Depersonalization	1M:2F

TABLE 3–3. Sex ratios for schizophrenic, mood, anxiety, adjustment, somatoform, dissociative, and sleep disorders in DSM-IV-TR *(continued)*

Disorder	Sex ratio
Eating disorders	
Anorexia nervosa	1M:9F
Bulimia nervosa	1M:9F
Sleep disorders	
Primary insomnia	M<F
Primary hypersomnia	3M:1F[f]
Narcolepsy	M=F
Breathing-related sleep	2–4M:1F
Circadian rhythm sleep	—
Nightmare disorder	1M:2–4F
Sleep terror disorder	M=F[g]
Sleepwalking disorder	M>F[h]

Note. F = female; M = male; — = no information provided.
[a]Jealous type more common in males.
[b]Equal sex ratio in childhood.
[c]More females present for treatment.
[d]In clinical settings, sex ratio is equal or more males with disorder.
[e]Munchausen variant occurs more often in males.
[f]This sex ratio refers to the Kleine-Levin variant.
[g]In children, disorder occurs more often in males.
[h]In children, disorder occurs more often in females.

quency in males and females, DSM-IV-TR stated that it occurs more often in males. Delirium was said to occur more often in females in DSM-IV, but males are described as being more at risk in DSM-IV-TR. Cocaine use disorders were said to occur equally in males and females in DSM-IV but were noted in DSM-IV-TR to occur more commonly in males, with a male-to-female ratio of 1.5–2.0 to 1. DSM-IV-TR also expanded the discussion of different expressions of disorders in males and females (e.g., oppositional defiant disorder, alcohol use disorders, and schizophrenia). In addition, DSM-IV-TR included possible explanations for some of the reported sex ratios. For example, some findings could be due to inaccurate assessments (e.g., reading disorder and histrionic personality disorder); differences between males and females in the reporting of symptoms or seeking of treatment (e.g., cyclothymic disorder, nightmare disorder, gender identity disorder, and pathological gambling); differences in the setting in which studies were done (e.g., attention-deficit/hyperactivity disorder, separation anxiety disorder, social phobia, generalized anxiety disorder, and adjustment disorder); differences in culture (e.g.,

TABLE 3–4. Sex ratios for sexual, gender identity, impulse-control, and personality disorders in DSM-IV-TR

Disorder	Sex ratio
Sexual disorders	
Hypoactive sexual desire	—
Sexual aversion disorder	—
Female sexual arousal	F only
Male erectile disorder	M only
Female orgasmic disorder	F only
Male orgasmic disorder	M only
Premature ejaculation	M only
Dyspareunia	M<F
Vaginismus	F only
Exhibitionism	M>F[a]
Fetishism	M>F[a]
Frotteurism	M>F[a]
Pedophilia	M>F[a]
Sexual masochism	20M:1F
Sexual sadism	M>F[a]
Transvestic fetishism	M>F[a]
Voyeurism	M>F[a]
Gender identity disorder	2–3M:1F[b]
Impulse-control disorders	
Intermittent explosive	M>F
Kleptomania	1M:2F
Pyromania	M>F
Pathological gambling	2M:1F[c]
Trichotillomania	M<F[d]
Personality disorders	
Paranoid personality disorder	M>F[e]
Schizoid personality disorder	M>F[e]
Schizotypal personality disorder	M>F[e]
Antisocial personality disorder	M>F
Borderline personality disorder	1M:3F
Histrionic personality disorder	M<F[f]
Narcissistic personality disorder	1–3M:1F

TABLE 3–4. Sex ratios for sexual, gender identity, impulse-control, and personality disorders in DSM-IV-TR *(continued)*

Disorder	Sex ratio
Personality disorders *(continued)*	
Avoidant personality disorder	M=F
Dependent personality disorder	M<F[g]
Compulsive personality disorder	2M:1F

Note. F= female; M = male; — = no information provided.
[a]These paraphilias are rarely diagnosed in females.
[b]In children, boys referred much more frequently than girls, due perhaps to referral bias involving greater stigmatization for boys.
[c]Females might be underrepresented due to greater stigma of gambling in females.
[d]Sex ratio is M=F in children.
[e]Disorders are said to occur slightly more commonly in males.
[f]Sex ratio not different than base rate of females in clinical setting, and no sex differences have been reported when structured assessments were used.
[g]Some studies report no differences in sex ratio.

nicotine and somatization); or differences in age (e.g., alcohol use disorders, schizophrenia, dysthymic disorder, adjustment disorder, sleepwalking disorder, sleep terror disorder, gender identity disorder, and pathological gambling).

Conclusions

In sum, the authors of DSM-IV-TR made tremendous progress in expanding the breadth, depth, and accuracy of the gender-related information included within the text of the diagnostic manual. What we need now are studies to capitalize on this opportunity as well those that address the limitations in the existing data currently identified within the text of DSM-IV-TR. Much of the research proposed in the chapters in this section of the present volume provides useful data that can ultimately inform gender-related information that will be included in the text of future editions of DSM. More specifically, it is evident that there is considerable inconsistency across disorders in the breadth and depth of the information that is provided. A considerable amount of information concerning the impact of sex/gender on the expression and course of the disorder is provided for some disorders, whereas for other disorders there is no information even on gender ratio. In addition, it is also apparent that the quality of the research must improve if this information can be considered to be sufficiently informative to include within the diagnostic manual. Gender ratio data can be quite sensitive to biases in assessment instruments, differences between males and females in the willingness to report symptoms, the setting or population in which the data are sampled, and the age of the participants who are studied. Finally, it is recommended that the authors of future editions of DSM follow a consistent and explicit set of guidelines for the provision of gender-related information so that a minimal and uniform standard is used and provide a published documentation of the empirical bases for the statements that are made within the text.

References

American Psychiatric Association: Diagnostic and Statistical Manual: Mental Disorders. Washington, DC, American Psychiatric Association, 1952

American Psychiatric Association: Diagnostic and Statistical Manual of Mental Disorders, 2nd Edition. Washington, DC, American Psychiatric Association, 1968

American Psychiatric Association: Diagnostic and Statistical Manual of Mental Disorders, 3rd Edition. Washington, DC, American Psychiatric Association, 1980

American Psychiatric Association: Diagnostic and Statistical Manual of Mental Disorders, 3rd Edition Revised. Washington, DC, American Psychiatric Association, 1987

American Psychiatric Association: Diagnostic and Statistical Manual of Mental Disorders, 4th Edition. Washington, DC, American Psychiatric Association, 1994

American Psychiatric Association: Diagnostic and Statistical Manual of Mental Disorders, 4th Edition, Text Revision. Washington, DC, American Psychiatric Association, 2000

First MB, Pincus HA: The DSM-IV Text Revision: rationale and potential impact on clinical practice. Psychiatr Serv 53:288–292, 2002

Frances AJ, First MB, Pincus HA: DSM-IV Guidebook. Washington, DC, American Psychiatric Press, 1995

Hartung CM, Widiger TA: Gender differences in the diagnosis of mental disorders: conclusions and controversies of DSM-IV. Psychol Bull 123:260–278, 1998

Ross R, Frances AJ, Widiger TA: Gender issues in DSM-IV, in American Psychiatric Press Review of Psychiatry, Vol 14. Edited by Oldham JM, Riba MB. Washington, DC, American Psychiatric Press, 1995, pp 205–226

Spitzer RL, Williams JBW, Skodol AE: DSM-III: The major achievements and an overview. Am J Psychiatry 137:151–164, 1980

Spitzer RL, Severino SK, Williams JBW, et al: Late luteal phase dysphoric disorder and DSM-III-R. Am J Psychiatry 146:892–897, 1989

Widiger TA: Deletion of the self-defeating and sadistic personality disorder diagnoses, in The DSM-IV Personality Disorders. Edited by Livesley WJ. New York, Guilford, 1995, pp 359–373

4

GENDER AND THE PREVALENCE OF PSYCHIATRIC DISORDERS

Bridget F. Grant, Ph.D., Ph.D.
Myrna M. Weissman, Ph.D.

Psychiatric epidemiology provides an invaluable starting point and foundation for the study of gender differences and psychopathology. Epidemiology is the study of the occurrence, distribution, and determinants of disorders in the population. Variations in the prevalence of psychiatric disorders across important population subgroups can provide important clues about their etiology. For example, a frequent finding in epidemiological studies is a female predominance in most anxiety and mood disorders (with the exception of bipolar I and bipolar II disorders) and a male predominance in substance use disorders and antisocial personality disorder.

In this section we review sex differences in the prevalence of psychopathology emerging from three large epidemiological surveys of the U.S. general population as well as cross-national studies conducted since 1980. We also identify major determinants of gender differences. For this purpose, we consider separately the artifactual and genuine determinants first proposed and considered in detail by Weissman and Klerman (1977). On the basis of this review, we identify gaps in our knowledge of gender differences in psychiatric disorders and set the stage for the development of an epidemiological research agenda for DSM-V and beyond.

TABLE 4–1. Comparison between the Epidemiologic Catchment Area (ECA) Study, National Comorbidity Survey (NCS), and National Epidemiologic Survey on Alcohol and Related Conditions (NESARC)

	ECA	NCS	NESARC
Date conducted	1980–1984	1990–1992	2001–2002
Sample size	18,571	8,089	43,093
Oversampling	Yes[a]	No	Yes[b]
Site	5 U.S. sites	48 U.S. states	50 U.S. states
Response rate	76%	83%	81%
Age range, *years*	18+	15–54	18+
Female	59%	52%	52%
Instrument	DIS	CIDI	AUDADIS-IV
Diagnosis	DSM-III	DSM-III-R	DSM-IV
Interviews	Lay	Lay	Lay

Note. AUDADIS-IV=Alcohol Use Disorder and Associated Disabilities Interview Schedule–DSM-IV version; CIDI = Composite International Diagnostic Interview; DIS = Diagnostic Interview Schedule.

[a]Blacks, Hispanics, the elderly, and rural poor at different sites.

[b]Blacks, Hispanics, and 18–24 year olds.

Epidemiological Surveys of the General Population

To enhance understanding of the epidemiology data discussed later in the chapter, we first briefly describe the major studies that generated these data. Table 4–1 presents a summary of the characteristics of the first three studies.

EPIDEMIOLOGIC CATCHMENT AREA STUDY

The Epidemiologic Catchment Area (ECA) study, conducted from 1980 to 1984, was an epidemiological survey of representative samples from five U.S. catchment area centers: New Haven, Connecticut; Baltimore, Maryland; St. Louis, Missouri; Durham, North Carolina; and Los Angeles, California (Robins and Regier 1991). The ECA was the first comprehensive epidemiological survey on psychiatric disorders in the United States. Blacks, Hispanics, the elderly, and the rural poor were oversampled at specific ECA sites.

The ECA program was designed to obtain accurate and uniform, and comparable-across-sites prevalence data on mental disorders in selected areas in the United States and to assess the adequacy of services to the mentally ill. The design required representative samples from both community and institutional settings at two different time points 1 year apart (wave 1 and wave 2). In wave 1, prevalence data were gathered for lifetime, past year, 6-month, 1-month, and 2-week periods. Wave 2 was a follow-up to ascertain rates of relapse and remission as well as incidence rates (Eaton et al. 1989). A total of 18,571 persons in the noninstitutionalized sample were interviewed by lay interviewers who used the Diagnostic Interview Schedule (DIS; Robins et al. 1981). Diagnostic criteria were from DSM-III (American Psychiatric Association 1980), Research Diagnostic Criteria (Spitzer et al. 1978), and the Feighner diagnostic system (Feighner et al. 1978).

THE NATIONAL COMORBIDITY SURVEY

The National Comorbidity Survey (NCS) was conducted between 1990 and 1992, 10 years after the ECA. It was based on a probability sample of 8,089 individuals ages 15–54 in the noninstitutionalized population of the 48 contiguous states. Unlike the ECA, which was based on five geographic sites, the NCS included a representative sample of the U.S. population. Subjects were interviewed by lay interviewers using the University of Michigan Composite International Diagnostic Interview (CIDI; Wittchen and Kessler 1994; World Health Organization 1990), which made DSM-III-R diagnoses (American Psychiatric Association 1987; Kessler et al. 1994). The rates of disorders were adjusted for nonresponse and weighted to the sociodemographic characteristics of the target population of the 1989 U.S. National Health Interview Survey.

NATIONAL EPIDEMIOLOGIC SURVEY ON ALCOHOL AND RELATED CONDITIONS

The National Epidemiologic Survey on Alcohol and Related Conditions (NESARC) was conducted in 2001–2002 (Grant et al. 2003, 2004). The target population consisted of civilian noninstitutionalized individuals (supplemented by a sample of group quarters—e.g., college dorms, rooming houses) who were 18 years and older and residing in all 50 states. Face-to-face computerized personal interviews were conducted with 43,093 respondents. Blacks, Hispanics, and young adults (ages 18–24 years) were oversampled. The data were weighted to reflect the design characteristics of the NESARC survey, to account for oversampling, and to adjust for nonresponse at the household and person levels. The weighted data were then adjusted to be representative of the United States civilian population for a variety of socioeconomic variables, including region, age, sex, race, and ethnicity, using the 2000 Decennial Census. Psychiatric disorders were assessed using the National Institute on Alcohol Abuse and Alcoholism's Alcohol Use Disorder and Associated Disabilities Interview Schedule–DSM-IV version (Grant et al. 2001), a fully structured diagnostic interview that yields DSM-IV diagnoses (American Psychiatric Association 1994).

CROSS-NATIONAL COLLABORATIVE GROUP

The publication of the ECA data in the United States in the 1980s spawned similar studies using the DIS in different countries. However, it was difficult to make cross-national comparisons, even when studies used the same diagnostic assessment, because there was variability in the data presentation. In the 1990s, 10 countries (see Table 4–2) formed the Cross-National Collaborative Group to directly compare rates and risk of DIS-diagnosed DSM-III psychiatric disorders across countries and to overcome some of the problems of disparate presentation of data (Weissman et al. 1994, 1996a, 1996b, 1997). With this approach, real differences in rates by country that were not due to different analytic methods could emerge. Not all 10 countries provided data on all the disorders; thus, there are missing data in the tables that follow. Nonetheless, the sites span diverse geographical, political, and cultural areas in North America, the Caribbean, Europe, the Middle East, Asia, and the Pacific Rim. Statistical analyses of these data standardize the rates at each site to the age and sex distribution of the ECA (Breslow and Day 1987).

WORLD MENTAL HEALTH STUDY 2000

The beginning of a new generation of cross-national comparisons of mental disorders was published by the World Health Organization's (2000) International Consortium of Psychiatric Epidemiology. This effort covered countries and geographic areas not included in the previous cross-national studies (more information on the International Consortium of Psychiatric Epidemiology can be obtained from www.hcp.med.harvard.edu/ICPE). The first prevalence rates using the CIDI that generated DSM-IV diagnoses came from 29,644 persons participating in population surveys in North America (Canada and the NCS in the United States), Latin America (Brazil and Mexico), and Europe (Germany, The Netherlands, and Turkey). The published rates that are available aggregate mood, anxiety, and substance abuse disorders, and they do not present rates separately for each sex. The first estimates from this consortium show that mental disorders are highly prevalent throughout the world (World Health Organization 2000). Additional surveys are being planned that will include the United States, Mexico, Colombia, Brazil, Germany, France, Italy, The Netherlands, Belgium, the Ukraine, South Africa, Indonesia, China, and New Zealand (Kessler, personal communication 2004).

Sex Differences in Psychiatric Disorders As Assessed in the ECA, NCS, and NESARC

Despite methodological differences among the ECA, NCS, and NESARC, including differences in sampling design, sample size, diagnostic criteria, diagnostic assessment instruments, and the years in which each survey was conducted (Table 4–1),

TABLE 4–2. Comparisons between sites in the Cross-National Collaborative Group by sample size, and response rate and gender

	United States[a]	Edmonton, Alberta[b]	Puerto Rico[c]	Paris, France[d]	West Germany[e]	Florence, Italy[b]	Beirut, Lebanon[g]	Taiwan[h]	Korea[i]	Christchurch, New Zealand[j]
Sample size	18,571	3,258	1,513	1,746	481[f]	1,000	526	11,004	5,100	1,498
Response rate, %	76	72	91	63	76	100	77	90	83	70
Female, %	59	59	57	62	52	53	57	48	52	66

Note. Percentages given as raw percentages.

[a]Data derived from five sites (New Haven, CT; Baltimore, MD; St. Louis, MO; the Piedmont region of North Carolina; Los Angeles, CA). Population figure to 1980 census.

[b]Population figures to 1981 census.

[c]Population figure to 1980 census.

[d]Data derived from Savigny, a newly built city near Paris. Population figure to 1987 census.

[e]Data derived from former Federal Republic of Germany. Population figures to 1974 census.

[f]Data derived, in 1981 from a random sample of 1,366 subjects first ascertained in 1974.

[g]Data determined in 1986 from counties in Beirut.

[h]Data derived from Taipei and eight areas in rural Taiwan. Population figure to 1980 census.

[i]Data derived from samples in urban Seoul and rural regions. Population figure to 1980 census.

[j]Population figures to 1986 census.

Source. Weissman et al. 1996a.

the observed sex differences are remarkably similar across major mood, anxiety, and substance use disorders and antisocial personality disorder (Table 4–3).

As shown in Table 4–3, the lifetime prevalences of major depression were greater among females than among males in the ECA, NCS, and NESARC studies, yielding female:male ratios of 2.2, 1.7 and 1.9, respectively. Similarly, the rates of dysthymia were greater for females than for males, with female:male ratios of 1.9 in the ECA, 1.7 in the NCS, and 2.0 in the NESARC study. However, this was not the case for bipolar I disorder in any study (all sex ratios approach 1.0). Sex differences in bipolar II disorder also were minimal in the ECA (female:male ratio, 1.3) and NESARC (female:male ratio, 1.1) studies. Interestingly, the prevalence of hypomania, only assessed in NESARC, was greater among males than among females (male:female ratio, 1.7).

The prevalences of panic disorder, social phobia, specific phobia, and generalized anxiety disorder were consistently greater for females than for males in all three studies, yielding female:male ratios of approximately 2.0–2.5 for panic disorder, 2.0 for specific phobia and generalized anxiety disorder, and 1.2–1.4 for social phobia.

In contrast, the lifetime prevalences of alcohol and drug use disorders were consistently greater for males than for females in the NCS and NESARC studies, with male:female ratios between 1.5 and 2.5. Similar sex differences were observed in the ECA study, with the exception of alcohol abuse and dependence, which had much greater male:female ratios (5.7 and 4.9, respectively). Antisocial personality disorder was associated with male:female ratios of 5.6 in the ECA, 4.8 in the NCS, and 2.9 in the NESARC.

The NESARC was the only national epidemiological survey to measure DSM-IV personality disorders other than antisocial personality disorder (Table 4–4). Avoidant, dependent, and paranoid personality disorders were significantly greater among females than among males, with female:male sex ratios of about 1.5. Of interest, there were no gender differences observed for obsessive-compulsive, schizoid, and histrionic personality disorders.

Sex Differences in Mood and Anxiety Disorders in Selected Cross-National Sites

Table 4–5 presents data from the Cross-National Collaboration on major depression and bipolar disorder; Table 4–6 shows data on panic disorder, social phobia, and obsessive-compulsive disorder (OCD). Despite the breadth of geographic areas and time periods that are represented, as well as cultural differences and differences in rates of disorders, the sex ratios are generally similar among countries and to the data published in the three U.S. studies. The female:male sex ratio for major depression is about 2 (1.6–3.1), whereas there are no consistent sex differences in bipolar disorder. Panic disorder is approximately threefold higher in females than

TABLE 4–3. Lifetime prevalence of psychiatric disorders in the Epidemiologic Catchment Area (ECA) Study, National Comorbidity Survey (NCS), and National Epidemiologic Survey on Alcohol and Related Conditions (NESARC) by sex

	ECA			NCS			NESARC		
Disorder	Male, % (SE)	Female, % (SE)	Sex ratio[a]	Male, % (SE)	Female, % (SE)	Sex ratio	Male, % (SE)	Female, % (SE)	Sex ratio
Mood disorders									
Major depressive	2.7 (0.22)	6.8 (0.36)	2.2	12.7 (0.09)[b]	21.3 (0.09)	1.7	9.0 (0.27)	17.1 (0.44)	1.9
Bipolar I	0.8 (0.13)	0.9 (0.13)	1.1	1.6 (0.28)	1.7 (0.28)	1.1	3.2 (0.16)	3.4 (0.18)	1.1
Bipolar II	0.4 (0.11)	0.5 (0.08)	1.3	—	—	—	1.0 (0.09)	1.2 (0.65)	1.1
Dysthymia	2.3 (0.27)	4.1 (0.25)	1.9	4.8 (0.40)	8.0 (0.60)	1.7	2.1 (0.13)	4.2 (0.18)	2.0
Hypomania	—[c]	—	—	—	—	—	1.5 (0.11)	0.9 (0.07)	1.7
Anxiety disorders									
Panic	1.0 (0.16)	2.1 (0.20)	2.1	2.0 (0.30)	5.0 (1.40)	2.5	3.3 (0.10)	6.7 (0.39)	2.0
Social phobia	2.5 (0.31)	3.1 (0.24)	1.2	11.1 (0.80)	15.5 (1.00)	1.4	4.2 (0.22)	5.7 (0.25)	1.4
Specific phobia	6.6 (0.37)	13.0 (0.44)	2.0	6.7 (0.50)	15.7 (1.10)	2.3	6.2 (0.28)	12.3 (0.41)	2.0
Generalized anxiety	2.4 (—)	4.9 (—)	2.0	3.6 (0.50)	6.6 (0.50)	1.8	2.8 (0.18)	5.3 (0.23)	1.9
Substance use disorders									
Alcohol abuse only	9.7 (0.47)	1.7 (0.17)	5.7	12.5 (0.80)	6.4 (0.60)	1.9	24.6 (0.70)	11.5 (0.44)	2.1
Alcohol dependence	13.6 (0.59)	2.8 (0.19)	4.9	20.1 (1.00)	8.2 (0.70)	2.5	17.4 (0.50)	8.0 (0.31)	2.2
Any drug abuse only	3.1 (0.28)	2.1 (0.21)	1.5	5.4 (1.00)	3.5 (0.40)	1.5	10.6 (0.36)	5.1 (0.24)	2.1
Any drug dependence	4.5 (0.32)	2.6 (0.22)	1.7	9.2 (0.70)	5.9 (0.50)	1.6	3.3 (0.19)	2.0 (0.12)	1.7
Personality disorder									
Antisocial	4.5 (0.32)	0.8 (0.10)	5.6	5.8 (0.60)	1.2 (0.30)	4.8	5.5 (0.25)	1.9 (0.11)	2.9

[a]Sex ratio = larger sex-specific prevalence divided by smaller sex-specific prevalence.

[b]Reported only as major depressive episode. [c]Specific estimate (or standard error) not assessed or available.

TABLE 4–4. Prevalence of DSM-IV personality disorders by sex from the National Epidemiologic Survey on Alcohol and Related Conditions

Personality disorders	Male, % (SE)	Female, % (SE)	Sex ratio[a]
Avoidant	1.9 (0.14)	2.8 (0.16)	1.5
Dependent	0.4 (0.07)	0.6 (0.06)	1.5
Obsessive-compulsive	7.9 (0.28)	7.9 (0.27)	1.0
Paranoid	3.8 (0.20)	5.0 (0.20)	1.3
Schizoid	3.2 (0.18)	3.1 (0.14)	1.0
Histrionic	1.9 (0.13)	1.8 (0.11)	1.1

[a]Sex ratio = larger sex-specific prevalence divided by smaller sex-specific prevalence.

in males, with greater variation in rates than for major depression. As in the three U.S. surveys, the female rates for social phobia exceed the male rate, but the sex ratio is lower. Data on OCD show patterns similar to social phobia, with a smaller sex difference in rates.

Determinants of Gender Differences in Psychopathology

Numerous reviews of the literature (Frank 2000; Gavranidou and Rosner 2003; Hartung and Widiger 1998; Kuehner 2003; Leibenluft 1999; Nolen-Hoeksema 1987; Piccinell and Wilkinson 2000; Weissman and Klerman 1977) have identified an array of factors that may account for the female predominance in unipolar depression, dysthymic disorder, and anxiety disorders and the male predominance in substance use disorders and antisocial personality disorder. These determinants can be artifactual or genuine. Artifactual determinants include gender-specific differences in recall, self-report, response to symptomatology, interviewer effects, treatment seeking, and sex-biased diagnostic criteria. Developmental pathways also may differ by gender, with females having preexisting mood and anxiety disorders and males experiencing more externalizing disorders such as substance use disorders and antisocial personality disorder.

Several genuine explanatory factors also have been proposed to account for sex differences in psychopathology. As discussed elsewhere in this section, psychosocial and sociocultural factors include differential coping styles, sex roles, poverty, educational status, marital status, income, social support, social isolation, childhood adversity, societal change, cultural norms, and vulnerability to exposure and reactivity to stressful life experiences. Other determinants point to sex differences in prior comorbidity, genetic predisposition, personality traits, sex hormones, endocrine stress reactivity, neurotransmitter systems, and neuropsychological determinants (e.g., rumination).

TABLE 4–5. Lifetime prevalence of major depression and bipolar disorder, among subjects ages 18–64 years, by sex in cross-national sites

	Major depression,[a] LP/100 (SE)			Bipolar disorder,[a,b] LP/100 (SE)		
	Females	Males	Female:Male ratio	Females	Males	Female:Male ratio
United States	7.4 (0.39)	2.8 (0.26)	2.6 (0.11)	1.0 (0.15)	0.8 (0.14)	1.2 (0.22)
Edmonton, Alberta	12.3 (0.93)	6.6 (0.73)	1.9 (1.3)	0.5 (0.21)	0.7 (0.25)	0.7 (0.51)
Puerto Rico	5.5 (0.91)	3.1 (0.72)	1.8 (0.29)	0.5 (0.27)	0.8 (0.38)	0.6 (0.74)
Paris, France	21.9 (1.80)	10.5 (1.39)	2.1 (0.16)	—	—	—
West Germany	13.5 (2.46)	4.4 (1.56)	3.1 (0.39)	1.0 (0.71)	—	—
Florence, Italy	18.1 (2.16)	6.1 (1.40)	3.0 (0.26)	—	—	—
Beirut, Lebanon	23.1 (2.63)	14.7 (2.25)	1.6 (0.19)	—	—	—
Taiwan	1.8 (0.19)	1.1 (0.16)	1.6 (0.17)	0.3 (0.07)	0.3 (0.09)	1.0 (0.36)
Korea	3.8 (0.38)	1.9 (0.29)	2.0 (0.18)	0.2 (0.09)	0.6 (0.16)	0.3 (0.53)
Christchurch, New Zealand	15.5 (1.51)	7.5 (1.14)	2.1 (0.18)	1.2 (0.45)	1.7 (0.56)	0.7 (0.50)

Note. LP = lifetime prevalence; — = data not available.

[a]Weissman et al. 1996a.

[b]Figures standardized to the 1980 U.S. age and sex distribution. Data from West Germany based on ages 26–64 years. Data from all other sites based on ages 18–64.

TABLE 4–6. Lifetime prevalence of panic disorder, social phobia, and obsessive-compulsive disorder by sex in cross-national sites

	Panic disorder,[a] LP/100 (SE)			Social phobia,[b] LP/100 (SE)			Obsessive-compulsive disorder,[c] LP/100 (SE)		
Site[d]	Females	Males	Female:Male ratio	Females	Males	Female:Male ratio	Females	Males	Female:Male ratio
United States	2.3 (0.22)	1.0 (0.15)	2.3 (0.18)	2.1 (0.26)	3.1 (0.30)	2.6 (0.20)	2.8 (0.22)	1.7 (0.20)	1.6
Edmonton, Alberta	1.9 (0.38)	0.9 (0.28)	2.1 (0.37)	1.3 (0.34)	2.1 (0.41)	1.7 (0.27)	2.7 (0.45)	2.0 (0.46)	1.3
Puerto Rico	1.8 (0.54)	1.4 (0.50)	1.3 (0.45)	0.8 (0.37)	1.1 (0.42)	1.0 (0.28)	2.7 (0.62)	2.3 (0.68)	1.2
Savigny, France	3.0 (0.74)	1.3 (0.50)	2.3 (0.47)	—	—	—	—	—	—
West Germany	3.8 (1.38)	1.4 (0.88)	2.7 (0.73)	—	—	—	1.9 (0.86)	2.5 (1.02)	0.8
Florence, Italy	3.9 (0.96)	1.2 (0.70)	3.2 (0.62)	—	—	—	—	—	—
Beirut, Lebanon	3.1 (1.65)	1.1 (1.02)	2.8 (1.09)	—	—	—	—	—	—
Taiwan	0.6 (0.10)	0.2 (0.07)	3.0 (0.37)	—	—	—	0.9 (0.16)	0.5 (0.11)	1.8
Korea	2.9 (0.34)	0.5 (0.15)	5.8 (0.32)	0.1 (0.06)	1.0 (0.20)	0.5 (0.11)	2.0 (0.31)	1.7 (0.30)	1.2
Christchurch, New Zealand	3.3 (0.74)	0.7 (0.37)	4.7 (0.55)	—	—	—	3.4 (0.65)	0.9 (0.46)	3.8

Note. LP = lifetime prevalence; — = data not available.

[a]Weissman et al. 1997. [b]Weissman et al. 1996b. [c]Weissman et al. 1994. [d]All values standardized to the age and sex distribution of the 1980 census. Data from West Germany based on age 26–64 years, data from all other sites based on ages 18–64. Epidemiologic Catchment Area data derived from five sites (New Haven, CT; Baltimore, MD; St. Louis, MO; the Piedmont region of North Carolina; Los Angeles, CA).

The consensus in the literature is that artifactual determinants may attenuate a female predominance in mood and anxiety disorders and a male predominance in substance use disorders and antisocial personality disorders; however, artifactual determinants are unlikely to account for all the differences in rates and for the sex differences. Given the consistency of findings across cultures, we conclude that the sex differences in rates of psychiatric disorders are genuine. The epidemiological data and recent reviews of the literature on sex differences in psychopathology also highlight the gaps in our knowledge and provide a blueprint for the development of a research agenda for DSM-V and further revisions of the classification.

A Research Agenda for DSM-V and Beyond

Take sex/gender into account in the design and analysis of psychosocial and biological studies.

Determinants of sex differences in psychopathology are far from established. However, the epidemiological data clearly show that sex differences in rates of many disorders exist across different cultures. It is critical that psychosocial as well as biological studies, including genetic and neuroimaging studies, take sex into account in their design and analysis and also covary gender with age and with pubertal and/or menopausal status of the samples. For example, biological studies of depression that mix samples of prepubertal and adolescent girls and boys are likely to obscure results.

Conduct large, representative longitudinal surveys of children and adolescents to determine at what age sex differences begin to emerge.

Different factors may contribute to the sex differences in psychopathology at different points across the life span. There is some suggestion that puberty is a critical point for an increase in rates of mood and anxiety disorders in females. There is also variation two other biological events in the female life cycle—i.e., pregnancy and menopause. Given that most psychiatric disorders begin early in life, large, representative longitudinal surveys of children and adolescents are needed to determine the age at which sex differences emerge. This type of epidemiological data would usefully inform designs of experimental prevention and intervention programs (Li et al. 2004). For example, if prepubertal phobias are an early sign of adolescent major depression in girls, as suggested by clinical studies, then a rational target for intervention is suggested.

Conduct cross-cultural epidemiological studies with consistent assessment instruments and diagnostic criteria to explore interactions between biological and cultural influences on sex differences.

Cross-cultural epidemiological studies using consistent assessment instruments and diagnostic criteria are needed to help answer questions about interactions between biological and cultural influences on sex differences in psychopathology and the effects of cross-national gender differences in social position and resources. The emerging data from the World Health Organization International Surveys, begun in 2000, are of critical importance in determining the universality of sex differences in rates of disorders. The full data from these surveys, which include developing as well as developed countries, should rapidly become a public use data set so that investigators from around the world can explore these issues.

Determine the impact of social and cultural traumatic events on gender differences in rates of disorders as well as on the resiliency of women from some cultures.

The World Health Organization study is a landmark study, but surveys of Africans may yield insights on some puzzling observations. The high rates of major depression in both men and women reported in small studies in Uganda and Rwanda are at variance with rates in African American individuals from the ECA, NCS, and a recent, as-yet unpublished U.S. national survey conducted by James Jackson. These international studies may provide information on the impact of social and cultural traumatic events on gender differences in rates of disorders as well as on the resiliency of women from some cultures.

Explore the contribution of race, ethnicity, socioeconomic, sociodemographic, and other putative risk factors to sex differences in a variety of psychiatric disorders.

In contrast to the amount of epidemiological research on psychopathology, few studies have taken gender and gender-related characteristics such as masculinity and femininity into account (see Chapter 6). Moreover, very little is known regarding the contribution of race, ethnicity, socioeconomic, sociodemographic, and other putative risk factors (e.g., discrimination, acculturation, social networks, social support, sexual orientation, and prior comorbidity) to the sex differences in a variety of psychiatric disorders. The possibility that the sex differences observed in psychopathology rates may be substantially attenuated or disappear altogether once these factors are controlled argues for the inclusion of a wide variety of such determinants in future epidemiological research. This research will benefit from large epidemiological surveys of the general population of sufficient size (perhaps on the order of 40,000 subjects) suitable for cross-tabulation of important determinants of the sex differentials and multivariate analyses.

Increase the coverage of psychiatric disorders assessed in representative samples of the general population.

Although the epidemiological surveys we reviewed have been highly informative, they have included only a limited number of disorders. The ECA provided data on only about one-fourth of the 101 disorders for which information on differential sex prevalence is provided in DSM-IV. The NCS's and NESARC's coverage was also limited (14 and 40 disorders, respectively). To date, only limited data are available about sex differences in posttraumatic stress disorder, eating disorders, somatoform disorders, sexual and gender identity disorders, and many other disorders. Future epidemiological research should strive to increase the coverage of psychiatric disorders assessed in representative samples of the general population.

Conduct further large-scale epidemiological research on personality disorders.

The NESARC was the first national epidemiological survey to assess DSM-IV Axis II personality disorders. The need for further epidemiological research on personality disorders is warranted because of their often-severe clinical presentation and implications for the treatment of Axis I disorders (Widiger and Anderson 2003).

Collect data on the proposed spectrum of bipolar disorders, in part, to identify possible sex differences.

The rates of bipolar I disorder in the ECA and NCS and of bipolar II disorder in a cross-national epidemiological study were quite low (0.3%–1.6%), precluding reliable estimation of gender differences (Kessler et al. 1994; Robins and Regier 1991; Weissman et al. 1996a). However, these studies used narrow definitions of bipolar disorder (i.e., those of DSM-III and DSM-III-R). More recent epidemiological data based on DSM-IV diagnoses (Angst 1998; Lewinsohn et al. 1995; Szadoczky et al. 1998) have challenged the foregoing figures. In these studies, the concept of bipolar disorders was expanded to include hypomania, brief hypomania (i.e., less than 4 days), and cyclothymia. These expanded definitions yielded much higher prevalence rates of 5.0%–8.3%. Future epidemiological surveys should collect data on this proposed bipolar spectrum using DSM-IV criteria and identify possible sex differences.

Focus on the empirical identification of gender-biased diagnostic criteria.

A failure to consider possible gender differences in how psychiatric disorders manifest and/or are expressed can substantially complicate the estimation of valid prevalence rates in epidemiological studies because of possible biases in the diagnostic criteria. Future epidemiological research should focus on the empirical identification of gender-biased diagnostic criteria. This can most fruitfully be accomplished through traditional psychometric research on individual diagnostic criteria, various taxometric methods, item response theory, and structural equation modeling and its recently developed variants (Muthén and Muthén 2002). In the final analysis, such information can be used to support revisions to existing criteria to eliminate any bias that may exist.

References

Angst J: The emerging epidemiology of hypomania and bipolar II disorder. J Affect Disord 50:143–151, 1998

American Psychiatric Association: Diagnostic and Statistical Manual of Mental Disorders, 3rd Edition. Washington, DC, American Psychiatric Association, 1980

American Psychiatric Association: Diagnostic and Statistical Manual of Mental Disorders, 3rd Edition Revised. Washington, DC, American Psychiatric Association, 1987

American Psychiatric Association: Diagnostic and Statistical Manual of Mental Disorders, 4th Edition. Washington, DC, American Psychiatric Association, 1994

Breslow NE, Day NE: Statistical Methods in Cancer Research: The Design and Analysis of Cohort Studies, Vol 2. Lyon, France, International Agency for Research on Cancer, 1987

Eaton WW, Kramer M, Anthony A, et al: The incidence of specific DIS/DSM-III mental health disorders: data from the NIMH Epidemiologic Catchment Area Program. Acta Psychiatr Scand 79:163–178, 1989

Feighner JP, Robins E, Guze SB, et al: Diagnosis criteria from the Saint Louis school (Missouri-USA). Encephale 4:323–339, 1978

Frank E: Gender and Its Effects on Psychopathology. Washington, DC, American Psychopathological Association, 2000

Gavranidou M, Rosner R: The weaker sex? Gender and post-traumatic stress disorder. Depress Anxiety 17:130–139, 2003

Grant BF, Dawson DA, Hasin DS: The Alcohol Use Disorder and Associated Disabilities Interview Schedule, DSM-IV Version. Bethesda, MD, National Institute on Alcohol Abuse and Alcoholism, 2001

Grant BF, Moore TC, Shepard J, et al: Source and Accuracy Statement: Wave 1 National Epidemiologic Survey on Alcohol and Related Conditions (NESARC). Bethesda, MD, National Institute on Alcohol Abuse and Alcoholism, 2003

Grant BF, Stinson FS, Hasin DS, et al: Co-occurrence of 12-month alcohol and drug use disorders and personality disorders in the United States: results from the National Epidemiologic Survey on Alcohol and Related Conditions (NESARC). Arch Gen Psychiatry 61:361–368, 2004

Hartung CM, Widiger TA: Gender differences in the diagnosis of mental disorders: conclusions and controversies of the DSM-IV. Psychol Bull 123:260–278, 1998

Kessler RC, McGonagle KA, Zhao S, et al: Lifetime and 12-month prevalence of DSM-III-R psychiatric disorders in the United States: results from the National Comorbidity Survey. Arch Gen Psychiatry 51:8–19, 1994

Kuehner C: Gender differences in unipolar depression: an update of epidemiological findings and possible explanations. Acta Psychiatr Scand 108:163–174, 2003

Leibenluft E: Gender Differences in Mood and Anxiety Disorders: From Bench to Bedside. Washington, DC, American Psychiatric Press, 1999

Li TK, Grant BF, Hewitt BG: Alcohol use disorders and mood disorders: A National Institute on Alcohol Abuse and Alcoholism perspective. Biol Psychiatry 56:718–720, 2004

Lewinsohn PM, Klein DL, Seeley JR: Bipolar disorders in a community sample of older adolescents: prevalence, phenomenology, comorbidity and course. J Am Acad Child Adolesc Psychiatry 34:454–463, 1995

Muthen LK, Muthen BO: Mplus: Statistical Analysis With Latent Variables, 2nd Version. Los Angeles, CA, Muthen and Muthen, 2002

Nolan-Hoeksema S: Sex differences in unipolar depression: evidence and theory. Psychol Bull 2:259–282, 1987

Piccinell M, Wilkinson G: Gender differences in depression: critical review. Br J Psychiatry 177:486–492, 2000

Robins LN, Regier DA (eds): Psychiatric Disorders in America: The Epidemiologic Catchment Area Study. New York, The Free Press, 1991

Robins LN, Helzer JE, Croughan J, et al: National Institute of Mental Health Diagnostic Interview Schedule: its history, characteristics, and validity. Arch Gen Psychiatry 38:381–389, 1981

Spitzer RL, Endicott J, Robin E: Research Diagnostic Criteria: rationale and reliability. Arch Gen Psychiatry 35:773–782, 1978

Szadoczky E, Papp Z, Vitrai J, et al: The prevalence of major depressive and bipolar disorders in Hungary: results from a national epidemiologic survey. J Affect Disord 50:153–162, 1998

Weissman MM, Klerman GL: Sex differences and the epidemiology of depression. Arch Gen Psychiatry 34:98–111, 1977

Weissman MM, Bland R, Canino G, et al: The cross national epidemiology of obsessive compulsive disorder. The Cross National Collaborative Group. J Clin Psychiatry 55(suppl):5–10, 1994

Weissman MM, Bland RC, Canino GJ, et al: Cross-national epidemiology of major depression and bipolar disorder. JAMA 276:293–299, 1996a

Weissman MM, Bland RC, Canino GJ, et al: The cross national epidemiology of social phobia: a preliminary report. J Int Clin Psychopharmacol 11:9–14, 1996b

Weissman MM, Bland RC, Canino GJ, et al: The cross national epidemiology of panic disorder. Arch Gen Psychiatry 54:305–309, 1997

Widiger TA, Anderson KG: Personality and depression in women. J Affect Disord 74:59–66, 2003

Wittchen H-U, Kessler R: Modifications of the CIDI in the National Comorbidity Study: the development of the UM-CIDI. NCS Working Paper #2. Ann Arbor, MI, 1994

World Health Organization: Composite International Diagnostic Interview (CIDI), Version 1.0. Geneva, Switzerland, World Health Organization, 1990

World Health Organization: Cross-national comparisons of the prevalences and correlates of mental disorders. Bull World Health Organ 78:413–426, 2000

5

NEUROBIOLOGY AND SEX/GENDER

Margaret Altemus, M.D.

As the knowledge base in neurobiology and relevant research technology continues to expand, we expect that neurobiology will play an increasing role in the definition and validation of diagnostic categories and biobehavioral dimensions of psychopathology that may cut across diagnostic categories. Charney et al. (2002), in *A Research Agenda for DSM-V,* outlined the importance of neurobiology and how neuroscience research should be applied to the DSM-V process and to longer-term efforts to refine our psychiatric diagnostic system. However, their chapter did not address sex differences in neurobiology that may contribute to sex differences in the prevalence, symptom patterns, and treatment response of psychiatric disorders. The aim of the present chapter is to provide a broad overview of research that examines sex differences in neurobiology and to identify lines of research that may provide useful information for further revisions of DSM.

Although there has been relatively little study of sex differences in neurobiology, there is emerging evidence across vertebrate species that differences between the sexes include brain anatomy, cell differentiation, synaptic density, neurochemistry, and patterns of activation and response to environmental stimuli (Cooke et al. 1998). Gender differences in the physiology and pathophysiology of other bodily systems have also been identified that may have an impact on the etiology and course of psychiatric disorders.

One of the major challenges in this effort will be to sort out which sex differences arise from purely biological determinants and which arise from interactions between biology and the environment. There is important evidence for many complex biological–environmental interactions. As reviewed later, there is evidence that sex modulates the effects of acute and chronic stress on neural systems. In addition, as detailed in other chapters in this volume, compared with men, women have greater exposure to and reactivity to sexual abuse. Other gender-specific economic, cultural, and psychosocial stressors may contribute to sex differences in neurobiology. Gender-specific environmental factors include culturally determined behaviors and experiences, such as dieting and exposure to toxins, as well as more biologically determined behaviors, such as sleep disruption associated with infant care. For example, food restriction is known to suppress thyroid hormone activity (Gingras et al. 2000) and to alter brain serotonergic function (Attenburrow et al. 2003), both of which may increase risk of depression in women who diet.

Another major challenge will be to determine whether neurobiological findings associated with particular diagnoses are consequences of the illness process or play more of an etiological role. Some biological measures, such as genetic polymorphisms or mitral valve prolapse, are more likely to be markers of vulnerability to psychiatric disorder. Other biological measures, such as functional neuroimaging or measures of autonomic nervous system regulation, may function as markers of higher-level systems dysregulation. Longitudinal clinical studies and animal models of psychiatric disorders will be needed to address this important issue.

Effects of specific reproductive hormones such as estrogen on gene expression, brain structure, neurochemistry, and behavior are receiving increasing research attention. Changes in reproductive hormones in utero and during puberty, the estrus cycle, pregnancy, and menopause clearly alter brain structure and function and are likely to play a role in the etiology and clinical presentation of psychiatric disorders.

Mechanisms of Sexual Differentiation

Sexual differentiation is influenced by both genetic and hormonal factors, and this process can be divided into several separate stages (Sobel and Imperato-McGinley 2004). First, the genotype (XX for female, XY for male) establishes the genetic sex. Second, the gonadal sex is established by differentiation of the gonad into either ovaries or testes. Development of the male genital phenotype is dependent on exposure to testosterone and hormones produced by the fetal testes. Third, during puberty, testosterone and estradiol promote the development of secondary sexual characteristics. Finally, fluctuations in circulating sex hormones and sex-specific environmental influences during postnatal development, adulthood, and aging contribute to sexual differentiation.

Exposure to gonadal steroid hormones clearly plays a major role in sexual differentiation. Gonadal steroids have physiological effects in a multitude of tissue and organs, including the brain, cardiovascular system, reproductive organs, breast, bone, and muscle. It is now known that gonadal steroids can act in the nucleus to affect gene transcription and act at the cell membrane and other areas within the cell to modulate a wide variety of cell functions. The distribution of cofactors that modulate gonadal steroid actions enable gonadal steroids to have tissue-specific effects. For example, estradiol enhances corticotropin-releasing hormone (CRH) gene expression in uterine tissue, but suppresses it in the hypothalamus. Some gene products differentially expressed in males and females are independent of gonadal steroid exposure and are more directly dependent on sex chromosome genotype (Arnold et al. 2003). Examples include *SRY,* a gene on the Y chromosome thought to initiate testes formation by control of transcription of other genes on autosomal chromosomes, including *SOX9* (Sobel and Imperato-McGinley 2004).

Animal studies have clearly demonstrated biological mechanisms involved in sexual differentiation of sexual phenotype, social and sexual behaviors, and brain circuits that promote sexual behavior. However, we have a relatively poor understanding of the time course and biological mechanisms involved in sexual differentiation of other aspects of brain and behavior.

Sex Differences in Brain Anatomy

A large number of sex differences in the central nervous systems of vertebrates have been identified at the levels of tissue organization as well as gross brain structure and functional organization. Many of these identified sex differences can be reversed by manipulating testosterone or its metabolites during prenatal life and also can be modulated by manipulating gonadal steroid exposure during adulthood. Sex differences in rates of cell death during development and adulthood have been shown to play a major role in sex differences in cell density in many, but not all, sexually dimorphic brain areas (Forger et al. 2004). Many sexually dimorphic brain areas have high concentrations of estrogen and androgen receptors as well as aromatase, the enzyme that converts testosterone to estrogen (Cooke et al. 1998).

A smaller number of sex differences in brain neuroanatomy have been identified in humans, and few findings have been replicated by separate research groups. One converging set of findings, however, suggests that language functions are less lateralized in women. Positron emission tomography (PET) and functional magnetic resonance imaging studies have demonstrated that during phonological language processing, brain activation is lateralized to the left inferior frontal gyrus in men but diffusely involves both the left and right inferior frontal gyri in women (Shaywitz et al. 1995). During recognition of visual and auditory emotional stimuli, men show unilateral frontal activation, whereas women exhibit bilateral frontal and limbic activation (Hall et al. 2004). The anterior commissure and massa intermedia, structures that connect the right and left hemispheres, have been reported to be larger in females (Allen and Gorski 1991), and there are conflicting reports regarding females having a larger corpus callosum (Bishop and Wahlsten 1997; Dubb et al. 2003), which also connects the hemispheres. Larger interhemispheric structures in women may play a role in reported sex differences in cerebral lateralization of cognitive function. Women have larger left cortical language regions (Gur et al. 2002; Harasty et al. 1997) and smaller reductions in volume of the temporal lobes over the course of adulthood (Cowell et al. 1994; Murphy et al. 1996). At the level of tissue organization, there is evidence for a sex difference in the relative number of input and output neurons in the layers of the temporal cortex (Witelson et al. 1995) and in the percentage of grey matter in the left hemisphere (Schlaepfer et al. 1995). These areas are important for language processing, leading investigators to hypothesize that the reported differences may play a role in sex differences in verbal abilities.

Neuroanatomical sex differences should be investigated in humans more thoroughly because sexual dimorphisms in brain structure and function may contribute to sex differences in prevalence, clinical features, and treatment response of psychiatric disorders. In addition, there is emerging evidence that abnormalities in brain structure and function associated with specific disorders may be different in men and women (Amin et al. 2005; Gur et al. 2004), and these findings may also point to a need for sex-specific treatments.

Sex Differences in Brain Neurochemistry

Many sex differences in brain neurochemistry have been identified in animals, but it remains to be determined whether these findings will extend to humans. In rodents, sex differences have been reported in almost all neurochemical systems, including γ-aminobutyric acid (GABA)–expressing neurons in the amygdaloid nuclei (Stefanova 1998), and dopaminergic, serotonergic, and cholinergic systems in the basal forebrain (McEwen and Alves 1999). Some, but not all, of these sex differences are obliterated by castration in males or ovariectomy in females. A much larger and growing body of literature has outlined the effects of estrogen, testosterone, and progesterone on these neurochemical systems and associated behaviors.

Receptor imaging, postmortem, and cerebrospinal fluid studies to date have identified few sex differences in brain neurochemistry in humans. There has been speculation, however, that sex differences in psychopathology may be related to sex differences in neurotransmitter and neuropeptide systems, including opiates, oxytocin, vasopressin, and CRH. Although animal studies have shown that many neuropeptide systems are substantially modulated by sex steroids and are sexually dimorphic, there are large species differences in these systems, so extrapolation from the few available animal studies to humans is difficult. Future research will be facilitated by development of improved methods for studying these systems in humans. One recent study found that in the amygdala, mu-opioid receptor binding potential was higher in women than in men but declined in postmenopausal women to levels below those of men (Zubieta et al. 1999). In another study from the same research group, single photon emission computed tomography showed that the number of years postmenopausal women used hormone replacement therapy correlated positively with vesicular acetylcholine transporter binding indexes in multiple cortical areas (Smith et al. 2001). This finding is consistent with preclinical evidence that estrogen promotes cholinergic activity and suggests that hormone replacement therapy may thereby enhance cognitive function.

Investigators have speculated that sex differences in the oxytocin system play a role in behavioral sex differences in response to stress. Animal studies have shown that oxytocin reduces fear, pain, and stress response and enhances parental, sexual, and social behaviors. However, organization and distribution of brain oxytocin systems vary widely among species. For example, in rodents oxytocin is released into the bloodstream in response to stress and promotes adrenocorticotropic hormone (ACTH) release from the pituitary; in humans, however, oxytocin is not released in response to psychological or physical stressors (except from hypoglycemia), and circulating oxytocin suppresses ACTH release at the pituitary (reviewed in McCarthy and Altemus 1997). We do know that in humans, stress responses are suppressed during pregnancy and lactation, when circulating levels of oxytocin are elevated. However, one study in humans found no sex difference in oxytocin neuron morphometry in the periventricular nucleus (Ishunina and Swaab 1999).

In contrast, sex differences in vasopressin-producing neurons have been found in the supraoptic and paraventricular nuclei of the hypothalamus. Vasopressin neurons are larger and have increased markers of neuronal activity in men compared with women (Ishunina and Swaab 1999; Ishunina et al. 1999). The finding of greater vasopressin production in the hypothalamus in males is consistent with reports that vasopressin may play a greater role in the hypothalamic-pituitary-adrenal (HPA) responses to stress in males versus females (Rubin et al. 1999; Viau et al. 2005).

Sex Differences in Genetic Vulnerability

Sex differences modulate genetic vulnerabilities in several ways. The first and most obvious pertain to X-linked traits or conditions—that is, traits whose genes are located on the X chromosome. Because women carry two X chromosomes, and men only one, X-linked recessive conditions are many orders of magnitude more prevalent in males than in females. X-linked recessive conditions range from mild or harmless (e.g., color blindness, G6PD deficiency) to severe or life-threatening (e.g., hemophilia, Duchenne muscular dystrophy, fragile X syndrome). X-linked dominant conditions are more rare but do exist. For example, hypophosphatemic (vitamin D–resistant) rickets follows this inheritance pattern. These conditions are approximately twice as prevalent in women as in men. More intense expression of X-linked traits can occur in women, because there can be incomplete inactivation of the second X chromosome that may carry the same trait.

Second, sex-specific traits may arise from genes on autosomal chromosomes that have differential effects in men and women due to interactions with other aspects of male versus female anatomy and physiology. Gene expression may be controlled by a sex-specific factor, such as sex steroid hormone levels. Alternatively, the function of the protein produced by the gene may be modulated by sex-specific factors. For example, inherited testicular or uterine defects can be expressed in only one sex. Male-limited precocious puberty (familial testotoxicosis) is an autosomal dominant condition that occurs only in boys but can be genetically transmitted by women. A less obvious but common example is male-pattern baldness, which is inherited as autosomal dominant in men but as autosomal recessive in women. There have been several reports of associations between particular genetic polymorphisms and specific psychiatric disorders that are found in one sex but not the other (Karayiorgou et al. 1997; Zubenko et al. 2002). These reports are preliminary, and need to be replicated, but could provide a new window into the pathophysiology of psychiatric disorders.

Third, parent-of-origin effects may cause a gene to be expressed differently if the gene was inherited from the father versus the mother. These effects can arise for several biological reasons, including genomic imprinting, trinucleotide repeats (e.g., Huntington disease), mitochondrial inheritance, or maternal uterine effects during fetal development (e.g., maternal phenylketonuria). Fourth, in humans and higher primates, mutation rates are several-fold higher in males compared with females (Makova and Li 2002). Finally, Y-linked inheritance probably does not play a role in psychiatric disease, but it should still be mentioned. As far as is known, the Y chromosome carries very few genes that express in humans, and most of those are involved in determining maleness. However, whatever genes are on the Y chromosome are expressed only in men, because women do not carry a Y chromosome.

Sex Differences in Stress Responses: Implications for Psychiatric Disorders

Recent work has demonstrated sex differences in multiple dimensions of neurobiology and behavior in response to stress, underscoring the importance of gender in determining vulnerability to stress. Stressful life events, ongoing stress, and emotional trauma are major risk factors for many psychiatric disorders, particularly when experienced early in life (see Chapter 7, "A Developmental Perspective, With a Focus on Childhood Trauma," of this volume). It has been hypothesized that increased rates of several mood, anxiety, and somatoform disorders in women may arise from increased stress exposure and increased biological stress responsiveness in women.

This hypothesis was initially supported by findings of increased HPA axis responsiveness in female rodents (Young 1998). However, findings in humans suggest that males have greater HPA axis responses to stress (Kudielka et al. 2004). Despite enhanced HPA responses to stress in female rodents, accumulating evidence in both animals and humans suggests that females are resistant to many of the neurobiological and behavioral effects of acute and chronic stress experienced by males. For example, although chronic stress over 21 days produces reversible atrophy of apical dendrites of hippocampal pyramidal neurons in males (Conrad et al. 1999), this effect is not seen in females (Galea et al. 1997). Similarly, repeated swim stress over 30 days decreased CA3 and CA4 pyramidal cell number in gonadectomized male rats but not in females (Mizoguchi et al. 1992). Similar results were found in a study of chronic stress in male and female vervet monkeys subjected to chronic social stress (Uno et al. 1989). Consistent with these sex differences in structural responses to chronic stress, female rats do not show the impairment of spatial memory or object recognition memory after chronic restraint stress that is characteristic of males (Luine 2002). In addition, after an acute stressor, males show enhancement of fear behaviors and impairment of escape learning (learned helplessness), but these effects of acute stress are attenuated in females (Heinsbroek et al. 1991; Steenbergen et al. 1990). In addition, although acute stress in males enhances eyeblink conditioning, a reflex learning that does not involve fear, in females acute stress impairs eyeblink conditioning (Shors and Miesegaes 2002). Finally, in response to acute stress, males and females show opposite patterns of dendritic spine responses on hippocampal neurons (Shors et al. 2001).

Activation of another major stress response system, the sympathetic nervous system, plays a role in the development of hypertension, particularly in its early stages. Essential hypertension is thought to be caused by both genetic and environmental factors, including exposure to chronic stress. Studies that have examined this phenomenon in both sexes have found that women are relatively resistant to the effects of stress on blood pressure. For example, job strain has been linked to higher blood pressure, but this association occurs only in men, not in women (Pickering 1997). In another study, depression was associated with increased blood pressure during sleep and a reduction of the normal diurnal variation of blood pressure in men, but not in women (Kario et al. 2001). On the other hand, blood pressure and pulse are more reactive to anxiety in women compared with men (Kario et al. 2001).

One way to potentially reconcile this evidence for female resistance to neurobiological effects of stress with the increased prevalence of affective illness and anxiety disorders in women is to consider the stress-induced neurobiological changes in males as adaptive, potentially preventing development of depression and anxiety symptoms. In contrast, females may be more susceptible to HPA axis dysregulation once depression develops. Impaired feedback control of the HPA axis in depression was observed in depressed women but not in depressed men (Young et al. 2001). Although animal studies suggest that females are protected from neurobiological and behavioral effects of stress, neurobiological and behavioral changes seen in males following acute and chronic stress may be adaptive in the long run. For example, impaired memory in response to 3 weeks of restraint stress may enable men to forget the stress more quickly when the stress is relieved. Women are twice as likely as men to ruminate about aversive experiences, which is a risk factor for depression (Nolan-Hoeksema 1987).

The role of circulating sex hormones in these sex-specific responses to chronic stress remains to be determined. Estrogen is suspected to contribute to female resistance to stress because of its neuroprotective effects. Estrogen enhances proliferation of neural progenitor cells in the dendate gyrus (Tanapat et al. 1999), increases density of CA1 hippocampal synapses (Woolley et al. 1997), and enhances hippocampal-dependent learning (Luine et al. 1998; Packard and Teather 1997). Estrogen also has been shown to be neuroprotective in brain injury models (Wise et al. 2001). In addition, estrogen has been shown to modulate activity of the two major stress response systems, the HPA axis and the autonomic nervous system. Estrogen effects on the HPA axis are dose-related, with HPA axis suppression occurring at physiological doses of estrogen in women (Roca et al. 2003) and rodents (Young et al. 2001). However, androgens suppress (Lund et al. 2004) and progesterone enhances HPA axis reactivity and may contribute to sex differences in HPA axis responses to stress.

Sex Differences in Physiology and Vulnerability to Medical Illness and Pain

Sex dimorphisms have been identified in the morphology, metabolic regulation, and function of numerous tissues, including bone, muscle, immune cells, and adipose tissue. Women have longer life spans, but greater levels of medical disability, than men. Women have an increased incidence of autoimmune disease, arthritis, and other inflammatory disorders. As our understanding of the interplay between mind and body grows, physiological differences such as these will be important to consider as contributors to sex differences in the prevalence, clinical features, and course of psychiatric disorders. For example, increased tendency toward autoimmune and inflammatory disorders in women many contribute to sex differences in depressive and anxiety disorders. Recent work indicates that immune activation and inflammation may increase risk of depression. Acute stress raises circulating levels of inflammatory cytokines, and individuals with depression and anxiety disorders have been shown to have elevated circulating levels of inflammatory cytokines (A.H. Miller 1998; G.E. Miller et al. 2005).

Sex differences have been found in perceived pain from stimuli such as heat, hypertonic saline injection, and deep-tissue pain. Although few studies have addressed the underlying mechanisms, emerging evidence suggests sex differences in patterns of inhibitory control in central pain systems (Ge et al. 2004; Staud et al. 2003), cognitive network activation, and μ-opioid receptor activation. Specifically, women appear to have decreased diffuse noxious inhibitory control, a mechanism of pain inhibition in which certain neurons in the dorsal horn of the spinal cord are inhibited in response to nociceptive stimuli applied to any part of the body.

There are also marked sex differences in the magnitude of μ-opioid activation following pain stimulus in the anterior thalamus, ventral basal ganglia, amygdala, and nucleus accumbens (Zubieta et al. 2002). During noxious heat stimulation, PET scans showed similar responses between men and women in bilateral premotor cortex and anterior cingulate cortex activation. However, women had significantly greater activation of contralateral prefrontal cortex and thalamus (Paulson et al. 1998).

PET scans of men and women with irritable bowel syndrome also indicated sex differences in brain activation in response to both visceral and anticipated pain (Naliboff et al. 2003). Whereas activation of the ventral prefrontal cortex, right anterior cingulate cortex, and left amygdala was greater in women, the dorsolateral prefrontal cortex, insula, and dorsal pons were more activated in men.

Currently, if a general medical cause can be identified, the DSM-IV diagnosis of "mood disorder due to a general medical condition" or "anxiety disorder due to a general medical condition" is assigned. This approach to diagnosis may need to be modified as increasing numbers of physiological factors that contribute to vulnerability are identified.

Sex Differences in the Effects of Drugs and Alcohol

Sex differences have been found in brain sensitivity to alcohol, which is thought to modulate brain glucose metabolism via GABAergic neurotransmission. For the same blood alcohol levels, brain metabolism is increased more in males, whereas self-reports of intoxication and cognitive impairments are greater in females (Wang et al. 2003). A recent report also suggests that brain GABA content is suppressed in female but not male smokers, potentially contributing to higher rates of depression in women after smoking cessation (Epperson et al. 2005). In another study, sex differences have been found in perfusion abnormalities of cocaine-dependent individuals. Men have decreased perfusion in the anterior cingulate and frontal regions, similar to that associated with withdrawal and impaired inhibition, whereas women have increased perfusion in the posterior cingulate region, which is correlated with a heightened stress response. It is possible that these differences contribute to different neural mechanisms for relapse in cocaine-dependent men and women (Tucker et al. 2004).

Gaps in the Literature and a Proposed Research Agenda

The primary gap in the literature on gender and neurobiology is a lack of knowledge of potential sex differences in human neurobiological systems and disease processes. Improved understanding of the sex-related biological processes that contribute to illness vulnerability and modulate clinical features of particular disorders will ultimately enhance the validity of DSM-V and subsequent editions of DSM.

Sex differences can be a window that provides new perspectives on biological mechanisms. For example, the finding that increased risk of depression at puberty is limited to girls with a family history of depression as they reach Tanner stage III (Angold et al. 1999) should lead to new understanding of how the effects of particular genetic alleles that increase risk for depression are amplified by increased production of estrogen or other reproductive hormones as girls reach Tanner stage III.

Additional research on neurobiology should also help to define and inform a number of sex-related diagnostic issues. The first, and clearest, example concerns disorders that are gender specific due to unambiguous and complete biological sex differences. These include premenstrual dysphoric disorder and some sexual dysfunctions such as vaginismus and premature ejaculation. Another relevant diagnostic issue is whether to include gender-specific syndromes within one diagnosis. For example, girls with conduct disorder demonstrate more impulsive sexual behavior and boys engage in more interpersonal violence (Fergusson et al. 1994). If these behaviors are linked to similar biological processes, it would strengthen the argument for having a single criteria set that incorporates both behavioral profiles. On the other hand, if gender-specific biological mechanisms are found to underlie phenotypically similar clinical syndromes, and to be associated with response to distinct treatments, this will raise the issue of creating separate diagnoses or diagnostic subgroups for men and women with similar symptoms. For example, episodic obsessive-compulsive disorder associated only with pregnancy and the postpartum period may arise from biological processes distinct from more chronic forms of the disorder and may respond to different treatments. Animal studies have shown that males and females can have distinct biological mechanisms underlying similar physiological and behavioral responses (De Vries and Boyle 1998). For example, in male voles, parental behavior is dependent on vasopressin but not on oxytocin, as in female voles (Insel et al. 1998). Another example discussed earlier is a greater role in males for vasopressin in activating the HPA axis responses to stress (Rubin et al. 1999; Viau et al. 2005). More careful attention to sex differences may extend our recognition of such phenomena.

More specifically, the following are some of the more salient research gaps that need to be addressed by future research.

1. *Develop experimental designs that allow meaningful consideration of gender as a variable in clinical studies.* Gender should be incorporated as a variable in clinical studies of phenomenology, genetics, neuroimaging, neuroendocrinology, pharmacokinetics, and treatment response. Gender should be considered in postmortem studies as well. Consideration of gender in experimental designs will need to include controls for reproductive stage of males and females

(puberty, menstrual cycle phase, menopausal status), hormonal treatments, and age. Study designs incorporating effects of gender will likely require increased numbers of subjects to provide adequate statistical power.

2. *Study potential neuroanatomical sex differences throughout the life span in healthy humans and individuals with psychiatric disorders.* Such investigations will include structural neuroimaging, magnetic resonance spectroscopy to detect sex differences in brain neurochemistry, and functional neuroimaging to detect potential sex differences in brain activation patterns in response to different stimuli and tasks. Postmortem studies examining brain structure, neurochemistry, and gene expression should also be designed to detect potential sex differences. Some sex differences may be evident in healthy adults, but others may emerge only among individuals with psychiatric disorders or at particular developmental stages. Neuropsychological studies should also be designed to detect potential sex differences.
3. *Include gender comparisons in preclinical studies of neurobiology and behavior.* A recent review by Becker et al. (2005) outlined a number of experimental design guidelines and experimental methods to facilitate meaningful comparison of males and females, to investigate the behavioral implications of sex differences, and to determine the endocrine and/or genetic factors that contribute to sex differences. A particularly striking gap in the field is knowledge of the potential interaction of gender and sexual maturation with genetic manipulations in transgenic mice. Typically, male and female animals are combined in one group for examination of the effects of genetic manipulations on neurobiology and behavior. In the majority of studies, genes are altered at the start of prenatal development, maximizing the opportunity for modulation by gonadal steroids of gene expression and downstream effects.
4. *Undertake more detailed study of the effects of reproductive transitions and hormonal treatments on neurobiology in healthy humans and on the neurobiology and phenomenology of psychiatric disorders.* Changes in reproductive hormones occur during puberty in boys and girls, across the menstrual cycle, and during pregnancy, lactation, and menopause, and with aging in men. However, naturalistic studies of the effects of reproductive events such as pregnancy or menopause on the course of psychiatric illness can only provide correlational data regarding hormonal effects. Experimental studies using specific hormone manipulations in human and animal models are necessary to determine the role of sex chromosomes and sex hormones in psychiatric disorders. Large numbers of men receive anti-androgen treatments for prostate cancer, and many women receive selective estrogen receptor antagonists during treatment for breast cancer. Women also undergo surgical or pharmacologically induced menopause for treatment of a variety of conditions. In addition, women are exposed to high levels of estrogen during some infertility treatments. Although the effects of these agents on cognitive function have received some attention, little is known

about their effect on the course of psychiatric disorders. Hormonal manipulations can also be performed in healthy volunteers and patient volunteers to clarify the effects of steroid hormones on neurobiology, behavior, and clinical features of psychiatric disorders.

5. *Conduct additional research on medical conditions characterized by disruption of the normal process of sexual differentiation or gonadal steroid regulation.* Studies of individuals with disorders of gonad steroid function can be used to help clarify the differential effects of genetic sex and hormonal exposure on sexual differentiation of brain and behavior. For example, women with congenital adrenal hyperplasia have an XX genotype but produce excessive levels of androgens in utero and postnatally if treatment is delayed or interrupted. This disorder is associated with masculinized genitalia, and there is evidence of masculinization of some behavioral traits during childhood (Hines and Kaufman 1994). Similar behavioral changes have been noted in women whose mothers received androgenic progestins during pregnancy (Collaer and Hines 1995). Men with complete androgen insensitivity syndrome have an XY genotype and produce androgens, but androgen receptor function is impaired. This disorder is characterized by feminization of external genitalia and development of female secondary sexual characteristics at puberty in males (Hines et al. 2003; Sultan et al. 2002). Preliminary evidence suggests a female pattern of cognitive function in males with this disorder (Imperato-McGinley et al. 1991). However, because men with the disorder are typically raised as females, and their gender role behavior and gender identity are similar to that of genetic females, it is not possible to sort out the contribution of sex-specific postnatal environmental influences on sexual differentiation of brain and behavior. In contrast, genetic males with a 5-alpha-reductase deficiency have female genitalia at birth but can respond to testosterone at puberty and develop male secondary sex characteristics. Women with polycystic ovarian syndrome also have elevated levels of circulating androgen hormones that can be controlled with treatment, but potential effects of this disorder on the prevalence or course of psychiatric illness has not been studied.
6. *Study the interaction between gender and acute and chronic stress.* Experimental animal studies and, in humans, age-cohort studies and longitudinal studies should be conducted to scrutinize the effects of different developmental stages and reproductive transitions (e.g., puberty and menopause) on stress-induced risk for psychopathology. Such studies may help elucidate the interrelationship among stressful life experiences, gender, and genotype in determining risk for psychiatric disorders as well as the underlying mechanisms across the life span. Insights gained from these studies might help identify developmental periods of particular risk for women versus men and might lead toward prevention and treatment strategies that directly target the involved mechanisms.

7. *Pay attention to species-specificity of sex differences.* Concentration of work in rodents may limit understanding of human sex differences. For example, models of the menstrual cycle may be better developed in primates, which have estrus cycles of more similar length to the human menstrual cycle.

Conclusions

The research agenda for sex differences in neurobiology has two primary points of focus: 1) to characterize sex differences in neurobiology, and 2) to determine the clinical relevance of these differences. It is unlikely that increased research on sex differences in neurobiology will substantially inform the empirical data base in time for the development of DSM-V. Unfortunately, there is a scarcity of adequate biological data sets that could be reexamined to detect effects of gender or sex hormones. In addition, it will be difficult to make definitive statements about the role of gender in psychopathology and relevance for DSM until there is a better understanding of the biological pathogenesis of psychiatric disorders. Instead, increased attention to sex differences in neurobiology should become long-term and highly prioritized goals of psychiatric research. Such research will undoubtedly enhance clinical understanding and improve the validity of our classification system. Because great progress is currently being made in clarifying the biological mechanisms contributing to psychopathology, it should be possible to make substantial progress toward these goals in the coming decades.

References

Allen L, Gorski R: Sexual dimorphism of the anterior commissure and massa intermedia of the human brain. J Comp Neurol 312:97–104, 1991

Amin Z, Canli T, Epperson CN: Effect of estrogen-serotonin interactions on mood and cognition. Behav Cogn Neurosci Rev 4:43–58, 2005

Angold A, Costello EJ, Erkanli A, et al: Pubertal changes in hormone levels and depression in girls. Psychol Med 29:1043–1053, 1999

Arnold AP, Rissman EF, De Vries GJ: Two perspectives on the origin of sex differences in the brain. Ann NY Acad Sci 1007:176–188, 2003

Attenburrow MJ, Williams C, Odontiadis J, et al: Effect of a nutritional source of tryptophan on dieting-induced changes in brain 5-HT function. Psychol Med 33:1381–1386, 2003

Becker JB, Arnold AP, Berkley KJ, et al: Strategies and methods for research on sex differences in brain and behavior. Endocrinology 146:1650–1673, 2005

Bishop K, Wahlsten D: Sex differences in the human corpus callosum: myth or reality. Neurosci Biobehav Rev 21:581–601, 1997

Charney DS, Barlow DH, Botteron K, et al: Neuroscience research agenda to guide development of a pathophysiologically based classification system, in A Research Agenda for DSM-V. Edited by Kupfer DJ, First MB, Regier DA. Washington DC, American Psychiatric Association, 2002, pp 31–83

Collaer M, Hines M: Human behavioral sex differences: a role for gonadal hormones during early development? Psychol Bull 118:55–107, 1995

Conrad CD, LeDoux JE, Magarinos AM, et al: Repeated restraint stress facilitates fear conditioning, independently of causing hippocampal CA3 dendritic atrophy. Behav Neurosci 113:902–913, 1999

Cooke BC, Hegstrom CD, Villeneuve LS, et al: Sexual differentiation of the vertebrate brain: principles and mechanisms. Front Neuroendocrinol 19:323–362, 1998

Cowell PE, Turetsky BI, Gur RC, et al: Sex differences in aging of the human frontal and temporal lobes. J Neurosci 14:4748–4755, 1994

De Vries GJ, Boyle PA: Double duty for sex differences in the brain. Behav Brain Res 92:205–213, 1998

Dubb A, Gur R, Avants B, et al: Characterization of sexual dimorphism in the human corpus callosum. Neuroimage 20:512–519, 2003

Epperson CN, O'Malley S, Czarkowski KA, et al: Sex, GABA, and nicotine: the impact of smoking on cortical GABA levels across the menstrual cycle as measured with proton magnetic resonance spectroscopy. Biol Psychiatry 57:44–48, 2005

Fergusson DM, Horwood LJ, Lynskey MT: The comorbidities of adolescent problem behaviors: a latent class model. J Abnorm Child Psychol 22:339–354, 1994

Forger NG, Rosen GJ, Waters EM, et al: Deletion of Bax eliminates sex differences in the mouse forebrain. Proc Natl Acad Sci USA 101:13666–13671, 2004

Galea LA, McEwen BS, Tanapat P, et al: Sex differences in dendritic atrophy of CA3 pyramidal neurons in response to chronic restraint stress. Neuroscience 81:689–697, 1997

Ge HY, Madeleine P, Arendt-Nielsen L: Sex differences in temporal characteristics of descending inhibitory control: an evaluation using repeated bilateral experimental induction of muscle pain. Pain 110:72–78, 2004

Gingras JR, Harber V, Field CJ, et al: Metabolic assessment of female chronic dieters with either normal or low resting energy expenditures. Am J Clin Nutr 71:1413–1420, 2000

Gur RC, Gunning-Dixon F, Bilker WB, et al: Sex differences in temporolimbic and frontal brain volumes of healthy adults. Cereb Cortex 12:998–1003, 2002

Gur RE, Kohler C, Turetsky BI, et al: A sexually dimorphic ratio of orbitofrontal to amygdala volume is altered in schizophrenia. Biol Psychiatry 55:512–517, 2004

Hall GB, Witelson SF, Szechtman H, et al: Sex differences in functional activation patterns revealed by increased emotion processing demands. Neuroreport 15:219–223, 2004

Harasty J, Double KL, Halliday GM, et al: Language-associated cortical regions are proportionally larger in the female brain. Arch Neurol 54:171–176, 1997

Heinsbroek RP, Van Haaren F, Van de Poll NE, et al: Sex differences in the behavioral consequences of inescapable footshocks depend on time since shock. Physiol Behav 49:1257–1263, 1991

Hines M, Kaufman F: Androgen and the development of human sex-typical behavior: rough-and-tumble play and sex of preferred playmates in children with congenital adrenal hyperplasia (CAH). Child Dev 65:1042–1053, 1994

Hines M, Ahmed SF, Hughes IA: Psychological outcomes and gender-related development in complete androgen insensitivity syndrome. Arch Sex Behav 32:93–101, 2003

Imperato-McGinley J, Pichardo M, Gautier T, et al: Cognitive abilities in androgen-insensitive subjects: comparison with control males and females from the same kindred. Clin Endocrinol 34:341–347, 1991

Insel TR, Winslow JT, Wang Z, et al: Oxytocin, vasopressin, and the neuroendocrine basis of pair bond formation. Adv Exp Med Biol 449:215–224, 1998

Ishunina TA, Swaab DF: Vasopressin and oxytocin neurons of the human supraoptic and paraventricular nucleus: size changes in relation to age and sex. J Clin Endocrinol Metab 84:4637–4544, 1999

Ishunina TA, Salehi A, Hofman MA, et al: Activity of vasopressinergic neurones of the human supraoptic nucleus is age- and sex-dependent. J Neuroendocrinol 11:251–258, 1999

Karayiorgou M, Altemus M, Galke BL, et al: Genotype determining low catechol-O-methyltransferase activity as a risk factor for obsessive-compulsive disorder. Proc Natl Acad Sci 94:4572–4575, 1997

Kario K, Schwartz JE, Davidson KW, et al: Gender differences in associations of diurnal blood pressure variation. Hypertension 38:997–1002, 2001

Kudielka BM, Buske-Kirschbaum A, Hellhammer DH, et al: HPA axis responses to laboratory psychosocial stress in healthy elderly adults, younger adults, and children: impact of age and gender. Psychoneuroendocrinology 29:83–98, 2004

Luine V: Sex differences in chronic stress effects on memory in rats. Stress 5:205–216, 2002

Luine VN, Richards ST, Wu VY, et al: Estradiol enhances learning and memory in a spatial memory task and effects levels of monoaminergic neurotransmitters. Horm Behav 34:149–162, 1998

Lund TD, Munson DJ, Haldy ME, et al: Dihydrotestosterone may inhibit hypothalamo-pituitary-adrenal activity by acting through estrogen receptor in the male mouse. Neuroscience Lett 365:43–47, 2004

Makova K, Li WH: Strong male-driven evolution of DNA sequences in humans and apes. Nature 416:624–626, 2002

McCarthy MM, Altemus M: Central nervous system actions of oxytocin and modulation of behavior in humans. Mol Med Today 3:269–275, 1997

McEwen BS, Alves SE: Estrogen actions in the central nervous system. Endocrine Rev 20:279–307, 1999

Miller AH: Neuroendocrine and immune system interactions in stress and depression. Psychiatr Clin North Am 21:443–463, 1998

Miller GE, Rohleder N, Stetler C, et al: Clinical depression and regulation of the inflammatory response during acute stress. Psychosom Med 67:679–687, 2005

Mizoguchi K, Kunishita T, Chui DH, et al: Stress induces neuronal death in the hippocampus of castrated rats. Neurosci Lett 138:157–160, 1992

Murphy DG, DeCarli C, McIntosh AR, et al: Sex differences in human brain morphometry and metabolism: an in vivo quantitative magnetic resonance imaging and positron emission tomography study on the effect of aging. Arch Gen Psychiatry 53:585–594, 1996

Naliboff BD, Berman S, Chang L, et al: Sex-related differences in IBS patients: central processing of visceral stimuli. Gastroenterology 124:1738–1747, 2003

Nolan-Hoeksema S: Sex differences in unipolar depression: evidence and theory. Psychol Bull 2:259–282, 1987

Packard MG, Teather LA: Post-training estradiol injections enhance memory in ovariectomized rats: cholinergic blockade and synergism. Neurobiol Learn Mem 68:172–188, 1997

Paulson PE, Minoshima S, Morrow TJ, et al: Gender differences in pain perception and patterns of cerebral activation during noxious heat stimulation in humans. Pain 76:223–229, 1998

Pickering TG: The effects of environmental and lifestyle factors on blood pressure and the intermediary role of the sympathetic nervous system. J Human Hypertension 11 (suppl):S9–S18, 1997

Roca CA, Schmidt PJ, Altemus M, et al: Differential menstrual cycle regulation of hypothalamic-pituitary-adrenal axis in women with premenstrual syndrome and controls. J Clin Endocrinol Metab 88:3057–3063, 2003

Rubin RT, Abbasi SA, Rhodes ME, et al: Pituitary-adrenal cortical responses to low-dose physostigmine and arginine vasopressin administration in normal women and men. Neuropsychopharmacology 20:434–446, 1999

Schlaepfer TE, Harris GJ, Tien AY, et al: Structural differences in the cerebral cortex of healthy female and male subjects: a magnetic resonance imaging study. Psychiatry Res 61:129–135, 1995

Shaywitz BA, Shaywitz SE, Pugh KR, et al: Sex differences in the functional organization of the brain for language. Nature 373:607–609, 1995

Shors TJ, Chua C, Falduto J: Sex differences and opposite effects of stress on dendritic spine density in the male versus female hippocampus. J Neurosci 21:6292–6297, 2001

Shors TJ, Miesegaes G: Testosterone in utero and at birth dictates how stressful experience will affect learning in adulthood. Proc Natl Acad Sci USA 99:13955–13960, 2002

Smith YR, Minoshima S, Kuhl DE et al: Effects of long-term hormone therapy on cholinergic synaptic concentrations in healthy postmenopausal women. J Clin Endocrinol Metab 86:679–684, 2001

Sobel V, Imperato-McGinley J: Fetal hormones and sexual differentiation. Obstet Gynecol Clin North Am 31:837–856, 2004

Staud R, Robinson ME, Vierck CJ Jr, et al: Diffuse noxious inhibitory controls (DNIC) attenuate temporal summation of second pain in normal males but not in normal females or fibromyalgia patients. Pain 10:167–174, 2003

Steenbergen HL, Heinsbroek RP, Van Hest A, et al: Sex-dependent effects of inescapable shock administration on shuttlebox-escape performance and elevated plus-maze behavior. Physiol Behav 48:571–576, 1990

Stefanova N: Gamma-aminobutyric acid-immunoreactive neurons in the amygdala of the rat: sex differences and effect of early postnatal castration. Neurosci Lett 255:175–177, 1998

Sultan C, Lumbroso S, Paris F, et al: Disorders of androgen action. Semin Reprod Med 20:217–228, 2002

Tanapat P, Hastings NB, Reeves AJ, et al: Estrogen stimulates a transient increase in the number of new neurons in the dentate gyrus of the adult female rat. J Neurosci 19:5792–5801, 1999

Tucker KA, Browndyke JN, Gottschalk PC, et al: Gender-specific vulnerability for rCBF abnormalities among cocaine abusers. Neuroreport 15:797–801, 2004

Uno H, Tarara R, Else JG, et al: Hippocampal damage associated with prolonged and fatal stress in primates. J Neurosci 9:1705–1711, 1989

Viau V, Bingham B, Davis J, et al: Gender and puberty interact on the stress-induced activation of parvocellular neurosecretory neurons and corticotropin-releasing hormone messenger ribonucleic acid expression in the rat. Endocrinology 146:137–146, 2005

Wang GC, Volkow ND, Fowler JS, et al: Alcohol intoxication induces greater reductions in brain metabolism in male than in female subjects. Alcohol Clin Exp Res 27:909–917, 2003

Wise PM, Dubal DB, Wilson ME, et al: Estrogens: trophic and protective factors in the adult brain. Frontiers in Neuroendocrinology 22:33–66, 2001

Witelson SF, Glezer II, Kigar DL: Women have greater density of neurons in posterior temporal cortex. J Neurosci 15:3418–3428, 1995

Woolley CS, Weiland NG, McEwen BS, et al: Estradiol increases the sensitivity of hippocampal CA1 pyramidal cells to NMDA receptor-mediated synaptic input: correlation with dendritic spine density. J Neurosci 17:1848–1859, 1997

Young EA: Sex differences and the HPA axis: implications for psychiatric disease. J Gend Specif Med 1:21–27, 1998

Young EA, Altemus M, Parkison V, et al: Effect of estrogen antagonists and agonists on the ACTH response to restraint stress in female rats. Neuropsychopharmacology 25:881–891, 2001

Zubenko GS, Hughes HB 3rd, Maher BS, et al: Genetic linkage of region containing the CREB1 gene to depressive disorders in women from families with recurrent, early onset, major depression. Am J Med Genet 114:980–987, 2002

Zubieta JK, Dannals RF, Frost JJ: Gender and age influences on human brain mu opioid receptor binding measured by PET. Am J Psychiatry 156:842–848, 1999

Zubieta JK, Smith YR, Bueller JA, et al: mu-opioid receptor-mediated antinociceptive responses differ in men and women. J Neurosci 22:5100–5107, 2002

6

SOCIOCULTURAL FACTORS AND GENDER

Katherine Shear, M.D.
Katherine A. Halmi, M.D.
Thomas A. Widiger, Ph.D.
Cheryl Boyce, Ph.D.

Environmental and sociocultural factors are risk factors for psychopathology that interact in complex ways with neurobiological factors. Culture and its relationship with psychopathology have been more extensively reviewed and discussed elsewhere (Alarcón et al. 2002). Here, we discuss additional aspects of sociocultural factors as they pertain to gender.

Culture has been defined in various ways, one of which is "broad collective patterns of thinking, feeling and acting that have important consequences for the functioning of societies, of groups within those societies and of individual members of such groups" (Arrindell et al. 2004). Culture has also been more colloquially referred to as "mental software" (Hofstede 1980). There is solid evidence that environmental and sociocultural factors contribute to gender differences in health and mental health. Attributes and experiences that may differ by gender and contribute to vulnerability, onset, or maintenance of illness include such variables as coping styles, personality traits, sex roles, demographic groups (e.g., age, marital status, educational status, income), social support, social isolation, childhood adversity, societal change, and cultural norms.

As groups, men and women have different degrees of demographic burden, such as poverty, unemployment, and caregiving responsibilities. Marital status has a different effect on men and women, and the two sexes differ in their reactivity to marital and other interpersonal difficulties. Men and women have different risks for experiencing common life stressors, and there is evidence for gender differences in reactivity to stressors (see Chapter 5). Much of the available data on sociocultural risk in mental health pertain to anxiety and/or depression in adults (e.g., Bebbington 1999). Thus, in this section we focus on these disorders, as well as suicide, eating disorders, and personality traits and disorders. The review provided here is not comprehensive. Instead, it focuses on selected aspects of this large topic in order to convey the importance of sociocultural factors and their influence on various types of gender differences. In addition, this summary provides the basis for our recommendations regarding the type of information researchers need to collect for future diagnostic classifications.

Depression, Anxiety Disorders, and Suicide

Marital status, child care, employment status, and income all contribute to risk for depression. However, studies suggest that marriage may affect men and women differently. Specifically, it appears that married men have lower rates of minor depression than their unmarried counterparts, whereas the reverse is true for women (Bebbington et al. 1981). A possible reason for this difference is that marital discord appears to affect women more than men. Kiecolt-Glaser and Newton (2001) provided an informative review of the relationship between marital functioning and physical health, with an emphasis on gender differences. They reviewed 64 published studies that addressed this topic and concluded that the evidence is mounting that gender influences the relationship between marital disharmony and physical ill health. Across studies, women show more pronounced and persistent physiological reactions to marital conflict, and several studies show a relationship between physical health and marital functioning for women but not for men. For example, a survey of social role functioning was conducted among a random sample of patients drawn from a large health maintenance organization (Hibbard and Pope 1993). Over a 15-year period following the survey, respondents' medical records were reviewed for data on serious morbidity and mortality. Among women, equality in decision making in their marriages and a sense of companionship were associated with a significant reduction in death rate (although no difference in other morbidity) over the study period. For men, no marital characteristics were related to morbidity or mortality. For women, support at work was associated with a lower death rate and lower rate of stroke at 15-year follow-up and lower rate of malignancy at 10-year follow-up. Among men, work stress predicted a greater incidence of myocardial infarction.

Kiecolt-Glaser and Newton's (2001) study of distressed marital couples provides parallel findings that may be related to these health outcomes. Her group found that wives responded to negative marital interaction with greater depression, hostility, and systolic blood pressure increase than their husbands. Also of interest, wives showed reduced lymphocyte proliferative response to phytohemaglutin, evidence of reduced immune function, and a possible mediator of stress-related illness. By contrast, lymphocyte phytohemaglutin increased in husbands following marital conflict (Mayne et al. 1997). Of interest, one study found that men who had divorced or separated had a higher incidence of major depression in the first year after divorce than did women (Bruce and Kim 1992). In fact, men's ratings of happiness and life satisfaction are positively correlated with being married, whereas this is not true for women. Also, when married men are asked to identify their best friend and confidante, they tend to pick their wives, whereas married women tend to choose other women, rather than their husband.

Severe marital conflict that results in domestic violence is also likely to affect women more than men because women are more likely to be the victims of violence. Domestic violence is a known risk factor for depressive and anxiety disorders (e.g., Hegarty et al. 2004) across cultures (e.g., Hicks and Li 2003). Child care, usually the province of women, is regularly found to be associated with increased rates of depression (Bebbington 1999). Women also have lower levels of employment, less education, and lower income, each of which is also a risk factor for depression. Unemployment, however, generally has a more severe impact on men than women.

As was discussed in Chapter 4 ("Gender and the Prevalence of Psychiatric Disorders"), cross-cultural studies document consistent gender differences in rates of depression and anxiety disorders, although the magnitude of gender differences varies across psychiatric disorders and across cultures. Reasons for such variation are not necessarily obvious and have been the focus of much speculation and, more recently, empirical research. Weissman et al. (1996) suggested that different prevalences of major depression across countries may be due to different risk factor profiles or cultural differences. Risk factors may include environmental factors such as stability and strength of the economy and political structure, rates of marital separation and divorce, and exposure to war. Social experiences such as these may affect men and women differently.

As another example, posttraumatic stress disorder (PTSD) rates are higher in women. Sex differences in hypothalamic-pituitary-adrenal (HPA) axis function might contribute to differential risk for PTSD and other disorders in men and women, particularly in response to stress. However, sociocultural factors, such as poorer social supports and exposure to family violence, may also play a role. Women also show increased rates of comorbid substance abuse and PTSD, with women who are substance users more likely to have PTSD than women in general (Najavits et al. 1997).

Important gender differences have also been found in death by suicide. There is evidence that suicide rates can be substantially influenced by sociocultural factors. Although rates of depression are higher in women than in men across cultures (see Chapter 4), the World Health Organization reported that in 1995–1996, male deaths by suicide exceeded female deaths in 83 of 84 countries (all countries except China). Across nations, the median suicide rates were 6.1 per 100,000 for females and 20.5 for males, with a range of 0.2–30.5 for females and 1.1–79.1 for males across different countries. Suicide incidence also varied significantly across age groups, from a low of 0.3 per 100,000 for young girls to 47.5 per 100,000 for older males (Rudmin et al. 2003; World Health Organization 1995, 1996).

Geert Hofstede (1980) analyzed data from a questionnaire survey administered to 88,000 people in 50 occupational groups in 66 countries. He initially developed a model that includes four dimensions of work-related cultural values:

1. *Power-distance,* a measure of social distance related to status, financial, and organizational power (higher power-distance reflects greater social distance between those low and high in status and power measures; the Philippines and Mexico are examples of countries high on power-distance, whereas Austria and Israel are low).
2. *Uncertainty-avoidance,* a measure of general preference for stability and predictability (Greece and Portugal are high on uncertainty–avoidance, whereas Denmark and Singapore are low).
3. *Individualism,* a measure of self-perception of being autonomous rather than defined by social groups (the United States and Australia are high on individualism whereas Venezuela and Colombia are low).
4. *Masculinity,* a measure of the degree to which social roles for men and women are distinct, with women having lower status; "masculine" societies tend to value performance, and "feminine" societies tend to value welfare and provide more opportunities for women (Japan and Austria are high on masculinity, and Norway and Sweden are low).

A fifth dimension, added later, was termed *long-term versus short-term orientation,* which refers to the degree to which a culture creates expectation of delayed gratification (http://www.geert-hofstede.com; accessed May 17, 2007).

A recent study of culture, age, and gender examined, using Hofstede's categories, the relationship of suicide to cultural values. Data on these cultural values, which were available for 39 countries, suggested that individualism correlated positively with suicidality, suggesting that this cultural orientation may facilitate or disinhibit suicide. Higher power-distance tends to be associated with lower suicidality. Greater preference for stability and predictability (uncertainty-avoidance) is associated with lower suicidality for people over 25, especially women. Higher masculinity was also weakly correlated with lower suicide rates. Overall, these cultural values explained a large proportion of the variance—25%—in reported suicide rates. Most of this effect was in the 34–54 age group, and the effect of these values appears stronger for women than for men.

There were some interesting gender-by-age interactions related to these cultural effects. For example, masculinity had no effect on suicide rates among males or females under 25 and a weak negative effect in older age groups (Rudmin et al. 2003).

The findings that suicide rates are consistently higher in men than in women across cultures but that suicide in women is more strongly predicted by cultural variables are both significant. Rudmin et al. (2003) hypothesized that women are more social and contextual in their moral reasoning and that suicide for women is more likely to entail social considerations. They suggested that suicide in women is less impulsive than in men and thus more influenced by context and culture. Despite this study's limitations, it suggests that cultural factors influence suicidality, that this influence is both qualitatively and quantitatively different in women and men, and that suicide rates differ within gender across the life span. These ideas are consistent with the *National Strategy for Suicide Prevention: Goals and Objectives for Action* (U.S. Public Health Service 2001), which calls for interventions tailored to cultural contexts as part of the plan to eliminate health disparities in suicide.

Additional research has focused on Hofstede's five cultural dimensions and their relationship to psychopathology. For example, a study of university students in 11 countries found that students from cultures with higher masculinity scores had higher scores on a measure of agoraphobia (Arrindell et al. 2003a). Cultures that score high on masculinity have more gender role differences and more rigid gender role expectations. In women especially, assertiveness is less accepted, and low assertiveness is associated with phobic symptoms. In another study, higher masculinity scores were strongly correlated with a broad range of phobic symptoms (excluding social fears); uncertainty-avoidance contributed further to the cultural variance in phobic symptom scores. In a study of 3,438 female and 2,091 male university students aged 17–30 from 21 countries (Arrindell et al. 2003b), cultural masculinity correlated strongly with Beck Depression Inventory scores. The authors suggested that cultures that are high on masculinity offer less opportunity for multiple role fulfillment and that sex role inequalities are associated with lower marital satisfaction. Masculine societies are less nurturing and associated with overall lower happiness. Thus, cultural values—in particular, those reflecting masculine/feminine traits—appear to be related to various aspects of psychopathology.

Cultural Aspects of Eating Disorders

Eating disorders offer an example of psychopathology that occurs primarily in women and whose prevalence and clinical features are clearly influenced by sociocultural factors (although biological factors are important as well). For example, identification of eating disorders, especially anorexia nervosa and bulimia nervosa or variations thereof, was rare in non-Western countries in the 1970s and 1980s, in contrast to the United States and Europe (Bebbington et al. 1981; Lee et al. 1989). Later studies published in the 1990s suggested that eating disorders did occur in Asiatic and Middle Eastern countries but did so predominately in families of higher socioeconomic status (Buhrich 1981; Mumford and Whitehouse 1988).

Several studies show that the stress of immigration and acculturation may be key factors for developing eating disorders. Arab college students in London (Ballot et al. 1981) and Greek and Turkish girls in Germany (Fichter et al. 1988) are more likely to develop eating disorders than their peers in their homeland. There is some indication that eating disorders increase in those migrating women who assimilate the values, such as the standard of thinness, of their new environment (Apter et al. 1994; Mukai et al. 1994; Mumford et al. 1992; Nasser 1986). The issue of wanting to be part of mainstream culture is not restricted to recent immigrants. One large survey in the United States showed that binge eating or vomiting is as likely among African American women as in white women (Striegel-Moore et al. 2000).

There are several problems and challenges in the study of sociocultural influences in the development of eating disorders. The first problem is the definition of eating disorders, given that our current definitions may not be equally relevant in all cultures. For example, a study of Asian individuals with anorexia nervosa showed that many of them do not have an excessive concern with body fat (Lee et al. 1989). In a retrospective study in Hong Kong (Furnham and Alibhai 1983), 41 of 70 Chinese anorectic patients stated they could not eat because of stomach bloating and lack of hunger. It is possible that in their culture, stomach bloating provides a better excuse for food refusal than wanting to be thin. Another possibility is that Chinese individuals may be more likely to have physiological attributions rather than psychosocial attributions for psychological problems.

A related problem in comparing eating disorders across cultures is the validity of the translated structured interviews and other research questionnaires. For example, if Chinese anorectic patients are not afraid of getting fat and do not have a fat phobia, they may be screened out as not having an eating disorder, even though all other aspects of their symptoms resemble those of classic anorexia in Europe or the United States. There is a need to develop appropriate diagnostic measures for different cultures, as has been done for anxiety and depressive disorders.

Personality, Personality Disorders, Gender, and Culture

The understanding of sex differences in personality functioning can be controversial (Eagly 1995). Nevertheless, consistent differences between males and females with respect to general personality functioning have been obtained. A predominant model of general personality functioning is the five-factor model, consisting of the five broad domains of neuroticism (affective instability versus emotional stability), extraversion versus introversion, conscientiousness (constraint) vs. disinhibition (impulsivity), agreeableness versus antagonism, and openness (unconventionality). Each of these broad domains can be differentiated into more specific facets. The most commonly used measure of the five-factor model is the NEO Personality Inventory–Revised (NEO PI-R; Costa and McCrae 1995), which identifies six facets within each domain. For example, some of the facets of agreeableness versus antagonism are trust (gullibility) versus mistrust (suspiciousness), straightforwardness versus deception (manipulation), altruism (self-sacrifice) versus exploitation, and compliance (submissiveness) versus defiance (aggression). Costa et al. (2001) reported consistent gender differences for the NEO-PI-R personality traits scales across 26 different cultures, ranging from quite traditional cultures (e.g., Pakistan) to relatively more modern cultures (e.g., The Netherlands). In particular, women scored higher than men in the domains of neuroticism (including the facets of anxiousness, depressiveness, and vulnerability) and agreeableness (including the facets of trust, altruism, and compliance). These sex differences obtained with the NEO-PI-R were consistent with a meta-analysis of gender differences reported for 13 different personality inventories across 36 independent normative samples (Feingold 1994). For example, Feingold reported that women scored higher than men on personality measures of depressiveness, anxiousness, vulnerability, and other components of neuroticism, as well as the facet of tendermindedness from the domain of agreeableness. These results are also consistent with earlier meta-analyses showing that women score higher on measures of helping and empathy, whereas men score higher on assertion and aggression (Ashmore 1990; Eagly and Steffen 1986).

These sex differences in general personality functioning have in turn been used to help explain gender differences in general psychopathology (Kendler et al. 2002; Widiger and Anderson 2003). For example, the higher rate of depression in women could be due, at least in part, to gender differences in neuroticism, which provides a vulnerability for the development of mood disorders (Kendler et al. 2002, 2004; Widiger and Anderson 2003). The higher proportion of females with borderline personality disorder could also be explained in part by the normatively higher rate of neuroticism in women. There is a considerable amount of research to suggest that all of the personality disorders are closely related to the domains and facets of the five-factor model, which can in turn help explain gender differences in personality disorders (Corbitt and Widiger 1995). For example, narcissistic and antisocial personality disorders represent, at least in part, maladaptively high levels of normative antagonism, whereas dependent personality disorder represents, in part, maladaptively high levels of agreeableness (Widiger and Costa 2002). Across cultures, males have consistently higher levels of antagonism, whereas females have consistently higher levels of agreeableness (Ashmore 1990; Costa et al. 2001; Eagly and Steffen 1986; Feingold 1994).

These gender differences in personality across cultures are also consistent with traditional sociobiological models of mate selection (Buss 1994). The cross-cultural finding that men tend to be relatively more assertive, domineering, and aggressive, whereas women tend to be relatively more empathic, compliant, and warm, is consistent to some extent with cross-cultural studies of mate selection (Buss 1996; Geary 1998; Mealey 2000). Across cultures, women (more so than men) have valued mates with higher earning capacity and industriousness, whereas men (more so than women) have valued youth, physical attractiveness, and chastity. Males have consequently developed qualities that increase their relative access to women (e.g., aggressiveness, competitiveness, assertiveness, and risk taking), and females have developed qualities associated with their higher parental investment (e.g., warmth, caring, empathy, and nurturance).

Nevertheless, an anomalous finding in the existing cross-culture studies of gender differences is the negative correlation between the extent to which a culture adheres to traditional mate selection preferences and gender differences in personality (Costa et al. 2001). The larger the gender differences in personality, the less likely the culture is adherent to traditional mate selection preferences. There is currently no clear explanation for this finding. One possible explanation for this anomaly is related to the self-report method of assessing personality. Costa et al. (2001) suggested that individuals in traditional cultures view their behavior as role bound, whereas people in cultures where there is more autonomy consider their behavior to be a manifestation of a psychological trait. In a culture that is strongly role bound, persons are perhaps more likely to explain their gender-related behavior as being due to their social role rather than to their personality (i.e., the more the culture enforces gender-role behavior, the less likely gender-role behavior reflects the apparent preferences, choices, or decisions of the individual). In more egalitarian societies, persons are perhaps more likely to understand and explain their behavior as being due to their own personal preferences, attitudes, and choices (i.e., their characteristic or personally preferred manner of thinking, feeling, and relating to others). McCrae and Terracciano (2005) replicated these cross-cultural findings in a more extensive study of 50 different cultures, this time having persons describe someone they knew well rather than describing their own personality. They suggested that the role-bound explanation would again be pertinent (i.e., persons from a role-bound culture explain the behavior of others in a manner consistent with their understanding of their own behavior): that even though subjects are describing someone other than themselves, they still exhibit an attributional style that is consistent with their own culture.

Both studies proposed that what is needed in future research are studies in which persons from different cultures are enlisted to assess and describe participants' behaviors. For instance, it would be of interest to determine whether persons from role-bound cultures describe other persons from egalitarian cultures as expressing role-bound behavior, and whether persons from egalitarian cultures describe persons from role-bound cultures as expressing their personal preferences, choices, and interests. This cross-cultural research would also be facilitated through the implementation of standardized semistructured interviews in multinational studies with interviewers who had been trained to provide consistent personality assessments. Intercultural reliability in personality assessments could then be assessed directly (Loranger et al. 1994), particularly if interviewers from different cultures are systematically compared with respect to their interviews and ratings of members of other, different cultures.

Although personality and personality disorders are widely thought to have both neurobiological and sociocultural roots, there has in fact been surprisingly little systematic research on the sociocultural contributions to gender differences in personality disorders (Bornstein 1993; Morey et al. 2005). A gender label at birth is thought to initiate a developmental gender socialization (Ruble and Martin 1998). Gender-typical play preferences in infancy are consistent with hormonally determined behavioral tendencies (Alexander 2003), but they can also be further shaped through social modeling and reinforcement (Bussey and Bandura 1999). The internalization of these social norms occurs with the formation of the individual's gender identity (Maccoby 1998). The identification early in life of the self as either male or female provides a relatively strong gender schema that guides subsequent perceptions, behaviors, and decisions in a manner consistent with respective gender roles and sociocultural expectations (Wood and Eagly 2002). Gender subcultures also occur in childhood (e.g., peer groups) that promote further sex differences in cognitive and emotional processing through gender-specific play and manner of interpersonal relatedness (Maccoby 1998). The close association of some personality disorders (e.g., dependent and histrionic) with sociocultural gender stereotypes is consistent with this perspective. As originally suggested by Kaplan (1983), women are encouraged by society to be compliant, submissive, chaste, faithful, and reliant but are then diagnosed with a dependent personality disorder when they conform too much to this expectation.

Summary and the Importance of Neurobiological/Environmental Interactions

There are both similarities and differences in psychopathology across different cultures (Draguns and Tanaka-Matsumi 2003). In addition, it appears that many sociocultural factors affect men and women differently. Such differences may be related to differential exposure to environmental experiences such as poverty, domestic violence, or rate of partner loss or to different role expectations and different attitudes regarding cultural values. In addition, women may react to stressors and other life events differently than do men.

It must be emphasized that sociocultural and neurobiological factors interact in complex ways to produce psychopathology, including gender differences in psychopathology (also see Chapters 2, 5, and 7). For example, as discussed earlier, the landmark study by Caspi et al. (2003) found that the influence of life stress on depression was moderated by a gene-by-environment interaction. Stressful life events predicted a diagnosis of major depression only among individuals with the short allele of the serotonin transporter promoter region gene. In contrast, stressful life events did not predict major depression in individuals with two copies of the long allele. Stressful life events also predicted the occurrence of suicidal ideation and suicide attempts among individuals who carried the short-form allele but not among long-form homozygotes. Although requiring replication, these results suggest that complex disorders, such as mental disorders, may result from variations in genes whose effects are conditional upon exposure to environmental risks.

Gaps in the Literature and Recommended Research Agenda

1. *Develop effective assessment strategies to identify relevant social and cultural characteristics and risk factors for psychopathology.* There are many gaps in our understanding of the influences of social and cultural forces on gender differences in psychopathology. Given that men and women may respond differently to a range of different cultural and interpersonal experiences, it is likely that mood and anxiety disorders, as well as suicidality, have different sociocultural risk factors for men and women. Good assessment strategies are needed to identify relevant social and cultural characteristics and risk factors for psychopathology, and studies characterizing people with DSM-defined conditions need to include sociocultural assessments.
2. *Include sociocultural factors in etiological models of DSM-defined disorders.* The role of factors such as role functioning and cultural values, and their interaction with neurobiological risk factors, need to be examined in relation to illness onset, course, and treatment response. Such studies need to examine interactions with gender, because sociocultural factors may have different effects on the development, expression, and treatment response of psychopathology in males and females. More generally, there is a need to move on from identifying sex differences, and trying to determine whether they are biologically or socioculturally generated, to trying to understand *which* of the complex biological and social components of sex/gender contribute to the differences that have already been documented.
3. *Design studies to evaluate the mechanism by which gender differences in response to marital conflict occur.* Mechanisms of the gender differences in health consequences of social support need to be elucidated.

4. *Explore sociocultural influences on the development and expression of psychiatric disorders and resulting impairment.* Increased knowledge of the sociocultural influences on the development and expression of psychiatric disorders and resulting impairment could enhance diagnosis and treatment among diverse populations across the developmental age span. Although we have learned much about the influence of biological processes and mechanisms such as the HPA axis, there is not a consensus on how these processes interact with sociocultural processes to increase risk of illness. Such understanding may create opportunities for the diagnosis, prevention, and treatment of psychiatric disorders for both women and men. The complex interactions of the environmental and biological experience unique to girls and women are still unknown for specific disorders.
5. *Conduct further prospective studies in developing countries to assess eating behavior and attitudes about body image.* There are few ongoing prospective studies in developing countries that are assessing eating behavior and attitudes about body image. Such research would be helpful to understand the effect of cultural influences and changes on the development of eating disorders and how these influences may affect men and women differently. As noted earlier, research is needed on cultural variations in the expression of eating disorders and how these variations should be reflected in diagnostic measures and future editions of DSM.
6. *Explore how risk factors for the development of eating disorders vary by sex/gender and culture.* Risk factors that mediate and moderate the development of eating disorders may vary in different cultures and may vary by gender. Increased knowledge of these factors would be helpful to more accurately define and diagnose eating disorders.
7. *Conduct research on sociocultural contributions to personality disorders and sex differences in personality disorders.* Although there is considerable empirical support for consistent gender differences in personality across cultures (Wood and Eagly 2002), and substantial empirical support for the relationship of general personality functioning to personality disorders (Widiger and Costa 2002), there is very little research that has explicitly addressed gender differences in personality disorders across cultures (Morey et al. 2005). Similarly, although there is substantial research on the sociocultural contributions to the development of general personality traits, there is little comparable research on the sociocultural contributions to the development of personality disorders or, specifically, to gender differences in personality disorders.

What is needed is an effort to integrate the scientific research on general personality functioning with our understanding of personality disorders, thereby facilitating the transfer of the considerable amount of basic science research on gender differences in personality to our understanding of gender differences in personality disorders. For example, it would be of interest to determine empirically whether the existing gender differences in personality disorders are consistent with the better-established gender differences in general personality functioning. Some of the gender differences in personality disorders are controversial (e.g., histrionic, dependent, and borderline; Morey et al. 2005), and it might be useful to determine empirically whether these controversial gender differences are in fact consistent with the existing scientific research on gender differences in personality structure.

With respect to our understanding of cultural differences in gender, what is needed are multinational studies of gender differences in personality (and personality disorders) whose methodology addresses effectively cross-cultural differences in the perception and attribution of normal and abnormal personality traits. For example, it would be useful to conduct a multinational study combining a self-report inventory and semistructured interview in which interviewers selected from different (egalitarian and role-bound) cultures would conduct interviews of males and females selected from cultures other than their own. One would then be able to address empirically the methodological concern that gender differences in personality and personality disorders across cultures are due (at least in part) to cultural differences in the attribution of personality traits.

References

Alarcón RD, Bell CC, Kirmayer LJ, et al: Beyond the funhouse mirrors: research agenda on culture and psychiatric diagnosis, in A Research Agenda for DSM-V. Edited by Kupfer DJ, First MB, Regier DA. Washington DC, American Psychiatric Association, 2002, pp 219–281

Alexander GM: An evolutionary perspective of sex-typed toy preferences: pink, blue, and the brain. Arch Sex Behav 32:7–14, 2003

Apter A, Abu Shah M, Iancu I, et al: Cultural effects on eating attitudes in Israeli subpopulations and hospitalized anorectics. Genet Soc Gen Psychol Monogr 120:83–99, 1994

Arrindell WA, Eisemann M, Richter J, et al: Cultural Clinical Psychology Study Group: masculinity–femininity as a national characteristic and its relationship with national agoraphobic fear levels: Fodor's sex role hypothesis revitalized. Behav Res Ther 41:795–807, 2003a

Arrindell WA, Steptoe A, Wardle J: Higher levels of state depression in masculine than in feminine nations. Behav Res Ther 41:809–817, 2003b

Arrindell WA, Eisemann M, Oei TPS, et al., Cultural Clinical Psychology Study Group: phobic anxiety in 11 nations, part II. Hofstede's dimensions of national cultures predict national-level variations. Pers Individ Dif 37:627–643, 2004

Ashmore RD: Sex, gender and the individual, in Handbook of Personality Theory and Research. Edited by Pervin LA. New York, Guilford, 1990, pp 486–526

Ballot NS, Delaney NE, Erskine PJ, et al: Anorexia nervosa: a prevalence study. S Afr Med J 59:992–993, 1981

Bebbington PE: Psychosocial causes of depression. J Gend Specif Med 2:52–60, 1999

Bebbington PE, Hurry J, Tennant C, et al: Epidemiology of mental disorders in Camberwell. Psychol Med 11:561–580, 1981

Bornstein RF: The Dependent Personality. New York, Guilford, 1993

Bruce ML, Kim KM: Differences in the effects of divorce on major depression in men and women. Am J Psychiatry 149:914–917, 1992

Buhrich N: Frequency of presentation of anorexia nervosa in Malaysia. Aust NZ J Psychiatry 15:153–155, 1981

Buss DM: The Evolution of Desire: Strategies of Human Mating. New York, Basic Books, 1994

Buss DM: Social adaptation and five major factors of personality, in The Five-Factor Model of Personality. Edited by Wiggins JS. New York, Guilford, 1996, pp 180–207

Bussey K, Bandura A: Social-cognitive theory of gender development and differentiation. Psychol Rev 106:676–713, 1999

Caspi A, Sugden K, Moffitt TE, et al: Influence of life stress on depression: moderation by a polymorphism in the 5-HTT gene. Science 301:386–389, 2003

Corbitt EM, Widiger TA: Sex differences among the personality disorders: an exploration of the data. Clinical Psychology: Science and Practice 2:225–248, 1995

Costa PT, McCrae RR: Domains and facets: hierarchical personality assessment using the Revised NEO Personality Inventory. J Pers Assess 64:21–50, 1995

Costa PT, Terracciano A, McCrae RR: Gender differences in personality traits across cultures: robust and surprising findings. J Pers Soc Psychol 81:322–331, 2001

Draguns JG, Tanaka-Matsumi J: Assessment of psychopathology across and within cultures: issues and findings. Behav Res Ther 41:755–776, 2003

Eagly AH: The science and politics of comparing women and men. Am Psychol 50:145–158, 1995

Eagly AH, Steffen VJ: Gender and aggressive behavior: a meta-analytic review of the social psychological literature. Psychol Bull 100:309–330, 1986

Feingold A: Gender differences in personality: a meta-analysis. Psychol Bull 116:429–456, 1994

Fichter MM, Elton M, Sourdi L, et al: Anorexia nervosa in Greek and Turkish adolescents. Eur Arch Psychiatry Neurol Sci 237:200–208, 1988

Furnham A, Alibhai N: Cross-cultural differences in the perception of female body shapes. Psychol Med 13:829–837, 1983

Geary DC: Male, Female: The Evolution of Human Sex Differences. Washington, DC, American Psychological Association, 1998

Hegarty K, Gunn J, Chondros P, et al: Association between depression and abuse by partners of women attending general practice: descriptive, cross sectional survey. Br Med J 328:621–624, 2004

Hibbard J, Pope C: The quality of social roles as predictors of morbidity and mortality. Soc Sci Med 36:217–225, 1993

Hicks MH, Li Z: Partner violence and major depression in women: a community study of Chinese Americans. J Nerv Ment Dis 191:722–729, 2003

Hofstede GH: Culture's Consequences: International Differences in Work-Related Values. Beverly Hills, CA, Sage, 1980

Kaplan M: A woman's view of the DSM-III. Am Psychol 38:786–792, 1983

Kendler KS, Gardner CL, Prescott CA: Toward a comprehensive developmental model for major depression in women. Am J Psychiatry 159:1133–1145, 2002

Kendler KS, Kuhn J, Prescott CA: The interrelationship of neuroticism, sex, and stressful life events in the prediction of episodes of major depression. Am J Psychiatry 161:631–636, 2004

Kiecolt-Glaser J, Newton TL: Marriage and health: his and hers. Psychol Bull 27:472–503, 2001

Lee S, Chiu HF, Chen CN: Anorexia nervosa in Hong Kong: why not more in Chinese? Br J Psychiatry 154:683–688, 1989

Loranger AW, Sartorius N, Andreoli A, et al: The International Personality Disorder Examination: the World Health Organization/Alcohol, Drug Abuse, and Mental Health Administration international pilot study of personality disorders. Arch Gen Psychiatry 51:215–224, 1994

Maccoby EE: The Two Sexes: Growing Up Apart, Coming Together. Cambridge, MA, Harvard University Press, 1998

Mayne TJ, O'Leary A, McCrady B, et al: The differential effects of acute marital distress on emotional, physiological and immune functions in maritally distressed men and women. Psychology and Health 12:277–288, 1997

McCrae RR, Terracciano A: Universal features of personality traits from the observer's perspective: data from 50 cultures. J Pers Soc Psychol 88:547–561, 2005

Mealey L: Sex Differences: Developmental and Evolutionary Strategies. San Diego, CA, Academic Press, 2000

Morey LC, Alexander GM, Boggs C: Gender, in American Psychiatric Press Textbook of Personality Disorders. Edited by Oldham JM, Skodol AE, Bender DS. Washington, DC, American Psychiatric Publishing, 2005, pp 541–560

Mukai T, Crago M, Shisslak CM: Eating attitudes and weight preoccupation among female high school students in Japan. J Child Psychol 35:677–688, 1994

Mumford DB, Whitehouse AM: Increased prevalence of bulimia nervosa among Asian schoolgirls. Br J Psychiatry 156:565–568, 1988

Mumford DB, Whitehouse AM, Choudry I: Survey of eating disorders in English medium schools in Lahore, Pakistan. Int J Eat Disord 11:173–184, 1992

Najavits LM, Weiss RD, Shaw SR: The link between substance abuse and posttraumatic stress disorder in women: a research review. Am J Addict 6:273–284, 1997

Nasser M: Comparative study of the prevalence of abnormal eating attitudes among Arab female students of both London and Cairo universities. Psychol Med 16:621–625, 1986

Ruble DN, Martin CL: Gender development, in Handbook of Child Psychology, Vol 3. Edited by Eisenberg N. New York, Wiley, 1998, pp 993–1016

Rudmin FW, Ferrada-Nolf M, Skolbekken J-A: Questions of culture, age, and gender in the epidemiology of suicide. Scand J Psychol 44:373–381, 2003

Striegel-Moore RH, Wilfley DE, Pike KM, et al: Recurrent binge eating in black American women. Arch Fam Med 9:83–87, 2000

U.S. Public Health Service National Strategy for Suicide Prevention: Goals and Objectives for Action. Rockville, MD, U.S. Department of Health and Human Services, 2001

Weissman M, Bland RC, Canino G, et al: Cross-national epidemiology of major depression and bipolar disorder. JAMA 276:293–299, 1996

Widiger TA, Anderson KG: Personality and depression in women. J Affect Disord 74:59–66, 2003

Widiger TA, Costa PT: Five factor model personality disorder research, in Personality Disorders and the Five Factor Model of Personality, 2nd Edition. Edited by Costa PT, Widiger TA. Washington, DC, American Psychological Association, 2002, pp 59–87

Wood W, Eagly AH: A cross-cultural analysis of the behavior of women and men: implications for the origins of sex differences. Psychol Bull 128:699–727, 2002

World Health Organization: World Health Statistics. Geneva, Switzerland, World Health Organization, 1995

World Health Organization: World Health Statistics. Geneva, Switzerland, World Health Organization, 1996

7

A DEVELOPMENTAL PERSPECTIVE, WITH A FOCUS ON CHILDHOOD TRAUMA

Adrian Angold, M.B., MRCPsych
Christine Marcelle Heim, Ph.D.

In this chapter, we discuss the importance of a developmental perspective in understanding the relationship between sex/gender and psychopathology. First, we address the importance of a time-varying developmental perspective. Then, we examine childhood trauma as a specific example of the role of early life experience in increasing risk for subsequent psychopathology. By focusing on childhood trauma, we emphasize the importance of considering interactions between neurobiological and sociocultural factors, as has been discussed in previous chapters (see Chapter 2 ["Why Gender Matters"], Chapter 5 ["Neurobiology and Sex/Gender"], and Chapter 6 ["Sociocultural Factors and Gender"]) in this volume.

Importance of a Developmental Perspective

Sex and gender are typically treated as fixed "demographic" factors in psychiatric research, but failure to regard sex as a time-varying, developmental phenomenon leads to substantial loss of analytic precision in many cases and missed opportunities for understanding the mechanisms by which psychopathology arises. The ontogeny of sex, even if we consider only its manifestations in genetic and hormonal effects, is a complex process that unfolds in a punctuated manner across the whole period of fetal, child, adolescent, and adult development. So we need to adopt a life span developmental approach if we are to fully appreciate and increase our understanding of its effects on psychopathology.

In arguing this case we need to consider the complex mechanisms by which sex differentiation arises and changes over time (also see Chapter 5), and in this chapter we illustrate how attending to these mechanisms provides a rich source for future research (using unipolar depression as a key example). First, however, we address some terminological considerations.

Sex Versus Gender

In a recent analysis of the titles of 30 million academic articles published between 1945 and 2001, Haig (2004) identified the introduction of the concept of "gender role" (Money 1955) as marking the beginning of a transition from a predominant use of the term *sex* to refer to the distinction between men and women to a two-to-one preference for *gender* over *sex.* The former term began to be used to distinguish between sociocultural aspects of differences between men and women, whereas the latter was limited to biological differences. More recently, the use of *gender* has expanded to encompass both sociocultural and biological differences, so that *sex* and *gender* have become pretty much synonymous. In other words, *gender* now means what *sex* always used to mean (Dunnett 2003). Attempts to preserve separate sociocultural and biological meanings for *gender* and *sex,* respectively (e.g., Pinn 2003; Wizemann 2001), have proved unsatisfactory for two reasons. First, there is, in reality, no necessary or even well-demarcated division between human biological and social functions and activities (Rutter et al. 2003). Second, as we have learned more about the developmental sociobiology of sex differentiation, it has become clear that more than two terms are needed to distinguish among the various processes involved. Throughout much of this chapter, we refer to *sex* rather than *gender* or *sex/gender* and now go on to distinguish a variety of constructs or components of sex that are relevant to a developmental perspective of sex differences in psychopathology.

Sex/Gender as a Multidimensional Developmental Construct

We are used to thinking of sex as a dichotomy and, in terms of its treatment as a risk factor for psychopathology, as what Kraemer et al. (1997) labeled a "fixed marker." However, this approach ignores the fact that sex is an inherently multidimensional and developmental process, not just a fixed state. Several conceptually (and biologically) distinguishable dimensions of sex need to be considered. In the vast majority of people, these dimensions all concur to produce our usual notion of sex as a dichotomy, but as we shall see, they do not *always* concur (despite powerful biological reasons to do so). This dimensional separability has important implications for understanding the possible mechanisms for effects of sex on psychiatric disorders. We first consider the multidimensionality of sex and then go on to illustrate the need to treat it as a developmental process. It is a truism to say that sex develops in embryogenesis, but we must recognize that sex remains a developmental process *throughout the life span.*

Dimensions of Sex/Gender

CHROMOSOMAL SEX

As is also discussed in Chapter 5, most humans have 46 chromosomes: 22 pairs of autosomes and two sex chromosomes. Typical females have two X chromosomes, and typical males have one X chromosome and one Y chromosome. However, we need to remember that not all "men" and "women" have this chromosomal complement. For instance, in Turner syndrome, an X chromosome is missing in individuals whose external genitalia identify them as females, whereas in Klinefelter syndrome additional X chromosomes may be present in individuals whose genitalia identify them as males. We are now familiar with the doctrine that the presence of a Y chromosome is required for male development. However, as we shall see, this doctrine is not universally true. Be that as it may, one possible mechanism for the generation of sex differences in psychiatric disorders is the differential "dose" of X chromosome genes in men and women. Even though one X chromosome is randomly "inactivated" in each female cell, it turns out that as many as 10%–15% of its genes may still be expressed (Willard 2000). The Y chromosome may also have direct effects, because the majority of the 78 protein coding genes on the nonrecombinant portion of the Y chromosome (which between them code for 27 discrete proteins) are expressed outside the gonads, including in the brain (Page 2004; Skaletsky et al. 2003).

GENETIC SEX

In 1990 a 0.9-kb region, the gene *SRY* (sex-determining region Y), responsible for the masculinization of the fetus, was identified (Berta et al. 1996; Jager et al. 1990). Deletion or dysfunction (resulting from mutations, of which several dozen have already been reported [http://archive.uwcm.ac.uk/uwcm/mg/search/125556.html]) of *SRY* results in failure to develop a typical male phenotype in XY individuals (e.g., *SRY* mutations can give rise to XY-apparent females with gonadal dysgenesis), whereas translocation (misplacement during meiosis) of the *SRY* gene onto an X chromosome results in the birth of an XX individual with apparently male genitalia. *SRY* is a 204–amino acid protein capable of binding to 1) two specific DNA base sequences, and 2) sequence nonspecific DNA four-way junctions. It thereby induces configurational changes in DNA, but how this translates into effects on sexual differentiation is unknown (Jordan and Vilain 2002). However, that is far from the end of genetic sex determination. *SRY* transcription is itself genetically regulated (e.g., by the Wilms tumor gene, *WT1,* on chromosome 11) (Hossain and Saunders 2001; Jordan and Vilain 2002), and hundreds of genes appear to be involved in sexual differentiation. For instance, in addition to *SRY,* the gene *DMRT1* on chromosome 9 is involved in testicular development (Dewing et al. 2002), and unlike *SRY,* it has to be present in two copies to work properly. XY humans who have lost one copy of the gene fail to develop testes and show gonadal sex reversal despite having a fully functional *SRY.* We do not know what other functions the cascade of genes involved in differential gonadal development might have, and so they represent a second possible source of neuropsychiatric differences between men and women.

GONADAL SEX

The sex-determinative genes just discussed initiate the development of ovaries or testes (and their associated structures). Thus, sex may also be defined by the nature of the gonads. Regardless of sex chromosome complement, until the seventh week of gestation the embryonic gonadal region remains undifferentiated, and the precursors of both male and female genital systems (the Wolffian and Müllerian ducts, respectively) are present, with the result that human embryos have sexual bipotential at all levels of differentiation (Jordan and Vilain 2002). Testicular differentiation occurs during the eighth and ninth weeks of gestation, but the ovary does not begin to differentiate until about the third month (Vilain 2000).

GENITAL SEX

It is now also well known that the "standard *anatomical* developmental plan" for the human embryo is female (Jost 1947). The development of male external genitalia requires the presence of a functional testis (and its hormonal products). Mullerian inhibiting substance, produced by Sertoli cells in the seminiferous tubules, causes apoptosis of the Mullerian ducts. Testosterone, produced by Leydig cells surrounding the seminiferous tubules, and its derivative, dihydrotestosterone, produced locally in the genital region, are responsible for the development of the male internal and external genitalia (Vilain 2000).

More importantly from our perspective, testosterone has also been identified as a key player in the masculinization of the brain. Until recently, gender differentiation of the brain was thought to be dependent entirely on testosterone production, and it was thought that the brain, like the gonads, would be female unless acted upon by testosterone. That, in itself, offers a mechanism by which sex differentiation of the development of psychopathology could be generated. However, it has now been found that, even in the absence of testosterone, genetically male and female mice exhibit substantial differences in gene expression in the brain (Dewing et al. 2003). It is therefore possible that some components of the genetic cascade that normally lead to anatomical masculinization may also have direct effects on brain function—providing a further possible route for gender differentiation in behavior and psychopathology.

Differences in hormonal milieu and gene expression could also lead to differential susceptibility to external threats to the fetus, such as nutritional deficiencies, environmental toxins, viral assaults, or placental deficits.

ASSIGNED SEX

Historically at birth, but more recently at ultrasound, the external genitalia of the newborn or fetus are observed, and the child is declared to be either a boy or a girl. However, it is also possible to manipulate the assigned sex of a child, as has been done in genetically and gonadally male children with cloacal exstrophy (who have often had their histologically normal testes removed), or in children who have had catastrophic penile damage, who have been raised as girls (Reiner and Gearhart 2004). The key point here is that the child enters a social world and that the social world treats boys and girls differently. Here we have another potential mechanism for generating psychopathological differences between males and females (see also Chapter 6).

Continuing Development of Sex/Gender Over the Life Span and Its Relation to Psychopathology

In most people, the assignment of sex at or before birth settles the issue. They will remain male or female, at first as a girl or a boy, growing up to be a woman or a man, and they will die as such. However, in considering this progress through life, it is immediately apparent that the meaning of being male or female changes dramatically across the life span—biologically, socially, and psychologically. Even the words we use to denote males and females are different in childhood and adulthood.

SEX/GENDER DIFFERENCES IN CHILDHOOD BEHAVIOR AND PSYCHOPATHOLOGY

There is a huge literature showing that the behavior of boys and girls differs in many ways from their earliest years. This is true in relation to psychopathology as well. Overall, male conceptuses appear to be more susceptible to a variety of biological hazards. It is also now well established that boys are more likely to have a variety of developmental disorders (such as autism), attention-deficit/hyperactivity disorder (ADHD), and antisocial behavior, suggesting that a broad range of neurodevelopmental mechanisms are more prone to be disrupted early in boys than girls (Rutter et al. 2003). However, there is little evidence that boys are more susceptible to *psychosocial* risk for psychiatric disorders overall (Rutter et al. 2003), so explanations of sex differences in this area have tended to concentrate on fetal and early life neurodevelopmental processes. The key point here is that the *timing* of the onsets of these disorders makes us consider certain classes of putative sex-differentiated causes. At different life stages, sex/gender is manifested in different ways, and so different classes of potential causes can be called into play. So, for example, concurrent testosterone level does not offer itself as a good candidate for explaining sex differences in the rates of ADHD, because ADHD is prevalent during developmental periods when both boys and girls have very low testosterone levels.

When it comes to childhood anxiety and depression, the most striking thing is their lack of sex differentiation. If there is any difference under age 13, it is in the direction of boys having higher rates of depression than girls (Angold and Costello 2001).

CONTINUING SEXUAL DEVELOPMENT IN CHILDHOOD

Although the hypothalamic-pituitary-gonadal (HPG) and hypothalamic-pituitary-adrenal (HPA) axes show a brief burst of activity in the first months after birth (Skuse 1984), circulating concentrations of gonadotropins and gonadal and adrenal steroids are very low in early to mid-childhood because of suppression of luteinizing hormone releasing hormone (LHRH, also known as gonadotropin releasing hormone, GnRH) secretion by GABA (γ-aminobutyric acid)-ergic (and perhaps neuropeptide Y) neural systems (Plant 2001; Terasawa and Fernandez 2001). An increase in adrenal androgen output (adrenarche) occurs at around 6–8 years in both boys and girls (DePeretti and Forest 1976; Ducharme et al. 1976; Lashansky et al. 1991; Parker et al. 1978; Reiter et al. 1977; Sizonenko and Paunier 1975). Adrenarche precedes the earliest changes of puberty on the HPG axis by about 2 years and was initially thought to act as a trigger for its onset (Collu and Ducharme 1975). We now know this to be untrue (Counts et al. 1987; Korth-Schutz et al. 1976; Wierman et al. 1986), but adrenarche is still suspected to play a facilitative role in the initiation of puberty. Leptin also appears to have a necessary permissive role in the onset of puberty (Clayton and Trueman 2000; Gueorguiev et al. 2001), but the ultimate "trigger" for puberty remains unknown (Terasawa and Fernandez 2001).

Despite the fact that these prepubertal changes in androgen levels are similar in boys and girls, they still have to be considered as possible factors in generating changes in the sex ratios for psychiatric disorders because they act on already sexually differentiated brains and patterns of behavior. It is also important to bear in mind that levels of the most abundant androgen of all, dehydroepiandrosterone

(DHEA, and its sulfated metabolite, DHEAS), increase enormously over this period (and continue to do so into the twenties), and that DHEA is a neurosteroid (Baulieu 1998) with reported protective effects against cortisol neurotoxicity (e.g., Gubba et al. 2000; Kaminska et al. 2000; Karishma and Herbert 2002; Kimonides et al. 1998). This serves as a reminder that there may be sex differences in responses to protective factors as well as risk factors. However, there is as yet little evidence for any important psychopathological effects of adrenarche.

PUBERTY: A TIME OF DRAMATIC CHANGE

Declining GABAergic LHRH suppression results in increases in release of glutamate (and other neurotransmitters), permitting the onset of puberty, manifested initially, beginning in late childhood, as closely sleep-entrained nighttime pulses of luteinizing hormone (Beck and Wuttke 1980; Dunkel et al.1990; Judd et al. 1977; Kulin et al. 1976; Wu et al. 1990). LHRH pulse amplitude and frequency increase across the late prepubertal to early and middle stages of puberty (Hale et al. 1998; Landy et al. 1990) and show progressive diminution of diurnal variation in early to mid-puberty. Pulse frequency decreases in late puberty as LHRH release becomes more sensitive to negative feedback control from gonadal steroids (Dunger et al. 1991; Marshall et al. 1991; Wennink et al. 1989). A critical sex difference established over the course of puberty is that females develop pulsatile GnRH release along with fluctuating estradiol and progesterone (Marshall et al. 1991). Maturation of this pattern extends from before menarche to several months or years beyond in the course of establishing regular ovulation and luteal function (Vihko and Apter 1980; Wennink et al. 1990). These changes are, of course, associated with enormous changes in cognitive, psychological, social, and sexual functioning. All of these have potential for changing the patterns of psychopathology manifested by females and males. Puberty also brings a whole new meaning to the word *sex*—as a libidinous act. As far as psychopathology is concerned, adolescence is a developmental period during which a variety of "female-typical" psychopathologies arise, the best documented examples being unipolar depression and eating disorders (Rutter et al. 2003).

Here, however, we focus on the continuing development of physiological sex (i.e., puberty) and its implications for sex differentiation in psychopathology. Indeed, space will allow us to consider only a few of the many manifestations of puberty. First, we need to distinguish among some possible *types* of effects.

Timing Effects

The age at which puberty occurs, relative to the norm, may be important. There is now very strong evidence that for conduct problems, early puberty is a substantial risk factor, but only in girls. The most likely mechanism involves young yet physically mature (but sociocognitively immature) girls making social contacts with behavior-disordered boys (Persson et al. 2004; Stattin and Magnusson 1990; Stattin et al. 2005). This pattern fits with the shrinkage in the sex ratio for adolescent-onset conduct disorder compared with early-onset conduct disorder (Moffitt et al. 2001).

Transition Effects

Here we need to consider the effects of changes from one state to another, in this case from prepuberty to adulthood. An example is the association between higher Tanner stage (a measure of secondary sex characteristics) levels and increased prevalence of unipolar depression (Angold et al. 1998). Prepubertal girls (and boys) are all in Tanner stage 1, whereas adult women (and men) are all in Tanner stage 5. There is no variability in Tanner stage within either group, so effects of Tanner stage can only be identified during the pubertal transition (Angold et al. 1998).

Level Effects

When there is within-group variability in a factor within a developmental period, effects of the level of that factor on psychopathology can be identified. For instance, it has been found that the effects of age and Tanner stage on rates of unipolar depression in girls are mediated statistically by the association of these factors with increasing levels of estradiol and testosterone. These hormone levels continue to show between-individual differences in adulthood (unlike Tanner stage), so one can ask whether the increase in rates of depression in girls in adolescence results from a pubertal transition effect or is better regarded as being a manifestation of a continuously variable hormone level effect. In the former case, we would expect to see no relationship between sex hormone levels and depression once adult levels had been obtained. In the latter case, we would find that individual differences in adult sex hormone levels are associated with the prevalence of adult depressive disorders. So far, there is little evidence that either hormone level (i.e., estradiol or testosterone) is strongly related to adult premenopausal rates of depression, so it may well be that there is an effect of crossing a certain threshold hormone level at puberty, which is maintained at least until the menopause (Angold et al. 1999). That would fit well with the finding that after age 12 or 13 the whole frequency distribution for depression scale scores is shifted to the right, indicating that the risk for depression increases in all (or most) women at puberty (Angold et al. 2002; Twenge and Nolen-Hoeksema 2002).

Cyclical Effects

The menstrual cycle, with its enormous monthly swings in neuroactive hormone levels, could also present a challenge to psychological well being. It may be that it is the repeated changes in hormonal levels, rather than any transition from one average level to another, that is the culprit in increasing risk for unipolar depression, for instance. At this point, there is no evidence that cycling *per se* is the key factor in relation to any psychopathology, but it must be admitted that this is a difficult parameter to separate from the others.

CONTINUING SEXUAL DEVELOPMENT IN ADULTHOOD

The development of sex as a biological phenomenon does not end at puberty. Only women become pregnant, and so only women can have postpartum depression. Only women breastfeed, and women still bear the brunt of childrearing, so sex continues to present newly differentiated challenges to males and females throughout the life span.

There is yet a final stage in sexual development that affects men and women rather differently. In both sexes, levels of androgens fall dramatically in later life (Labrie et al. 1997; D.G. Young et al. 1999), but women also experience menopause, with its much more rapid and dramatic hormonal change. Here again, we witness changes in the sex ratio for unipolar depression, with a falling prevalence in women over the age of 55 and perhaps even a reversal of the sex ratio (Bebbington et al. 2003). In other words, there appears to be a return to the sex distribution of depression reminiscent of that prior to puberty, perhaps representing the etiological inverse of the transition effect seen there.

If we suppose that to be the case, what implications does that have for how sex might operate as a risk factor for psychiatric disorders? First, it brings us back full circle to the genome from which we started, because the steroid hormones are transcription modulators. In other words, they can control the "output" of sections of the genome, turning genetic influences on and off (or, at least, affecting their "volume"). Second, it directs us to look at the brain regions in which steroid hormones function in the cytoplasm as allosteric receptor modulators ("neurosteroids"). Third, it leads us to consider the degree to which sex (or other) hormones might potentiate the psychopathological effects of other genetic, hormonal, and/or environmentally mediated sex differences (e.g., differences in affiliative behavior; Cyranowski et al. 2000) Fourth, because various steroid hormones are known to modulate components of the stress response system, it suggests that we should consider the environmental conditions under which sex differences are manifested. Finally, it reminds us that there may be *different* explanations for gender differences in psychiatric disorders at different developmental stages because, by definition, the developing organism *changes* over time. As a field we have hardly even begun the empirical task of differentiating among these potential mechanisms for generating sex differences.

Role of Gender in Childhood Trauma and Risk for Adult Psychopathology

We now turn to a specific example of the importance of early experiences in the development of subsequent psychopathology. Compelling evidence from a variety of studies suggests that early adverse experience constitutes a major risk factor for the development and persistence of a wide range of psychiatric and nonpsychiatric medical disorders, including major depression, anxiety disorders, and substance use disorders as well as cardiovascular, immune, and metabolic disorders (e.g., Agid et al. 1999; Edwards et al. 2003; Felitti et al. 1998; McCauley et al. 1997; Mullen et al. 1996; reviewed in Heim and Nemeroff 2001). The manifestation or worsening of these disorders in adulthood is often related to acute life events or ongoing stress. These stress-related disorders also frequently occur comorbidly. For example, there are high rates of comorbidity between depression and cardiovascular disease, and the risk of developing both disorders is increased by early life adversity (Felitti et al. 1998). It thus appears that early adverse experience causes biological "scars" that increase an individual's vulnerability to stress later in life and predispose an individual to develop a spectrum of disorders that are known to manifest or worsen in relation to stress (Heim and Nemeroff 2001).

Laboratory studies in animals have provided direct evidence that adverse experience early in life induces sensitization of the endocrine, autonomic, and behavioral stress responses. A multitude of central nervous system changes subsequently were identified as a consequence of early life stress in animal models that likely converge into sensitization to stress (reviewed in Heim et al. 2004; Sanchez et al. 2001). Remarkably similar changes have been reported for adult humans with a history of childhood adversity (e.g., Carpenter et al. 2004; Heim and Nemeroff 2001; Heim et al. 2001; Pruessner et al. 2004; Vythilingam et al. 2002). In fact, it appears that the risk of many of the classic features of depression and anxiety disorders is increased by early life stress (Heim et al. 2004). It has also been demonstrated that chronically depressed patients are differentially responsive to psychotherapy versus medication as a function of childhood trauma. For example, in a recent multicenter study, Nemeroff et al. (2003) evaluated whether the presence or absence of childhood trauma might moderate treatment responses of patients with chronic depression to either pharmacological treatment or psychotherapy or to a combination of both. It was found that patients with chronic depression who had a history of childhood trauma (e.g., parental loss, physical abuse, sexual abuse, or neglect) showed a superior response to psychotherapy alone compared with the antidepressant alone. In chronically depressed patients who did not report childhood trauma, the pattern was reversed, with an antidepressant superior to psychotherapy. The combination of psychotherapy and pharmacotherapy was only marginally superior to psychotherapy alone among the depressed patients with childhood stress. These results suggest that psychotherapy may be essential in the treatment of depression associated with early life stress. The results also suggest that there appear to be different biological subtypes of depression that reflect different developmental pathways (Heim et al. 2004; Nemeroff et al. 2003).

However, vulnerability to stress and disease is surely not exclusively determined by exposure to early life stress. It is also influenced by constitutional factors that may moderate the effects of early stress, in addition to other factors. One such factor may be sex/gender. Interestingly, many of the disorders that have been associated with childhood adversity—for example, depression and anxiety disorders, including posttraumatic stress disorder (PTSD)—are generally more prevalent in adult women than in men. For example, major depression is about twice as common in women as in men (see Chapter 4 and E.A. Young 1998). Piccinelli and Wilkinson (2000) noted that certain artifacts in the estimation of prevalence rates of depression in men and women may enhance a female preponderance. For example, gender differences in clinical presentation, reporting of symptoms, and preexisting conditions that increase risk for depression, as well as social and cultural norms, likely influence prevalence estimates (Piccinelli and Wilkinson 2000). However, a critical review of the literature suggests that the sexual dimorphism in depression is genuine (Piccinelli and Wilkinson 2000).

Several authors have suggested that the sexual dimorphism in the prevalence of depression and perhaps certain anxiety disorders could, in part, be influenced by sex differences in the *prevalence* of childhood adverse experience or different *types* of such experiences (Piccinelli and Wilkinson 2000; Weiss et al. 1999; also see Chapter 6). According to the latest report of the National Child Abuse and Neglect Data System, boys experience about 48% of all reported incidents of child maltreatment. Rates of physical abuse and neglect are virtually identical in boys and girls. There are almost identical rates of fatalities in boys and in girls, which may serve as a rough measure of severity of physical abuse and neglect. The rate of reported cases of sexual abuse is higher in girls than in boys, although sexual abuse in boys might be largely underreported (Holmes and Slap 1998). Interestingly, a recent population-representative study conducted by the Centers for Disease Control in 8,667 adult members of a large health maintenance organization in the San Diego, California, area confirmed significantly higher rates of sexual abuse in females compared with males, and more than 85% of these cases of sexual abuse remained unreported (Edwards et al. 2003). Taken together, higher rates or greater severity of sexual abuse in girls versus boys may contribute to the sexual dimorphism of depression and potentially anxiety disorders.

An additional contribution to the preponderance of women among patients with depression and anxiety disorders might involve sex differences in *responsiveness* to the pathogenic effects of childhood adversity (Weiss et al. 1999). Indeed, several studies suggest that the relationship between childhood abuse experience and adult depression is stronger for women than for men: Carmen et al. (1984) reported that women with a history of child abuse were more than twice as likely to have major depression than men with a history of child abuse (67% versus 27%). A reanalysis of data from a community study involving 3,132 adults found a higher lifetime prevalence and current incidence of major depression in female victims of child abuse versus nonvictims, but not in male victims versus nonvictims (Stein et al. 1988). In a community study that comprised more than 7,000 individuals, women—but not men—with a history of childhood physical abuse had significantly higher lifetime rates of major depression than nonvictims. A history of sexual abuse was related to several psychiatric disorders in women and in men, but the relationship was stronger for women. A similar gender-based susceptibility for the development of PTSD in relation to childhood trauma has also been reported (e.g., Kessler et al. 1995; Stein et al. 2000; Walker et al. 2004). In another recent study, 8,000 men and 8,000 women were interviewed in the National Violence Against Women Survey. Whereas men more frequently reported physical abuse, the adverse health consequences of the physical abuse were generally more detrimental in women (Thompson et al. 2004). On the basis of these findings, it can be hypothesized that early adverse experience interacts with gender to produce vulnerability to various syndromes. The moderating effect of gender on the long-term consequences of early adversity may be mediated through differential responses in neurobiological pathways regulating stress and emotion that are sexually dimorphic or influenced by sex steroids, in addition to genetic or other environmental factors.

Sex Differences in the Neurobiological Response to Childhood Adversity

As described in more detail in the chapter on neurobiology (Chapter 5), there are marked sex differences in the stress response. In particular, animal studies suggest increased HPA axis reactivity in females, whereas findings in humans are more inconsistent and warrant further investigation. As mentioned earlier, the observed sex differences in HPA axis reactivity are generally attributed to the effects of sex steroids, estradiol in particular, on HPA axis function, glucocorticoid receptors, and corticotropin-releasing factor neuronal activity. Other mechanisms may include sex steroid effects on brain regions such as the hippocampus and the amygdala (for reviews, see McEwen 2001; Rhodes and Rubin 1999; E.A. Young 1998; also see Chapter 5). Such processes, in addition to hormone-independent genetic and developmental differences in the brains of males and females, may eventually converge to form the basis of sex differences in neuroendocrine, autonomic, and behavioral responses to stress. Thus, it would not be surprising if early life stress were associated with sex-specific long-term neurobiological consequences that translate into differential risk for psychopathology.

However, there is only very limited evidence on potential sex-specific neurobiological effects of early life stress. Only a few animal studies have specifically targeted the investigation of interactions between early life stress and gender in shaping a stress-reactive phenotype. In one study, pregnant rats were exposed to restraint stress in the last week of gestation, and the offspring were exposed to restraint stress at 5 months of age. Prenatal stress induced increased adrenocorticotropic hormone and corticosterone responses to restraint stress in the adult offspring, but only in the female rats, whereas male rats were largely unaffected (McCormick et al. 1995). In contrast, Wigger and Neumann (1999), who studied sex differences in the effects of periodic maternal separation, observed more pronounced long-term neuroendocrine and behavioral reactivity to emotional stress in male rats than in female rats who were maternally deprived. These findings suggest that the timing and specific type of early stress may influence the direction of sex differences. Interestingly, there is also evidence from animal studies that early maternal care influences estrogen receptor alpha expression as well as estrogen sensitivity in the central nervous system, which might in turn influence gonadal steroid effects on stress responses and behavior (Champagne et al. 2004). Whether there are sex differences in the long-term neurobiological effect of childhood stress in humans is largely unknown, although sex differences in the development of certain brain regions have been noted in maltreated children. One study (De Bellis and Keshavan 2003) examined neuroanatomical changes using magnetic resonance imaging in male and female children with chronic PTSD due to childhood abuse, compared with control subjects. Analyses stratified by gender revealed that children with PTSD did not show a normal age-related increase in total corpus callosum size or the size of region 7 (splenium) of the corpus callosum. This finding was more prominent in males than in females. In addition, maltreated boys had smaller cerebral volumes and smaller corpus callosum regions 1 (rostrum) and 6 (isthmus) and greater lateral ventricular volume increases compared with maltreated females. De Bellis and Keshavan (2003) suggested that there are gender differences in the effects of maltreatment and/or PTSD on brain maturation in children. Taken together, the findings reviewed here suggest that a comprehensive investigation of sex differences in response to early life stress in humans is strongly warranted.

Gaps in the Literature and Research Recommendations

Early adverse experience appears to interact with the unfolding genetic blueprint to permanently program brain circuits involved in the mediation of stress and emotion, resulting in increased responsiveness to subsequent environmental events that persist throughout the life span. These changes likely underlie the increased risk for depression and certain anxiety disorders, as well as certain other disorders, after early life stress. There is evidence for sex differences in the prevalence of mental disorders related to child abuse. On the basis of our literature review, it can be postulated that this sexual dimorphism may be influenced by sex differences in exposure to different types of childhood adversity and/or by sex differences in the underlying neurobiological long-term responses to early adversity. Most likely, there is a complex interaction between these factors, and the nature of this interaction may vary over the life span. Such differences in neurobiological responsiveness might be due, in part, to the effects of sex steroids on stress-mediating neurobiological systems.

The lack of consideration of gender differences is a major gap in current research on the relationship between childhood adversity and risk for psychopathology in adulthood. In fact, most studies exclusively include women due to the assumption that childhood abuse mostly affects girls. Thus, men are a largely understudied population regarding potential sex-specific consequences of childhood trauma and their prevention or treatment.

Future research studies should scrutinize sex/gender differences in the effects of childhood adversity. Studies are also needed that examine sex differences more generally and their relationship to psychopathology over time. Such studies should include gender as an independent factor. Research on the following areas is recommended:

1. *Sex/gender differences in the nature or timing of childhood adverse experiences and their link to differences in psychopathological outcome.* For example, studies should identify whether different types of maltreatment experiences—and the age at which they occur—in girls versus boys predict gender differences in specific disease vulnerability.
2. *Sex/gender differences in the psychopathological consequences of comparable types of childhood adversity.* For example, research is needed on whether sexually abused girls have a different risk for depression and other disorders compared with sexually abused boys.
3. *Sex/gender-specific impact of childhood adversity on the clinical presentation, illness onset and course, and comorbidity rates within a given disorder.*
4. *Sex/gender differences in the effects of childhood adversity on neurobiological parameters, such as the HPA axis, the autonomic nervous system, and neural systems that have been implicated in mental disorders.*
5. *Sex/gender-specific effects of stress and life events in different developmental stages or during transitions between stages (e.g., puberty, menopause) on risk for psychopathology.* Age-cohort studies and longitudinal studies should be conducted to examine such effects. For example, studies assessing gender differences in the effects of stress before, during, or after puberty on psychopathological or neurobiological outcome are warranted.
6. *Interactions between stress response systems and sex steroids.* To further understand the mechanisms by which gender might moderate the effects of childhood stress on mental health and neurobiological function, studies on the interactions between stress response systems and sex steroids are important.
7. *Sex/gender and childhood stress interactions in the prediction of treatment response in stress-related disorders.* Gender should also be used for stratification when studying the reversibility of the effects of childhood trauma on the brain and endocrine function.
8. *Multidimensional developmental approach to the role of sex/gender.* There is no reason to suppose that the same components of sex/gender will be involved in all

disorders, or that the same components will be involved at each developmental stage. Thus, a multidimensional developmental approach will be required.

Studies such as these may help elucidate the fascinating and important interrelationship between developmental phase, stressful experiences, and sex/gender in determining risk for psychiatric disorders, as well as their underlying mechanisms across the life span. Insights gained from these studies might help identify developmental periods of particular risk for females versus males and might lead toward prevention and treatment strategies that directly target the involved mechanisms.

Such studies may also have an impact on future editions of the DSM. It has been argued that the current, purely descriptive classification system in DSM has obscured research and has failed to produce uniform neurobiological findings or predictors of treatment response in depression and other disorders (Charney et al. 2002). Therefore, new paradigms of mental disorders should be empirically tested using clinical, etiological, and biological variables. The findings summarized here would suggest that childhood adversity should be considered when deriving new disease models and diagnostic algorithms. A new typology of mental disorders, based on developmental pathways and neurobiological patterns, might indeed lead toward improved treatment and the identification of predictors of treatment response (Heim et al. 2004). Given the potential gender differences in exposure to risk factors such as early life stress, and in their behavioral and neurobiological responses, such a typology likely should be gender specific.

The complexity of this task is such that it will barely have been begun by the time the DSM-V is produced. Looking farther into the future, however, elucidating the mechanisms by which sex differences are produced is likely to be a productive means of investigating the etiology of psychiatric disorders in general. Developing such understanding will be an important part of the process of moving from our current purely phenomenological-descriptive nosology to a nosology based on etiopathology.

References

Agid O, Shapira B, Zislin J, et al: Environment and vulnerability to major psychiatric illness: a case control study of early parental loss in major depression, bipolar disorder and schizophrenia. Mol Psychiatry 4:163–172, 1999

Angold A, Costello EJ: Epidemiology of depression in children and adolescents, in The Depressed Child and Adolescent, 2nd Edition. Edited by Goodyear I. Cambridge, United Kingdom, Cambridge University Press, 2001, pp 143–178

Angold A, Costello EJ, Worthman CM: Puberty and depression: the roles of age, pubertal status, and pubertal timing. Psychol Med 28:51–61, 1998

Angold A, Costello EJ, Worthman CM: Pubertal changes in hormone levels and depression in girls. Psychol Med 28:51–61, 1999

Angold A, Erkanli A, Silberg J, et al: Depression scale scores in 8–17-year-olds: effects of age and gender. J Child Psychol Psychiatry 43:1052–1063, 2002

Baulieu EE: Neurosteroids: a novel function of the brain. Psychoneuroendocrinology 23:963–987, 1998

Bebbington PE, Dunn G, Jenkins R, et al: The influence of age and sex on the prevalence of depressive conditions: report from the National Survey of Psychiatric Morbidity. Int Rev Psychiatry 15:74–83, 2003

Beck W, Wuttke W: Diurnal variations of plasma luteinizing hormone, follicle-stimulating hormone, and prolactin in boys and girls from birth to puberty. J Clin Endocrinol Metab 50:635–639, 1980

Berta P, Hawkins JR, Sinclair AH, et al: Genetic evidence equating SRY and the testis-determining factor. Nature 348:448–450, 1996

Carmen EH, Rieker PP, Mills T: Victims of violence and psychiatric illness. Am J Psychiatry 141:378–383, 1984

Carpenter LL, Tyrka AR, McDougle CJ, et al: Cerebrospinal fluid corticotropin-releasing factor and perceived early life stress in depressed patients and healthy control subjects. Neuropsychopharmacology 29:777–784, 2004

Champagne FA, Weaver ICG, Diorio J, et al: Natural variations in maternal care are associated with estrogen receptor alpha expression and estrogen sensitivity in the medial preoptic area. Endocrinology 144:4720–4724, 2004

Charney DS, Barlow DH, Botteron K, et al: Neuroscience research agenda to guide development of a pathophysiologically based classification system, in A Research Agenda for DSM-V. Edited by Kupfer DA, First MB, Regier DA. Washington, DC, American Psychiatric Association, 2002, pp 123–199

Clayton P, Trueman J: Leptin and puberty. Arch Dis Child 83:1–3, 2000

Collu R, Ducharme JR: Role of adrenal steroids in the regulation of gonadotropin secretion at puberty. J Steroid Biochem 6:869–872, 1975

Counts DR, Pescovitz OH, Barnes KM, et al: Dissociation of adrenarche and gonadarche in precocious puberty and in isolated hypogonadotropic hypogonadism. J Clin Endocrinol Metab 64:1174–1178, 1987

Cyranowski JM, Frank E, Young E, et al: Adolescent onset of the gender difference in lifetime rates of major depression: a theoretical model. Arch Gen Psychiatry 57:21–27, 2000

De Bellis MD, Keshavan MS: Sex differences in brain maturation in maltreatment-related pediatric posttraumatic stress disorder. Neurosci Biobehav Rev 27:103–117, 2003

DePeretti E, Forest MG: Unconjugated dehydroepiandrosterone plasma levels in normal subjects from birth to adolescence in human: The use of a sensitive radioimmunoassay. J Clin Endocrinol Metab 43:962–969, 1976

Dewing P, Bernard P, Vilain E: Disorders of gonadal development. Semin Reprod Med 20:189–198, 2002

Dewing P, Shi T, Horvath S, et al: Sexually dimorphic gene expression in mouse brain precedes gonadal differentiation. Brain Res Mol Brain Res 118:82–90, 2003

Ducharme JR, Forest MG, DePeretti E, et al: Plasma adrenal and gonadal sex steroids in human pubertal development. J Clin Endocrinol Metab 42:468–476, 1976

Dunger DB, Villa AK, Matthews DR, et al: Pattern of secretion of bioactive and immunoreactive gonadotrophins in normal pubertal children. J Clin Endocrinol Metab 35:267–275, 1991

Dunkel L, Alfthan H, Stenman UH, et al: Gonadal control of pulsatile secretion of luteinizing hormone and follicle stimulating hormone in prepubertal boys evaluated by ultrasensitive time-resolved immunofluorometric assay. J Clin Endocrinol Metab 70:107–114, 1990

Dunnett S: Sex and gender in Brain Research Bulletin. Brain Res Bull 60:187–188, 2003

Edwards VJ, Holden GW, Felitti VJ, et al: Relationship between multiple forms of childhood maltreatment and adult mental health in community respondents: results from the adverse childhood experiences study. Am J Psychiatry 160:1453–1460, 2003

Felitti VJ, Anda RF, Nordenberg D, et al: Relationship of childhood abuse and household dysfunction to many of the leading causes of death in adults in The Adverse Childhood Experiences (ACE) Study. Am J Prev Med 14:245–258, 1998

Gubba EM, Netherton CM, Herbert J: Endangerment of the brain by glucocorticoids: experimental and clinical evidence. J Neurocytol 29:439–449, 2000

Gueorguiev M, Goth M, Korbonits M: Leptin and puberty: a review. Pituitary 4:79–86, 2001

Haig D: The inexorable rise of gender and the decline of sex: social change in academic titles, 1945–2001. Arch Sex Behav 33:87–96, 2004

Hale PM, Khoury S, Foster CM, et al: Increased luteinizing hormone pulse frequency during sleep in early to midpubertal boys. J Clin Endocrinol Metab 66:785–791, 1998

Heim C, Nemeroff CB: The role of childhood trauma in the neurobiology of mood and anxiety disorders: preclinical and clinical studies. Biol Psychiatry 49:1023–1039, 2001

Heim C, Newport DJ, Bonsall R, et al: Altered pituitary-adrenal axis responses to provocative challenge tests in adult survivors of childhood abuse. Am J Psychiatry 158:575–581, 2001

Heim C, Plotsky PM, Nemeroff CB: Importance of studying the contributions of early adverse experience to neurobiological findings in depression. Neuropsychopharmacology 29:641–648, 2004

Holmes WC, Slap GB: Sexual abuse of boys: definition, prevalence, correlates, sequelae, and management. JAMA 280:1855–1862, 1998

Hossain A, Saunders GF: The human sex-determining gene SRY is a direct target of WT1. J Biol Chem 276:16817–16823, 2001

Jager RJ, Anvret M, Hall K, et al: A human XY female with frame shift mutation in the candidate sex determining gene, SRY. Nature 348:452–454, 1990

Jordan B, Vilain E: Sry and the genetics of sex determination. Adv Exp Med Biol 511:1–14, 2002

Jost A: Recherches sur la differenciation sexuelle de l'embryon de lapin III: role des gonades foetales dans la differenciation sexuelle somatique. Archives d Anatomie Microscopique et de Morphologie Experimentale 36:271–315, 1947

Judd HL, Parker DC, Yen SSC: Sleep-wake patterns of LH and testosterone release in prepubertal boys. J Clin Endocrinol Metab 44:965–969, 1977

Kaminska M, Harris J, Gijsbers K, et al: Dehydroepiandrosterone sulfate (DHEAS) counteracts decremental effects of corticosterone on dentate gyrus LTP: implication for depression. Brain Res Bull 52:229–234, 2000

Karishma KK, Herbert J: Dehydroepiandrosterone (DHEA) stimulates neurogenesis in the hippocampus of the rat, promotes survival of newly formed neurons and prevents corticosterone-induced suppression. Eur J Neurosci 16:445–453, 2002

Kessler RC, Sonnega A, Bromet E, et al: Posttraumatic stress disorder in the National Comorbidity Survey. Arch Gen Psychiatry 52:1048–1060, 1995

Kimonides VG, Khatibi NH, Svendsen CN, et al: Dehydroepiandrosterone (DHEA) and DHEA-sulfate (DHEAS) protect hippocampal neurons against excitatory amino acid-induced neurotoxicity. Proc Natl Acad Sci USA 95:1852–1857, 1998

Korth-Schutz S, Levine LS, New MI: Serum androgens in normal prepubertal and pubertal children and in children with precocious adrenarche. J Clin Endocrinol Metab 42:117–124, 1976

Kraemer HC, Kazdin AE, Offord DR, et al: Coming to terms with the terms of risk. Arch Gen Psychiatry 54:337–343, 1997

Kulin HE, Moore RW, Satner SJ: Circadian rhythms in gonadotropin excretion in prepubertal and pubertal children. J Clin Endocrinol Metab 42:770–773, 1976

Labrie F, Belanger A, Cusan L, et al: Marked decline in serum concentrations of adrenal C19 sex steroid precursors and conjugated androgen metabolites during aging. J Clin Endocrinol Metab 82:2396–2402, 1997

Landy H, Beopple PA, Mansfield MJ, et al: Sleep modulation of neuroendocrine function: developmental changes in gonadotropin-releasing hormone secretion during sexual maturation. Pediatr Res 28:213–217, 1990

Lashansky G, Saenger P, Fishman K, et al: Normative data for adrenal steroidogenesis in a healthy pediatric population: age and sex-related changes after adrenocorticotropin stimulation. J Clin Endocrinol Metab 73:674–686, 1991

Marshall JC, Dalkin AC, Haisenieder DJ, et al: Gonadotropin-releasing hormone pulses: regulators of gonadotropin synthesis and ovulatory cycles. Recent Programs of Hormone Research 47:155–187, 1991

McCauley J, Kern DE, Kolodner K, et al: Clinical characteristics of women with a history of childhood abuse: unhealed wounds. JAMA 277:1362–1368, 1997

McCormick CM, Smythe JW, Sharma S, et al: Sex-specific effects of prenatal stress on hypothalamic-pituitary-adrenal responses to stress and brain glucocorticoid receptor density in adult rats. Brain Res Dev 84:55–61, 1995

McEwen BS: Invited review: Estrogens effects on the brain: multiple sites and molecular mechanisms. J Appl Physiol 91:2785–2801, 2001

Moffitt T, Caspi A, Rutter M, et al: Sex differences in antisocial behaviour: conduct disorder, delinquency, and violence, in Dunedin Longitudinal Study. New York, Cambridge University Press, 2001

Money J: Hermaphroditism, gender and precocity in hyperadrenocorticism: psychologic findings. Bull Johns Hopkins Hosp 96:253–264, 1955

Mullen PE, Martin JL, Anderson JC, et al: The long-term impact of the physical, emotional, and sexual abuse of children: a community study. Child Abuse Negl 20:7–21, 1996

Nemeroff CB, Heim CM, Thase ME, et al: Differential responses to psychotherapy versus pharmacotherapy in patients with chronic forms of major depression and childhood trauma. Proc Natl Acad Sci USA 100:14293–14296, 2003

Page DC: On low expectations exceeded; or, the genomic salvation of the y chromosome. Am J Hum Genet 74:399–402, 2004

Parker LN, Sack J, Fisher DA, et al: The adrenarche: prolactin, gonadotropins, adrenal androgens, and cortisol. J Clin Endocrinol Metab 46:396–404, 1978

Persson A, Kerr M, and Stattin H: Why a leisure context is linked to normbreaking for some girls and not others: personality characteristics and parent-child relations as explanations. J Adolesc 27:583–598, 2004

Piccinelli M, Wilkinson G: Gender differences in depression (review). Br J Psychiatry 177:486–492, 2000

Pinn VW: Sex and gender factors in medical studies: implications for health and clinical practice. JAMA 289:397–400, 2003

Plant T: Neurobiological bases underlying the control of the onset of puberty in the rhesus monkey: a representative higher primate. Front Neuroendocrinol 22:107–139, 2001

Pruessner JC, Champagne F, Meaney MJ, et al: Dopamine release in response to a psychological stress in humans and its relationship to early life maternal care: a positron emission tomography study using [11C] raclopride. J Neurosci 24:2825–2831, 2004

Reiner W, Gearhart J: Discordant sexual identity in some genetic males with cloacal exstrophy assigned to female sex at birth. N Engl J Med 350:333–341, 2004

Reiter EO, Fuldauer VG, Root AW: Secretion of the adrenal androgen, dehydroepiandrosterone sulfate, during normal infancy, childhood, and adolescence, in sick infants, and in children with endocrinologic abnormalities. J Pediatr 90:76–80, 1977

Rhodes ME, Rubin RT: Functional sex differences ("sexual diergism") of central nervous system cholinergic systems, vasopressin, and hypothalamic-pituitary-adrenal axis activity in mammals: a selective review. Brain Res Brain Res Rev 30:135–152, 1999

Rutter M, Caspi A, Moffitt T: Using sex differences in psychopathology to study causal mechanisms: unifying issues and research strategies. J Child Psychol Psychiatry 44:1092–1115, 2003

Sanchez MM, Ladd CO, Plotsky PM: Early adverse experience as a developmental risk factor for later psychopathology: evidence from rodent and primate models. Dev Psychopathol 13:419–449, 2001

Sizonenko PC, Paunier L: Hormonal changes in puberty III: correlation of plasma dehydroepiandrosterone, testosterone, FSH, and LH with stages of puberty and bone age in normal boys and girls and in patients with Addison's disease or hypogonadism or with premature or late adrenarche. J Clin Endocrinol Metab 41:894–904, 1975

Skaletsky H, Kuroda-Kawaguchi T, Minx PJ, et al: The male-specific region of the human Y chromosome is a mosaic of discrete sequence classes. Nature 423:825–837, 2003

Skuse D: Extreme deprivation in early childhood. J Child Psychol Psychiatry 25:543–572, 1984

Stattin H, Magnusson D: Pubertal Maturation in Female Development. Mahwah, NJ, Lawrence Erlbaum, 1990

Stattin H, Kerr M, Mahoney J, et al: Explaining why a leisure context is bad for some girls and not for others, in Organized Activities as Contexts of Development: Extracurricular Activities, After-School and Community Programs. Edited by Mahoney JL, Larson RW, Eccles JS. Mahwah, NJ, Lawrence Erlbaum, 2005

Stein JA, Golding JM, Siegel JM, et al: Long-term psychological sequelae of child sexual abuse, in Lasting Effects of Child Sexual Abuse. Edited by Wyatt GE, Powell GJ. Newbury Park, CA, Sage, 1988, pp 135–154

Stein MB, Walker JR, Forde DR: Gender differences in susceptibility to posttraumatic stress disorder. Behav Res Ther 38:619–628, 2000

Terasawa E, Fernandez D: Neurobiological mechanisms of the onset of puberty in primates. Endocr Rev 22:111–151, 2001

Thompson MP, Kingree JB, Desai S: Gender differences in long-term health consequences of physical abuse of children: data from a nationally representative survey. Am J Public Health 94:599–604, 2004

Twenge J, Nolen-Hoeksema S: Age, gender, race, socioeconomic status, and birth cohort differences on the Children's Depression Inventory: a meta-analysis. J Abnorm Psychol 111:578–588, 2002

Vihko H, Apter D: The role of androgens in adolescent cycles. J Steroid Biochem 12:369–373, 1980

Vilain E: Genetics of sexual development. Annu Rev Sex Res 11:1–25, 2000

Vythilingam M, Heim C, Newport J, et al: Childhood trauma associated with smaller hippocampal volume in women with major depression. Am J Psychiatry 159:2072–2080, 2002

Walker JL, Carey PD, Mohr N, et al: Gender differences in the prevalence of childhood sexual abuse and in the development of pediatric PTSD. Arch Women Ment Health 7:111–121, 2004

Weiss EL, Longhurst JG, Mazure CM: Childhood sexual abuse as a risk factor for depression in women: psychosocial and neurobiological correlates. Am J Psychiatry 156:816–828, 1999

Wennink JM, Delemarre-van de Waal HA, Schoemaker R, et al: Luteinizing hormone and follicle stimulating hormone secretion patterns in boys throughout puberty measured using highly sensitive immunoradiometric assays. J Clin Endocrinol 31:551–564, 1989

Wennink JM, Delemarre-van de Waal HA, Schoemaker R, et al: Luteinizing hormone and follicle stimulating hormone secretion patterns in girls throughout puberty measured using highly sensitive immunoradiometric assays. Clin Endocrinol 33:333–344, 1990

Wierman ME, Beardsworth DE, Crawford JD, et al: Adrenarche and skeletal maturation during luteinizing hormone releasing hormone analogue suppression of gonadarche. J Clin Invest 77:121–126, 1986

Wigger A, Neumann ID: Periodic maternal deprivation induces gender-dependent alterations in behavioral and neuroendocrine responses to emotional stress in adult rats. Physiol Behav 66:293–302, 1999

Willard HF: The sex chromosomes and X chromosome inactivation, in The Metabolic and Molecular Bases of Inherited Disease. Edited by Scriver CR, Sly WS, Childs B, et al. New York, McGraw Hill, 2000

Wizemann TM, Pardue M (eds) Exploring the Biological Contributions to Human Health: Does Sex Matter? Washington, DC, National Academies Press, 2001

Wu FC, Butler GE, Kelnar CJ, et al: Patterns of pulsatile luteinizing hormone secretion before and during the onset of puberty in boys: a study using an immunoradiometric assay. J Clin Endocrinol Metab 70:629–637, 1990

Young DG, Skibinski G, Mason JI, et al: The influence of age and gender on serum dehydroepiandrosterone sulphate (DHEA-S), IL-6, IL-6 soluble receptor (IL-6 sR) and transforming growth factor beta 1 (TGF-[beta]1) levels in normal healthy blood donors. Clin Exp Immunol 117:476–481, 1999

Young EA: Sex differences and the HPA axis: implications for psychiatric disease. J Gend Specif Med 1:21–27, 1998

8

THE LONGITUDINAL LABORATORY OF WOMEN'S REPRODUCTIVE HEALTH

Katherine L. Wisner, M.D., M.S.

This chapter continues the developmental perspective outlined in Chapter 7 ("A Developmental Perspective, With a Focus on Childhood Trauma"), extending it into adulthood, with a focus on women's reproductive health. Certainly, reproductive events have profound implications for women's lives and also for the psychopathology they may experience. Reproductive events are also reflected in DSM-IV-TR (American Psychiatric Association 2000) in a number of ways, and they are likely to be even further integrated into future editions of DSM as their relevance to psychiatric diagnosis and treatment becomes better understood.

In this chapter, the reproductive events in women's lives are conceptualized and presented as a natural "laboratory" for research hypothesis generation. Historically, women have been excluded from clinical trials, in part because of the physiological "noise" that menstrual cycling, pregnancy, lactation, and menopause create in the collection and interpretation of research data. At this juncture in the evolution of research paradigms, this perceived disadvantage of the past can be recast as an advantage. Research advances result from continually refining our understanding of psychiatric disorders by discovering new relationships between variables that explain aspects of illness (and wellness). As a field, we are poised to pursue the study of the importance of gender as a variable that impacts the etiology, epidemiology, symptomatic expression, and treatment response in psychiatric illness.

An increasing number of publications related to sex and gender have been included in our scientific literature (see Chapter 2, "Why Gender Matters," this volume). Stimulated by the need to interpret findings from brain imaging studies, the study of the developmental trajectories of normal brain development by age and gender is crucial (Durston et al. 2001). On average, the male brain is about 10% larger than the female brain. The caudate and possibly the globus pallidus and hippocampus are disproportionately larger in female brains, and the amygdala is disproportionately smaller than in the male brain (Durston et al. 2001). Striking gender differences in the pathophysiology and outcome of acute neurological injury have been reported. Greater neuroprotection in females versus males may be due to sex hormone–mediated antioxidant mechanisms (Bayir et al. 2004). Clarification of the genesis of these differences is an intriguing challenge. Do these gender differences play a role in differential rates of psychopathology between the genders?

Gender is a variable that is highly relevant to the clinical practice of psychiatry, and information about gender is included in DSM-IV-TR in the "Specific Culture, Age, and Gender Features" sections of the text for various disorders (see Chapter 3, "DSM's Approach to Gender," this volume). For example, the gender ratio of females to males for both anorexia and bulimia nervosa is approximately 10:1. Exploration of this striking gender predominance in females surely will allow investigators to elucidate biopsychosocial contributions to the as-yet-unknown etiology of eating disorders. Why do so many more women than men develop eating disorders? Is illness expression the same in men and women? Does brain structure or function differ between males and females with bulimia? Of those males who develop eating disorders, what are the commonalities with females? Are the natural history and treatment response the same? How might the fact that the prevalence increases as societies become more urbanized increase our understanding of etiological factors (Hsu 2004)?

Gender differences are also prominent in the presentation and course of schizophrenia (Seeman 2004). Women are more likely to have a later onset, more prominent mood symptoms, and a better prognosis than men. The median age at onset is in the early to mid-twenties for men and the late twenties for women. The age at onset may have both pathophysiological and prognostic significance. Males have less optimal premorbid adjustment, lower educational achievement, more evidence of structural brain abnormalities, more prominent negative signs, and a worse outcome than females. Women have less severe symptoms, fewer hospitalizations, briefer hospital admissions, a higher likelihood of returning to work, and more social support (Hafner 2003). Women with schizophrenia are much more likely to be married than men and are twice as likely to have children (Hafner 2003). If we can elucidate the factors that produce a more favorable course in women, can interventions be designed to improve the course of illness in men?

Gender-based differences in illness expression are more than curiosities. In psychiatric epidemiological research, variables that account for differences in disease expression between populations are the basis for hypothesis generation. Differences in psychiatric illness expression present an invitation to study the reasons that they occur. This is an opportunity for *variable partitioning*—that is, dividing groups of individuals along some variable (gender) and evaluating disease expression in the groups. This strategy is common in health research: categorize a population on the basis of a particular variable, such as smoking versus nonsmoking, and evaluate the risk for lung cancer. Partition a population according to intimate partner violence and evaluate rates of posttraumatic stress disorder. Partition a depressed population according to whether they received randomly assigned antidepressant or placebo and evaluate the rate of remission of depression. In these examples, the health implications of gender can be used to add to our knowledge base. For example, do female and male smokers have the same risk for the development of lung cancer or depression? Intimate partner violence is a social problem that affects more females than males. Is posttraumatic stress disorder in these women similar to that which occurs in male combat veterans? Do differences in presentations suggest different therapies? Do male and female combat veterans exposed to the same traumatic event differ in symptom development, time course of evolution of the illness, or comorbidity? The increasing number of gender-focused papers in our literature demonstrates the increasing application of this notion (see Chapter 2).

The Laboratory of Women's Reproductive Lives

The dramatic events of women's reproductive lives also provide a source of variable partitioning that creates immense potential for research advancements. For example, naturally occurring hormone fluctuations can be correlated with mood and behavior. Women can act as their own controls in research studies. For example, women with and without premenstrual dysphoric disorder can be compared for trait differences that can be explored for etiological significance. Why do about 5% of women have major functional impairment premenstrually? Why *don't* the remaining 95% have this illness, despite similar fluctuations in hormone levels? Women with premenstrual dysphoric disorder can be assessed during both the asymptomatic follicular phase and the symptomatic luteal phase for clues about pathophysiological state changes. If these mechanisms are clarified, preventive and therapeutic measures potentially can be developed. Clarification of the mechanisms by which hormones affect various aspects of brain and behavior relationships will improve our knowledge of psychiatric illness in both genders.

Postpartum-onset depression is another example of the profound effect of reproductive events on psychopathology. The hormonal milieu of parturition is distinct compared with any other time in a woman's life. Bloch et al. (2000) studied women with a history of postpartum-onset depression and those without a history of depression (the partitioning variable). They found evidence that reproductive hormones play a role in the development of postpartum depression. These researchers simulated the withdrawal of hormones at birth by inducing a hypogonadal state in women with leuprolide, adding back supraphysiological doses of estradiol and progesterone for 8 weeks, and then withdrawing both steroids under double-blind conditions. Five of eight women with a history of postpartum depression, compared with none of the eight women without a history of depression, developed significant mood symptoms. The women with previous postpartum-onset depression developed depressive symptoms at the end of the add-back phase (which simulated the end of pregnancy), and symptoms peaked in the withdrawal (postpartum simulation) phase. The implication of this finding is that women with postpartum depression are differentially sensitive to the mood-destabilizing effects of withdrawal from gonadal steroids compared with women with no history of depression. Some aspect of their neurophysiology creates a trait vulnerability that does not appear to be present in women with no history of depression. What is responsible for this vulnerability? Can the vulnerability be identified before childbirth? Do women with premenstrual dysphoric disorder evidence this same vulnerability, and is premenstrual dysphoric disorder a predictor of postpartum depression? Are all depressive syndromes that are associated with hormonal instability in women similar in presentation? Can we treat postpartum depression (or augment a poor antidepressant response) with estradiol, as was demonstrated in the United Kingdom (Gregoire et al. 1996)?

As would be predicted by a biopsychosocial disease model, postpartum-onset major depression has contributions from several risk factor domains. Women who have postpartum depression after one birth have a 25% risk of developing it after the subsequent birth (Wisner et al. 2001). Therefore, even women with known trait vulnerability do not consistently become depressed after giving birth. Some interaction of trait vulnerability and other proximal factors must occur for disease to result. Cumulative biological and psychosocial factors act independently and interactively to influence health in adult life (Kuh et al. 2003).

Menopause is characterized by a syndrome of somatic and psychological symptoms that are associated with a reduction in circulating levels of the female sex steroids. This natural laboratory has provided an opportunity to study central nervous system effects of decreasing sex steroids. Hormones have been studied as therapies for psychological symptoms, particularly depression (Epperson et al. 1999). Investigators have found that estradiol or other estrogenic agents may be effective for perimenopausal depression (Rasgon et al. 2002). Soares et al. (2001) studied the efficacy of 17 beta-estradiol (100 μg delivered *transdermally*) for the treatment of clinically significant depressive disorders in endocrinologically confirmed *peri*menopausal women. Fifty women were enrolled in the study; 26 had mood symptoms that met DSM-IV (American Psychiatric Association 1994) criteria for major depressive disorder, 11 for dysthymic disorder, and 13 for minor depressive disorder. Remission of depression was observed in 17 (68%) women treated with 17 beta-estradiol compared with 5 (20%) in the placebo group (P=0.001). Patients treated with estradiol sustained the antidepressant effect of treatment after the 4-week washout period, although somatic complaints increased in frequency and intensity. Treatment was well tolerated, and adverse events were rare in both groups. In contrast, estradiol patch (100 μg/day) was not effective as an antidepressant in *post*menopausal women (Morrison et al. 2004). Is estradiol effective for depression related to hormonal change at other reproductive change times in women?

Research with menopausal women has stimulated the question of whether a parallel syndrome occurs in men (Carnahan and Perry 2004). *Andropause*—the decline in sex steroid activity experienced by males as part of aging—may result in sexual dysfunction, loss of muscle and bone mass, depression, anxiety, and irritability (Bates et al. 2005; Carnahan and Perry 2004). Testosterone replacement therapy has been studied for treatment of depression in men and for augmentation of antidepressants in men with treatment-refractory illness (Carnahan and Perry 2004). Similarly, testosterone has also been used to improve sexual function in postmenopausal women (Alexander et al. 2004). Research about hormone–mood relationships in one gender has led to hypotheses about the efficacy of hormones in the other.

The Life Span Approach in Psychiatry

According to the National Institutes of Health Roadmap (nihroadmap.nih.gov), new conceptual approaches are needed to achieve meaningful gains in health outcomes. Evans and Stoddart (1990) and Misra et al. (2003) elaborated models of health with an emphasis on multiple etiological determinants across the life span. One way to conceptualize this model is along vertical and horizontal axes: the vertical axes are the multiple determinants of health that are dynamically active and interactive at all time points in life. Women's reproductive cycles through the life course are represented on the horizontal axis (Misra et al. 2003). Improving health requires an interdisciplinary approach that integrates the complex biological, physical environmental, and social environmental influences—as well as the individual biomedical and behavioral responses that shape it (the "vertical axes")—across the "horizontal" life course (Kuh et al. 2003; Misra et al. 2003).

The life course approach is well suited to psychiatry. Mental disorders are characterized by symptom development, disease consolidation, and the addition of other symptoms and/or disorders across time (comorbidities) that evolve as life unfolds. Returning to the concept of variable partitioning, these observations can be used for hypothesis generation. A major experience in the life course of most women is childbearing. For example, does the experience of pregnancy increase the probability that a woman with bipolar disorder will have more lifetime episodes of mania (Yonkers et al. 2004)? If she has multiple repeat pregnancies, is her chance of full recovery less, or is her requirement for multiple medications increased? Does her illness become more treatment resistant?

These concepts have been applied to perinatal health by Misra et al. (2003). They are readily applied to mental health, which is fundamental to health more generally (U.S. Department of Health and Human Services 1999). *Distal* (in time) risk factors place an individual or population at greater susceptibility to *proximal* (current) risk factors. For example, a woman who was sexually abused by a family member from early childhood brings different distal risks to adulthood than a woman from a family with clear and psychologically healthy interpersonal boundaries. Distal factors increase or decrease an individual's likelihood of developing health problems. *Proximal factors* have a direct impact on individual health status and are represented by behavioral and biomedical responses to the distal risk factors. Does the sexually abused woman develop posttraumatic stress disorder and withdraw from social interactions, or does she seek and accept support from friends and community resources? Does she welcome pregnancy by avoiding alcohol, or does she drink even more while pregnant? What determines such decisions? The interaction between distal and proximal risk factors determines an individual's overall health status. If pregnancy is the focal area of interest, it is the interrelationship between a woman's health status directly prior to conception and the demands of pregnancy that primarily influence perinatal health outcomes. In turn, the course of pregnancy itself has a major effect on a woman's life course. Outcomes can be understood as maternal, fetal/infant, familial, community, and societal. Health care professionals essentially seek to minimize distal and proximal risks in order to maximize positive outcomes. Application of this multiple-determinants life course model to psychiatric illnesses holds potential for new views and interventions at key impact points in the evolution of episodes, outcomes, and overall function.

Potential opportunities for interventions to improve perinatal health are included in this model. The crisis of the sexually abused pregnant patient described earlier could result in increased support from her partner, minister, and medical team, who provide education and encouragement to attend Alcoholics Anonymous meetings and a psychotherapy group to prepare for the birth. Although her depressive symptoms increase after the birth, she is treated immediately with an antidepressant, with remission of depressive symptoms. The patient and her partner remain engaged with their community and healthcare team and enjoy the infant, who meets normal developmental milestones. Each patient can be understood as coming to pregnancy with sets of malleable risks and assets that shape pregnancy outcome. To the extent that biopsychosocial exposures that have a negative impact upon pregnancy outcome can be diminished, eliminated, or replaced with positive factors, the risk of poor pregnancy outcome can be reduced.

DSM-IV-TR recognizes the importance of the natural history of psychiatric disorders as evidenced by the provision of course specifiers for many disorders. A number of specifiers for mood disorders are available to increase diagnostic specificity and create more homogeneous subgroups, assist in treatment selection, and improve the prediction of prognosis. Examples of specifiers for mood disorder are severity, remission, psychotic features, catatonic features, atypical features, melancholic features, and seasonal pattern. The postpartum onset specifier can be applied to the current or most recent major depressive episode in major depressive disorder; to the current or most recent major depressive episode, manic episode, or mixed episode in bipolar I or bipolar II disorder; or to a brief psychotic disorder. To qualify as having postpartum onset, the episode must begin within 4 weeks of birth.

Many investigators, however, use a broader definition for postpartum onset than 4 weeks—they consider episodes as postpartum if their onset is later than 4 weeks after birth (Elliott 2000)—and they apply the term *postpartum* to other disorders in addition to those listed earlier. The DSM-IV-TR text describes the symptomatology of postpartum episodes as being not different from non-postpartum mood episodes, and it notes that psychotic features may be present. However, mounting evidence indicates that acute-onset postpartum psychosis differs from psychosis in women that occurs outside this period. The presentation of postpartum psychoses is often characterized by alterations in cognition, manic symptoms, and confusion (Brockington et al. 1981). The confused, delirium-like, disorganized clinical picture of postpartum psychosis has been observed and reported repeatedly (Brockington et al. 1981; Hamilton 1982). Similarly, Wisner et al. (1994) found that postpartum women with acute-onset psychoses differed from psychotic episodes in non-childbearing women. Thought disorganization; bizarre behavior; lack of insight; delusions of reference, persecution, and jealousy; grandiosity, suspiciousness; impaired sensorium/orientation; and self-neglect were significantly more common in childbearing women. Thus, childbirth influences the presentation of psychotic symptoms. Research exploration of life course symptom changes will generate new hypotheses about etiology, prevention, and treatment that may have implications not only for future editions of DSM but also for clinical practice and social policy. For example, the case of Andrea Yates, a woman with postpartum psychosis who drowned her five children, generated ongoing discussions about whether the legal definitions of insanity are consistent with current concepts in mental health (Spinelli 2003).

Lifelong Implications of Pregnancy

Implicit in considering pregnancy outcomes is research about the importance of perturbations in the intrauterine environment and poor fetal health to long-term disease. An individual's susceptibility to cardiovascular disease cannot be explained completely by differences in lifestyle factors or genetic predispositions, but is also influenced by factors during intrauterine life (Dodic et al. 2003). Individuals who had low birth weight for gestational age (a broad index of suboptimal intrauterine environment) have an increased incidence of cardiovascular and metabolic diseases in adulthood. An environment that impairs growth in utero or during early childhood can influence an individual's metabolism and/or physiology in a way that increases the risk for cardiovascular disease in adult life.

Converging evidence from several areas of research supports a neurodevelopmental hypothesis of schizophrenia, which posits that a disruption of brain development (possibly from maternal viral infection, undernutrition, folate deficiency, and/or high life stress) plays an etiological role in a substantial proportion of cases of schizophrenia (Susser et al. 1999). Both early and late factors are thought to interact in complex ways. Mental and physical health outcomes are inseparable throughout the life course and, in fact, are a false dichotomy in need of reunification.

Antenatal maternal major depression increases risk to the gravid woman and her fetus. The physiological dysregulation of major depression is a suboptimal milieu for pregnancy. Maternal prenatal stress is significantly associated with low infant birth weight and premature birth in humans (Wadhwa et al. 1993, 1998). Major stressful events during the first trimester of pregnancy, such as the death of another child, increase the risk for fetal malformations, especially from the cranial neural crest (Hansen et al. 2000). The implication is that the physiological sequelae of extreme stress can create teratogenic effects that are typically conceptualized as the result of exposures such as drugs or radiation.

Research Opportunities and a Research Agenda

The potential of studying the longitudinal laboratory of women's lives is before us as investigators. In the life course epidemiology model, reproductive events are powerful natural perturbations that affect development and produce changes in the life course trajectory. The etiological contributions of these factors to the natural history of women's lives create numerous opportunities for research and for increasing our understanding of psychopathology, including its development and clinical expression. Examples of potential investigations include the following:

1. *Evaluate the predictive validity of illness at each point in the life cycle for the development of illness at a later reproductive transition.* Are women who develop depression at puberty at higher risk for developing premenstrual, prepartum, postpartum, and menopausal depression than women who remain well? Are the clinical features of a recurring illness similar across episodes? Why is our primary research attention limited primarily to depression? What variations in other psychiatric disorders occur during times of hormonal fluctuation?
2. *Conduct prospective investigations of women with established psychiatric episodes that are associated with reproductive events in their lives.* The study of the natural history of psychiatric disorders across pregnancy and the postpartum period has been limited to major depression and, to a lesser extent, bipolar disorder and eating disorders. Notably minimal is research on anxiety disorders, which are common in childbearing-aged women, as well as research on schizophrenia, dis-

sociative, somatoform, substance use, and personality disorders. Application of the multiple-determinants life course model to all disorders is timely. Such research is expected to generate new and more valid course specifiers in DSM.

3. *Include menstrual-cycle timing in studies of psychopathology, treatment outcome, and other types of investigations (for all disorders).* Such a focus will help to elucidate related changes in symptom presentation or effects on treatment response, as suggested by Leibenluft et al. (1994).
4. *Reconsider the definition of the DSM specifier "with postpartum onset" in view of new research and the operational definition used by investigators* (Elliott 2000; Munk-Olsen et al. 2006). The clinical value and validity of using longitudinal course qualifiers for reproductive events in addition to birth should be explored, for example, "with menopausal onset" or "with premenstrual exacerbation." Additional studies of disorders other than depression may allow more precise and clinically valuable specification of the clinical features of other disorders—for example, obsessive-compulsive disorder "with postpartum onset."
5. *Include in depression studies standard symptom measures that cover atypical symptoms.* Depression is a heterogeneous disorder, and women have more atypical depressive symptoms (such as hypersomnia and hyperphagia) that are associated with earlier age of onset as well as a higher frequency of suicidal thoughts and attempts, psychiatric comorbidity, disability and restricted activity days, and a history of childhood neglect and sexual abuse, than men (Matza et al. 2003). It is not known why atypical depressive symptoms are more frequent in women than in men and whether such symptoms are particularly characteristic of certain groups of women. The gold-standard Hamilton Depression Rating Scale is being reevaluated and its replacement debated; depression studies need to routinely use standard depression symptom measures that include atypical symptoms of depression. In addition, treatment studies of both men and women with prominent atypical depressive symptoms are needed to assess the relative efficacy of current modalities (particularly light therapy; Golden et al. 2005).
6. *Conduct studies of females and males with established psychiatric illnesses through the pubertal transition.* We consider people to have a primary diagnosis, and we also allow for comorbid diagnoses. However, if we take a life span approach, we must consider that diagnoses are essentially constellations of symptoms that represent psychophysiological states. Is there a developmental progression of diagnoses? Hypothetically, does a girl develop an anxiety disorder in early adolescence, an eating disorder in late adolescence, substance abuse (perhaps with a male partner) in her early twenties, and recurrent major depression and perhaps her first manic episode after she gives birth? Are there symptomatic expressions of the same brain dysfunction that interact with an evolving central nervous system developmental process and environmental factors to create different symptoms (and diagnoses) over the life span? Evaluation of children through the pubertal transition presents an opportunity for early identification of children with

psychiatric illness. With the life course model, the possibility of modifying risk factors at this transition may prevent episodes at later reproductive transitions. Studies are needed of females and males with established psychiatric illnesses (e.g., obsessive-compulsive disorder) through the pubertal transition. Although longer-term research strategies through multiple transitions over the lifetime are ideal, resource allocation may mean studying such transitions independently.

7. *Develop new, comprehensive conceptual approaches to achieve gains in psychiatric health outcomes.* In its Roadmap, the National Institutes of Health identified an interdisciplinary approach (as opposed to multidisciplinary) and recommended training for scientists in an area outside their primary educational emphasis. Because it is fundamental to health (U.S. Department of Health and Human Services 1999), mental health is positioned at the interface between behavior and every other medical discipline. Behavioral factors contribute to all disease processes. The ability of a physician to have an impact on behavior is critical to treatment. Basic science enriches our clinical research endeavors, including neurophysiology, pharmacology, genetics, teratology, toxicology, biostatistics, and epidemiology, to name a few. All science exists within the overall rubric of public health and within the complexities of the social, cultural, and political arenas of society. To enact these Roadmap-defined concepts, we must consider the most feasible approach to a new *interdisciplinary*, as opposed to *multidisciplinary*, mindset.

   Collaborative teams that include representatives from multiple specialties (e.g., psychiatrists, obstetricians, pediatricians, psychologists, pharmacologists, teratologists, representatives from the U.S. Food and Drug Administration, epidemiologists, biostatisticians, ethicists, anthropologists, advocacy group members) are needed to study issues related to psychotropic drug use during pregnancy and its development into public health policy. For example, what can we learn from comparable diagnostic systems, such as the ICD classification, about categorization concepts?

8. *Include both genders in ongoing research, and especially National Institute of Mental Health–funded studies, unless the scientific aims of the study preclude this strategy.* The publication of gender-specific analyses from such investigations must be prioritized, because such studies provide an invaluable opportunity to increase our understanding of gender similarities and differences across a broad range of research.

References

Alexander JL, Kotz K, Dennerstein L, et al: The effects of postmenopausal hormone therapies on female sexual functioning: a review of double-blind, randomized controlled trials. Menopause 11:749–765, 2004

American Psychiatric Association: Diagnostic and Statistical Manual of Mental Disorders, 4th Edition. Washington, DC, American Psychiatric Association, 1994

American Psychiatric Association: Diagnostic and Statistical Manual of Mental Disorders, 4th Edition, Text Revision. Washington, DC, American Psychiatric Association, 2000

Bates KA, Harvey AR, Carruthers M, et al: Androgens, andropause and neurodegeneration: exploring the link between steroidogenesis, androgens and Alzheimer's disease. Cell Mol Life Sci 62:281–292, 2005

Bayir H, Marion DW, Puccio AM, et al: Marked gender effect on lipid peroxidation after severe traumatic brain injury in adult patients. J Neurotrauma 21:1–8, 2004

Bloch M, Schmidt PJ, Danaceau M, et al: Effects of gonadal steroids in women with a history of postpartum depression. Am J Psychiatry 157:924–930, 2000

Brockington IF, Cernik AF, Schofield EM, et al: Puerperal psychosis, phenomena and diagnosis. Arch Gen Psychiatry 38:829–833, 1981

Carnahan RM, Perry PJ: Depression in aging men: the role of testosterone. Drugs and Aging 21:361–376, 2004

Dodic M, Moritz K, Wintour EM: Prenatal exposure to glucocorticoids and adult disease. Arch Physiol Biochem 111:61–69, 2003

Durston S, Hulshoff P, Hilleke E, et al: Anatomical MRI of the developing human brain: what have we learned? J Am Acad Child Adolesc Psychiatry 40:1012–1020, 2001

Elliott S: Report on the Satra Bruk workshop on classification of postnatal mental disorders. Arch Womens Mental Health 3:27–33, 2000

Epperson CN, Wisner KL, Yamamoto B: Gonadal steroids in the treatment of mood disorders. Psychosom Med 61:676–697, 1999

Evans RG, Stoddart GL: Producing health, consuming health care. Soc Sci Med 31:1347–1363, 1990

Golden RN, Gaynes BN, Ekstrom RD, et al: The efficacy of light therapy in the treatment of mood disorders: a review and meta-analysis of the evidence. Am J Psychiatry 162:656–662, 2005

Gregoire AJ, Kumar R, Everitt B, et al: Transdermal oestrogen for treatment of severe postnatal depression. Lancet 347:930–933, 1996

Hafner H: Gender differences in schizophrenia. Psychoneuroendocrinology 2:17–54, 2003

Hamilton JA: The identity of postpartum psychosis, in Motherhood and Mental Illness. Edited by Brockington IF, Kumar R. London, England, Academic Press, 1982, pp 1–17

Hansen D, Lou HC, Olsen J: Serious life events and congenital malformations: a national study with complete follow-up. Lancet 356:875–880, 2000

Hsu LK: Eating disorders: practical interventions. J Am Med Womens Assoc 59:113–124, 2004

Kuh D, Ben-Shlomo Y, Lynch J, et al: Life course epidemiology. J Epidemiol Community Health 57:778–783, 2003

Leibenluft E, Fiero PL, Rubinow DR: Effects of the menstrual cycle on dependent variables in mood disorder research. Arch Gen Psychiatry 51:761–781, 1994

Matza LS, Revicki DA, Davidson JR, et al: Depression with atypical features in the National Comorbidity Survey: classification, description, and consequences. Arch Gen Psychiatry 60:817–826, 2003

Misra DP, Guyer B, Allston A: Integrated perinatal health framework: a multiple determinants model with a life span approach. Am J Prev Med 25:65–75, 2003

Morrison MF, Kallan MJ, Ten Have T, et al: Lack of efficacy of estradiol for depression in postmenopausal women: a randomized, controlled trial. Biol Psychiatry 55:406–412, 2004

Munk-Olsen T, Laursen TM, Pedersen CB, et al: New parents and mental disorders: a population-based register study. JAMA 296:2582–2589, 2006

Rasgon NL, Altshuler LL, Fairbanks LA, et al: Estrogen replacement therapy in the treatment of major depressive disorder in perimenopausal women. J Clin Psychiatry 63:45–48, 2002

Seeman MV: Gender differences in the prescribing of antipsychotic drugs. Am J Psychiatry 161:1324–1333, 2004

Soares CN, Almeida OP, Joffe H, et al: Efficacy of estradiol for the treatment of depressive disorders in perimenopausal women: a double-blind, randomized, placebo-controlled trial. Arch Gen Psychiatry 58:529–534, 2001

Spinelli MG: The promise of saved lives: recognition, prevention, and rehabilitation, in Infanticide: Psychosocial and Legal Perspective on Mothers Who Kill. Edited by Spinelli MG. Washington, DC, American Psychiatric Publishing, 2003, pp 235–255

Susser E, Brown A, Matte T: Prenatal factors and adult mental and physical health. Can J Psychiatry 44:326–334, 1999

U.S. Department of Health and Human Services: Mental Health: A Report of the Surgeon General—Executive Summary. Rockville, MD, U.S. Department of Health and Human Services, Substance Abuse and Mental Health Services Administration, Center for Mental Health Services, National Institutes of Health, National Institute of Mental Health, 1999

Wadhwa PD, Sandman CA, Porto M, et al: The association between prenatal stress and infant birth weight and gestational age at birth: a prospective investigation. Am J Obstet Gynecol 169:858–865, 1993

Wadhwa PD, Porto M, Garite TJ, et al: Maternal corticotropin-releasing hormone levels in the early third trimester predict length of gestation in human pregnancy. Am J Obstet Gynecol 179:1079–1085, 1998

Wisner KL, Peindl KS, Hanusa BH: Symptomatology of affective and psychotic illnesses related to childbearing. J Affect Disord 30:77–87, 1994

Wisner KL, Perel JM, Peindl KS, et al: Prevention of recurrent postpartum depression: a randomized clinical trial. J Clin Psychiatry 62:82–86, 2001

Yonkers KA, Wisner KL, Stowe Z, et al: Management of bipolar disorder during pregnancy and the postpartum period. Am J Psychiatry 161:608–620, 2004

9

CLINICAL VALIDATORS OF DIAGNOSES

Symptom Expression, Course, and Treatment

Kimberly A. Yonkers, M.D.
William E. Narrow, M.D., M.P.H.
Katherine A. Halmi, M.D.

Although we assume that the phenomenology of a psychiatric disorder and its clinical course are parallel in men and women, this is not always the case. There is considerable face validity for potential sex differences in the expression of illnesses. Indeed, as discussed in previous chapters, sex differences in biological and societal factors can have a variety of influences on illness in various developmental periods and at different stages of illness. These differences interact with treatment and the delivery of services because variations in illness perception and the individual's sociocultural milieu may have effects on treatment seeking and response.

Although the literature exploring sex differences in psychiatric illness (both phenomenology and course), treatment seeking, and treatment response is nascent, findings can be broken down into two categories: 1) highly replicated and consistent results, and 2) investigations that either are not replicated or are mixed. Some sex differences in the phenomenology and course of psychiatric disorders are included in the diagnostic criteria and text descriptions of previous iterations of the DSM, whereas others are not. An exhaustive summary is beyond the scope of this chapter, but we highlight interesting research findings that are relevant to various disorders and summarize these findings by the strength of the data and the domain (phenomenology, course, treatment seeking, and treatment response). We also identify some areas that are in need of future research attention.

Phenomenology

Sex differences in the prevalence of selected psychiatric disorders are well documented and replicated (see Chapter 4, "Gender and the Prevalence of Psychiatric Disorders," this volume). Importantly, some illnesses are characterized by vast differences in prevalence but generally similar clinical symptom expression (e.g., agoraphobia, anorexia nervosa). Alternatively, other conditions occur approximately equally in men and women but differ in terms of the propensity for a man or woman to experience particular symptoms (e.g., bipolar disorder and schizophrenia).

Bipolar disorder is an example of an illness that has a similar prevalence in men and women but may be expressed differently in the two sexes (Arnold et al. 2000; Leibenluft 1996, 2000). Community studies find that women are more likely to experience the depressed pole of bipolar illness and less likely to have only manic episodes (Angst 1978; Kessler et al. 1997). Several studies show that women are at increased risk of expressing depressive symptoms in conjunction with manic symptoms (i.e., mixed mania; Bauer et al. 1994b), although discrepancies in such findings (Leibenluft 1996; McElroy et al. 1992) may relate to how mixed mania is operationalized (Arnold et al. 2000). For example, definitions of mixed mania that require a full major depressive syndrome in conjunction with mania have a more disproportionate sex ratio than definitions that stipulate the presence of only one or two symptoms of depression in conjunction with manic symptoms.

Schizophrenia, another disorder with approximately equal prevalence in men and women, may also be expressed somewhat differently in men and women, although there is some inconsistency among studies. A number of reports find that women with schizophrenia are more likely to have affective symptoms along with psychotic symptoms than are men (Goldstein and Tsuang 1990; Seeman and Lang 1990), although this finding has not been replicated in one cohort (Usall et al. 2001). In a similar vein, positive symptom expression may be more common among women with schizophrenia than among men with the disorder (Goldstein and Tsuang 1990) but again, data are not consistent (Usall et al. 2001, 2003). Variability in findings for schizophrenia may be a result of data collection methods. Because schizophrenia is relatively uncommon, with a prevalence of slightly less than 1%, our understanding of the presentation of the disorder is dependent upon clinical rather than community cohorts. The various clinical cohorts may differ depending on recruitment methods. Furthermore, substantial cohort sizes may be required to detect certain sex differences.

Major depressive disorder differs somewhat from previous examples in that the illness is more common in women than men. Possible sex differences in the expression of major depression are fairly controversial, and this is an area in need of greater research. Some community (Angst and Dobler-Mikola 1984; Angst et al. 2002b) and clinical studies (Frank et al. 1988; Perugi et al. 1990; Scheibe et al. 2003; Young et al. 1990) find that women are more likely to experience "atypical," or "reverse," neurovegetative symptoms (e.g., hypersomnia and weight gain), but not all studies find this (Kessler et al. 1993). Using data from the National Comorbidity Survey, one report noted a greater propensity for women to express "somatic" depression, which includes disturbances of sleep, appetite, and energy, whereas men and women are equally likely to experience major depression without these symptoms (Silverstein 1999). Other studies have also found that disturbances of sleep are more common in women (Frank et al. 1988; Kornstein et al. 2000a; Williams et al. 1995). A number of researchers have found an increased risk in women of anxious symptoms associated with depression (Frank et al. 1988; Kornstein et al. 2000a; Perugi et al. 1990; Scheibe et al. 2003; Silverstein 1999).

Several groups have noted that women with major depression endorse more symptoms associated with the disorder and that the disparity in illness rates for men and women increases when more symptoms are required by the disorder's definition (Angst and Dobler-Mikola 1984; Angst et al. 2002a; Kessler et al. 1993). This finding is less likely to be replicated in studies of clinical cohorts than community cohorts, possibly suggesting differences between individuals with depression in clinical settings and the community (Kornstein et al. 2000a; Scheibe et al. 2003). However, studies that recruit individuals who are not very ill may not be able to detect differences across a spectrum of severity, because a wide range of illness severity is needed to detect differences (Kornstein et al. 2000a; Scheibe et al. 2003). It is interesting that the gender disparity in illness rates for mixed mania also rises as the number of symptoms required for the illness increases. Thus there may be patterns to certain sex differences that are similar across diagnoses.

Finally, numerous studies have found a tendency for women with major depression to report greater illness severity and functional impairment. The sex difference in severity is more pronounced when self-report, rather than observer, measures are compared (Frank et al. 1988; Kornstein et al. 2000a; Perugi et al. 1990; Scheibe et al. 2003; Thase et al. 1994). This finding may reflect women's greater willingness to report problematic symptoms.

Despite large sex disparities in the rates of eating disorders, most studies have found the clinical profile of both anorexia nervosa and bulimia nervosa to be generally similar in males and females. However, several studies have found a tendency for the onset of eating disorders to occur later in men than in women (Carlat et al. 1997; Finkel et al. 1999). One study with an adequate sample size found a significant difference in age at onset, with a mean age at onset of 20.56 years for males compared with a mean age at onset of 17.15 years for females (Braun et al. 1999). The latter study also found that males were more likely to be involved in an occupation or sport in which weight control influences performance. In the same study, the prevalence of divorce was significantly higher in the parents of males with an eating disorder than those of females with an eating disorder. In this study, diet pills and laxatives were used more often by females than by males. Frequencies of comorbid mental disorders were identical. No other clinical characteristics differed between males and females. These findings suggest that societal factors (body appearance, childhood events) may increase risk similarly for men and women but that variations in men and women's exposure to these same factors (e.g., careers related to body appearance) may lead to differences in the prevalence of eating disorders.

Illness Course

An additional manner through which an illness is expressed is via the longitudinal course and long-term outcome of the condition. Understanding sex differences in the clinical course of illness is critical, because such knowledge may illustrate factors that allow us to predict which patients are more likely to experience remission and recover and which patients are more likely to stay ill. Course of illness has also long been considered an external validator of psychiatric disorders/diagnoses (Robins and Guze 1970)—that is, one of several variables that may help determine whether different syndromes constitute the same disorder or not. Again, when the framework described earlier is used, some disorders show well-defined differences in the longitudinal course of illness, whereas others show less consistent data for sex differences or no sex differences in illness course.

Bipolar illness is intriguing in that the risk of rapid cycling is higher in women than in men (Bauer et al. 1994a; Leibenluft 1996, 2000). Research in support of this finding is more consistent than, for example, the sex differences in risk of depression or mixed mania. Some authors have suggested that the risk of rapid cycling might be related to the increased likelihood of depression in bipolar women and their consequent greater exposure to antidepressants, which can trigger rapid cycling (Leibenluft 1996).

Sex differences in the course of illness and outcome of schizophrenia are well documented and show general agreement. Women tend to have a later onset of illness (Goldstein and Tsuang 1990; Szymanski et al. 1995; Usall et al. 2001, 2003) and a more benign course with better treatment response. It appears that the clinical course may worsen in women around menopause (Seeman 1983). Some authors have hypothesized that estrogen, through its effects on dopaminergic systems, blunts the severity of illness for some women but that the small amount of protection conferred is lost around menopause. This theory is largely based on women's superior response to typical antipsychotic agents that act as dopamine blockers and on findings that course worsens somewhat after menopause, although direct biological support for this theory does not exist.

Treatment Seeking

Consideration of the impact of treatment-seeking behavior is important when gender differences in illness course and symptom expression are being examined. Community surveys such as the Epidemiologic Catchment Area program (ECA) and the National Comorbidity Survey have shown that in any given year, fewer than half of adults with a mental or addictive disorder receive treatment of any kind for these disorders (Narrow et al. 2002). Given that service use is associated with factors such as severity (e.g., comorbidity) and functional impairment (Andrews et al. 2001; Bijl and Ravelli 2000; Wu et al. 1999), caution should be used when making nosologic conclusions strictly on the basis of findings from treated samples.

It is generally accepted that, overall, women with mental disorders seek mental health services at higher rates than men with mental disorders. Although the limited existing data support this statement, sex-specific rates of treatment seeking differ both by disorder and setting. In an analysis of ECA data for this chapter (see Table 9–1), females with mental or addictive disorders had higher rates of mental health service use than males in all sectors of the mental health service system. These differences were largely driven by substantial sex differences in service use among those with substance use disorders, in particular alcohol use disorders. When persons with substance use disorders (and no other mental disorder) were excluded from the analyses, rates of service use were more similar between men and women. There were still significant differences in use by sector: women were more likely to use general medical services, the human services sector (such as social service agencies and clergy), and support networks (such as support groups and social networks) for mental healthcare than were men. Strikingly, there was no difference in the use of specialty mental health services between men and women.

Several factors are thought to influence treatment seeking (Olfson et al. 1998), including clinical, demographic, attitudinal, cultural, social, and geographic factors. Many of these factors can interact with gender. Income differentials, different expressions of distress, and different manifestations of the "sick role" all may play a role in observed female/male differences in the decision to seek treatment. As noted earlier, women may be less likely to minimize the impact of their illness in terms of its severity and the effect it has on their lives. Hence, they may be more likely to seek treatment and to be offered treatment after visiting a physician. Personality factors also play a role in treatment seeking. Recent work by Goodwin et al. (2002) has shown that conscientiousness and extraversion are associated with treatment seeking in females but not in males.

Treatment Response

Response to pharmacological treatment for some conditions may differ between men and women. However, this is largely an understudied area and one that relies

TABLE 9–1. Use of services for mental and addictive problems by disorder and sex, Epidemiologic Catchment Area Program

	Percentage with disorder using services (mean [SD])									
	Any anxiety disorder		Any phobia		Social phobia		Simple phobia		Agoraphobia	
Sector	Male	Female	Male	Female	Male	Female	Male	Female	Male	Female
Specialty MH	16.2 (2.0)	14.5 (1.1)	14.4 (2.2)	14.0 (1.2)	30.4 (6.9)	31.1 (4.2)	12.9 (2.6)	14.3 (1.4)	23.8 (4.3)	19.2 (1.8)
General medical[a]	12.2 (1.7)	16.0 (1.1)	12.1 (1.9)	16.1 (1.1)	17.1 (5.2)	26.2 (4.4)	11.2 (2.1)[b]	17.2 (1.4)	17.6 (3.6)	21.7 (2.0)
Health systems[c]	23.9 (2.2)	26.7 (1.4)	22.6 (2.6)	26.1 (1.4)	43.5 (7.2)	49.0 (4.6)	20.5 (2.9)	27.0 (1.7)	35.4 (4.5)	35.0 (2.3)
Human services	4.5 (0.9)[d]	7.7 (0.9)	3.8 (0.8)[d]	7.2 (0.9)	5.2 (2.3)[b]	14.4 (3.4)	3.3 (1.0)[d]	7.8 (1.0)	6.5 (1.9)	9.8 (1.6)
Voluntary support networks	9.3 (1.4)	9.4 (1.0)	8.1 (1.4)	9.2 (1.1)	26.7 (6.1)	15.3 (3.4)	6.2 (1.4)	9.0 (1.2)	9.7 (2.8)	10.1 (1.5)
Any care	29.5 (2.3)	34.2 (1.4)	27.0 (2.6)[b]	33.0 (1.5)	52.0 (7.0)	56.6 (4.3)	24.4 (3.0)[d]	34.4 (1.7)	39.9 (4.6)	42.3 (2.3)

	Panic		Obsessive-compulsive		Any mood disorder		Major depressive episode		Unipolar major depressive disorder	
Sector	Male	Female	Male	Female	Male	Female	Male	Female	Male	Female
Specialty MH	38.6 (8.4)	31.6 (4.1)	26.4 (5.0)	24.7 (3.5)	26.0 (2.8)	22.3 (1.6)	30.7 (3.6)	28.9 (2.3)	30.5 (3.8)	27.5 (2.6)
General medical[a]	24.9 (8.1)	31.7 (4.3)	18.4 (4.5)	18.3 (3.1)	18.4 (2.4)	23.7 (1.7)	20.1 (2.8)[d]	29.9 (2.3)	19.2 (3.1)[b]	27.1 (2.5)
Health systems[c]	54.9 (8.5)	50.6 (4.6)	36.6 (5.4)	36.3 (3.9)	35.8 (3.2)	39.3 (2.0)	42.4 (3.8)	49.6 (2.6)	40.5 (4.1)	46.5 (2.9)
Human services	9.7 (3.7)	13.9 (3.2)	7.5 (2.5)	12.1 (2.8)	7.4 (1.6)	10.4 (1.2)	9.2 (2.2)	12.1 (1.7)	10.3 (2.7)	12.4 (1.9)
Voluntary support networks	10.2 (4.9)	14.3 (2.7)	14.2 (3.9)	8.6 (1.9)	12.3 (1.8)	13.2 (1.4)	13.2 (2.1)	17.5 (2.0)	15.4 (2.5)	17.8 (2.2)
Any care	59.9 (9.2)	58.3 (4.6)	46.8 (5.6)	44.0 (4.0)	42.4 (3.0)	47.9 (1.9)	47.8 (3.7)[d]	59.3 (2.5)	46.5 (3.9)[b]	56.9 (2.8)

TABLE 9–1. Use of services for mental and addictive problems by disorder and sex, Epidemiologic Catchment Area Program *(continued)*

	Dysthymia		Bipolar I		Bipolar II		Schizophrenia		Antisocial PD	
Sector	Male	Female	Male	Female	Male	Female	Male	Female	Male	Female
Specialty MH	22.3 (3.4)	18.1 (1.8)	38.2(10.6)	30.0 (6.6)	23.8 (9.8)	45.1 (8.5)	42.5 (7.8)	49.5 (5.4)	19.4 (3.9)	28.3 (8.3)
General medical[a]	16.1 (2.9)[b]	23.6 (2.2)	31.9 (9.6)	39.5 (7.8)	17.3 (9.5)[b]	42.9 (8.5)	17.3 (6.7)[b]	37.6 (5.6)	9.4 (2.9)	29.6(10.4)
Health systems[c]	31.2 (4.1)	36.5 (2.4)	56.7 (9.7)	56.7 (7.7)	35.1(12.1)[b]	68.2 (7.5)	52.1 (7.7)	66.3 (4.6)	21.5 (4.0)[d]	52.5(10.0)
Human services	6.2 (1.6)	9.2 (1.4)	5.3 (3.7)[b]	18.3 (5.2)	0.9 (0.7)	8.8 (4.1)	14.3 (5.5)	13.2 (3.6)	9.3 (3.3)	5.3 (3.9)
Voluntary support networks	11.6 (2.3)	8.8 (1.3)	0.2 (0.2)[d]	15.1 (4.8)	8.6 (6.5)	11.7 (5.0)	6.6 (3.1)	7.4 (2.5)	10.5 (4.1)	23.8(10.0)
Any care	38.7 (3.7)	43.7 (2.4)	57.0 (9.7)	69.3 (7.0)	42.2(13.0)	71.3 (7.3)	58.6 (7.4)	69.0 (4.6)	31.2 (4.9)[b]	58.7 (9.7)

	Anorexia nervosa		Somatization		Severe cognitive impairment		Any mental disorder (excluding SUDs)		Any SUD	
Sector	Male	Female	Male	Female	Male	Female	Male	Female	Male	Female
Specialty MH	19.7 (18.3)	39.5 (18.4)	33.7 (18.0)	45.2 (9.0)	8.8 (2.2)	5.9 (1.2)	15.8 (1.4)	14.3 (0.9)	10.1 (1.3)[d]	18.6 (2.4)
General medical[a]	16.4 (15.8)	43.1 (22.8)	19.3 (10.6)[b]	54.5 (8.5)	6.4 (1.7)	7.8 (1.3)	11.6 (1.2)[d]	16.2 (0.8)	7.8 (1.3)[e]	17.4 (2.2)
Health systems[c]	36.1 (22.7)	51.1 (19.9)	45.0 (17.4)	68.0 (7.1)	14.0 (2.3)	12.2 (1.7)	22.9 (1.7)[b]	26.6 (1.1)	15.0 (1.7)[f]	29.8 (2.8)
Human services	0.0 (0.0)	11.8 (11.6)	5.1 (3.7)	16.8 (7.0)	2.6 (1.1)	3.2 (0.9)	5.3 (0.8)[b]	7.7 (0.7)	3.6 (0.7)[b]	7.3 (1.5)
Voluntary support networks	19.7 (18.3)	8.0 (6.1)	23.7 (18.4)	15.3 (6.1)	4.1 (1.6)	4.3 (1.4)	8.8 (1.0)	10.0 (0.8)	5.5 (0.8)[f]	18.6 (2.7)
Any care	36.1 (22.7)	51.1 (19.9)	50.1 (17.5)	74.6 (6.2)	18.0 (2.5)	16.5 (2.2)	28.7 (1.6)[d]	34.3 (1.1)	19.3 (1.8)[f]	41.6 (3.2)

TABLE 9–1. Use of services for mental and addictive problems by disorder and sex, Epidemiologic Catchment Area Program *(continued)*

	Alcohol use disorders		Other drug use disorders		Any disorder	
Sector	Male	Female	Male	Female	Male	Female
Specialty MH	9.5 (1.4)[e]	21.7 (3.2)	15.4 (2.4)	15.2 (3.2)	11.7 (1.0)[b]	14.2 (0.8)
General medical[a]	7.3 (1.2)[e]	21.1 (3.1)	10.1 (3.2)	15.2 (3.7)	9.4 (1.0)[f]	15.7 (0.8)
Health systems[c]	14.0 (1.7)[f]	34.4 (3.8)	21.4 (3.5)	25.6 (4.3)	17.7 (1.2)[f]	26.2 (1.0)
Human services	2.8 (0.7)[d]	8.5 (1.9)	6.4 (1.7)	5.2 (1.8)	4.1 (0.6)[e]	7.5 (0.7)
Voluntary support networks	5.1 (0.9)[f]	21.3 (3.5)	6.9 (1.5)	13.6 (3.0)	7.1 (0.8)[d]	10.5 (0.8)
Any care	17.5 (1.7)[f]	46.0 (4.2)	27.5 (3.6)	37.7 (4.7)	22.8 (1.2)[f]	34.1 (1.1)

Note. MH = mental health; PD = personality disorder; SUD = substance use disorder.

[a]"General medical" refers to use of general medical services (e.g., primary care providers and emergency rooms) for mental or addiction problems.

[b]Male/female comparisons: $P<0.05$.

[c]"Health systems" refers to any use of specialty mental health or general medical services for mental or addiction problems.

[d]Male/female comparisons: $P<0.01$.

[e]Male/female comparisons: $P<0.001$.

[f]Male/female comparisons: $P<0.0001$.

on secondary analyses of datasets from studies not designed to directly address the question. Such analyses may not have adequate statistical power to detect gender differences. Most frequently studied with regard to sex differences in treatment response are the unipolar mood disorders. However, even for these conditions, data are limited and somewhat conflicting. Among the findings that are more consistent are studies showing that men and older women have a better response to imipramine than do younger women (Kornstein et al. 2000b; Raskin 1974). Also fairly consistent are comparisons of treatment response for monoamine oxidase inhibitors, which appear to be somewhat more efficacious in females regardless of the presence of atypical symptoms (Quitkin et al. 2002; Raskin 1974), Some studies (Bakish et al. 1993; Hellerstein et al. 1993; Kornstein et al. 2000b; Steiner et al. 1993) but not all (Hildebrandt et al. 2003; Lewis-Hall et al. 1997; Quitkin et al. 2002; Scheibe et al. 2003) have found that depressed women have a better response to serotonin reuptake inhibitors, although findings have varied somewhat for different agents. For example, data for sertraline consistently show higher response rates in women (Kornstein et al. 2000b), whereas no consistent differences have been found for fluoxetine (Lewis-Hall et al. 1997; Quitkin et al. 2002).

There are very few studies with adequate methodology to assess gender differences in response to psychotherapy. In one study comparing the responses of 40 men and 44 women treated with cognitive-behavioral therapy for the diagnosis of depression, interpretation of the results was complicated by the fact that the men attended significantly fewer therapy sessions than did the women. In spite of this, the men and women had comparable responses, with those patients with higher pretreatment levels of depression responding less well (Thase et al. 1994). Another study comparing the outcome of men and women who received analytical group psychotherapy found the proportion of dysphoric content (i.e., depressive content) in the narratives (transcripts of the group sessions) increased for men but not for women. Changes in narratives were not related to self-reported symptoms of depression (Staats et al. 1998). The social context and political consequences of various gender-related clinical responses have been described but not systematically studied (Knudson-Martin 1997). Likewise, conceptual issues of gender-specific response to psychotherapy have been discussed but not systematically studied (Frank et al. 1999).

Proposed Research Agenda

1. There are intriguing findings in the literature that show sex differences in the prevalence and phenomenology of a number of psychiatric illnesses. However, the overarching theme largely missing in the literature is the utility of studies that are specifically designed to explore sex differences in all of these clinically important domains of psychiatric illness, including phenomenology, illness course, and treatment response. Because the phenomenology of disorders is currently the

primary basis of the diagnostic criteria in DSM, this domain is of particular relevance to DSM-V, and while it is likely that our future diagnostic system will increasingly be based on etiopathology, phenomenology will remain of fundamental importance. In addition, domains such as illness course are highlighted in the text descriptions of DSM and may also be incorporated into the diagnostic criteria themselves. Furthermore, examining gender in relationship to illness course may shed light on the extent to which disorders are fundamentally the same or different in women and men. Thus, research that elucidates gender similarities and differences in etiopathology, phenomenology, and illness course is greatly needed to inform future editions of DSM.

2. The vast majority of research regarding sex differences in phenomenology in treatment response has relied on secondary analyses of databases that have been designed to address other issues. This approach has limitations, and studies are needed that are specifically designed—and have adequate statistical power—to examine sex/gender differences in numerous clinical domains.
3. It is not possible to develop a comprehensive picture of sex/gender differences in the expression of a psychiatric illness when the symptoms probed are limited to those that are listed in the current diagnostic criteria. Theoretical models need to inform and generate potential alternative diagnostic criteria that may reflect valid and meaningful sex differences in the phenomenology of psychiatric disorders.
4. Information on gender-related aspects of treatment seeking is very limited. Areas of research that are needed include basic information on rates of treatment seeking by patient sex and diagnosis and research on the causes of underlying sex differences that may be a window to understanding some of the cultural, societal, and system differences in treatment seeking. Research is also needed to better understand how treatment seeking may influence clinical information that is presented in DSM and reflected in its diagnostic criteria. It is important that diagnostic criteria are valid for illness presentations not only in clinical settings but also in community settings.
5. In exploring sex differences in the course of psychiatric illness, prospective cohort studies need adequate power to fully evaluate differences. Such analyses may require an exploration of the interaction of predictor variables by subject gender. Only when medicine moves to the explicit exploration of sex differences can we make the leap to understanding what sex differences exist and which are clinically meaningful.

References

Andrews G, Issakidis C, Carter G: Shortfall in mental health service utilization. Br J Psychiatry Suppl 179:417–425, 2001

Angst J: The course of affective disorders, II: typology of bipolar manic-depressive illness. Archives of Psychiatry and Neurological Sciences 226:65–73, 1978

Angst J, Dobler-Mikola A: Do the diagnostic criteria determine the sex ratio in depression. J Affect Disord 7:189–198, 1984

Angst J, Gamma A, Gastpar M, et al: Gender differences in depression. Eur Arch Psychiatry Clin Neurosci 252:201–209, 2002a

Angst J, Gamma A, Sellaro R, et al: Toward validation of atypical depression in the community: results of the Zurich cohort study. J Affect Disord 72:125–138, 2002b

Arnold L, McElroy S, Keck P: The role of gender in mixed mania. Compr Psychiatry 41:83–87, 2000

Bakish D, Lapierre YD, Weinstein R, et al: Ritanserin, imipramine, and placebo in the treatment of dysthymic disorder. J Clin Psychopharmacol 13:409–414, 1993

Bauer MS, Calabrese J, Dunner DL, et al: Multisite data reanalysis of the validity of rapid cycling as a course modifier for bipolar disorder in DSM-IV. Am J Psychiatry 151:506–515, 1994a

Bauer MS, Whybrow PC, Gyulai L, et al: Testing definitions of dysphoric mania and hypomania: prevalence, clinical characteristics and inter-episode stability. J Affect Disord 32:201–211, 1994b

Bijl RV, Ravelli A: Current and residual functional disability associated with psychopathology: findings from the Netherlands Mental Health Survey and Incidence Study (NEMESIS). Psychol Med 30:657–668, 2000

Braun D, Sunday S, Huang A, et al: More males seek treatment for eating disorders. Int J Eat Disord 25:415–424, 1999

Carlat D, Camargo C, Hertzog D: Eating disorders: a report of 135 patients. Am J Psychiatry 154:1127–1132, 1997

Finkel S, Richter E, Clary C, et al: Comparative efficacy of sertraline vs. fluoxetine in patients age 70 or over with major depression. Am J Geriatr Psychiatry 7:221–227, 1999

Frank E, Carpenter LL, Kupfer DJ: Sex differences in recurrent depression: are there any that are significant? Am J Psychiatry 145:41–45, 1988

Frank E, Thase M, Spanier C, et al: Gender-specific response to depression treatment. J Gend Specif Med 2:40–44, 1999

Goldstein JM, Tsuang MT: Gender and schizophrenia: an introduction and synthesis of findings. Schizophr Bull 16:179–183, 1990

Goodwin RD, Hoven CW, Lyons JS, et al: Mental health service utilization in the United States: the role of personality factors. Soc Psychiatry Psychiatr Epidemiol 37:561–562, 2002

Hellerstein DJ, Yanowitch P, Rosenthal J, et al: A randomized double-blind study of fluoxetine versus placebo in the treatment of dysthymia. Am J Psychiatry 150:1169–1175, 1993

Hildebrandt MG, Steyerberg EW, Stage KB, et al: Are gender differences important for the clinical effects of antidepressants. Am J Psychiatry 160:1643–1650, 2003

Kessler RC, McGonagle KA, Swartz M, et al: Sex and depression in the National Comorbidity Survey I: lifetime prevalence, chronicity and recurrence. J Affect Disord 29:85–96, 1993

Kessler R, Rubinow D, Holmes C, et al: The epidemiology of DSM-III-R bipolar I disorder in a general population survey. Psychol Med 27:1079–1089, 1997

Knudson-Martin C: The politics of gender in family therapy. J Marital Fam Ther 23:421–437, 1997
Kornstein S, Schatzberg A, Thase M, et al: Gender differences in chronic major and double depression. J Affect Disord 60:1–11, 2000a
Kornstein S, Schatzberg A, Thase M, et al: Gender differences in treatment response to sertraline versus imipramine in chronic depression. Am J Psychiatry 157:1445–1452, 2000b
Leibenluft E: Women with bipolar illness: clinical and research issues. Am J Psychiatry 153:163–173, 1996
Leibenluft E: Women and bipolar disorder: an update. Bull Menninger Clin 64:5–13, 2000
Lewis-Hall FC, Wilson MG, Tepner RG, et al: Fluoxetine vs tricyclic antidepressants in women with major depressive disorder. J Womens Health 6:337–343, 1997
McElroy SL, Keck PE, Pope HG, et al: Clinical and research implications of the diagnosis of dysphoric or mixed mania or hypomania. Am J Psychiatry 149:1633–1644, 1992
Narrow WE, Rae DS, Robins LN, et al: Revised prevalence estimates of mental disorders in the United States: using a clinical significance criterion to reconcile 2 surveys' estimates. Arch Gen Psychiatry 59:115–123, 2002
Olfson M, Kessler RC, Berglund PA, et al: Psychiatric disorder onset and first treatment contact in the U.S. and Ontario. Am J Psychiatry 155:1415–1422, 1998
Perugi G, Musetti L, Simonini E, et al: Gender-mediated clinical features of depressive illness. the importance of temperamental differences. Br J Psychiatry 157:835–841, 1990
Quitkin F, Stewart J, McGrath P, et al: Are there differences in women's and men's antidepressant response? Am J Psychiatry 159:1848–1854, 2002
Raskin A: Age-sex differences in response to antidepressant drugs. J Nerv Ment Dis 159:120–130, 1974
Robins E, Guze SB: Establishment of diagnostic validity in psychiatric illness: its application to schizophrenia. Am J Psychiatry 126:983–987, 1970
Scheibe S, Preuschhof C, Cristi C, et al: Are there gender differences in major depression and its response to antidepressants? J Affect Disord 75:223–235, 2003
Seeman MV: Interaction of sex, age, and neuroleptic dose. Compr Psychiatry 24:125–128, 1983
Seeman MV, Lang M: The role of estrogens in schizophrenia gender differences. Schizophr Bull 16:185–194, 1990
Silverstein B: Gender difference in the prevalence of clinical depression: the role played by depression associated with somatic symptoms. Am J Psychiatry 156:480–482, 1999
Staats H, May M, Herrmann C, et al: Different patterns of change in narratives of men and women during analytical group psychotherapy. Int J Group Psychother 48:363–380, 1998
Steiner M, Wheadon DE, Kreider MS, et al: Antidepressant response to paroxetine by gender, in 1993 Annual Meeting Syllabus and Proceedings Summary. Washington, DC, American Psychiatric Association, 1993, p 176
Szymanski S, Lieberman J, Alvir J, et al: Gender differences in onset of illness, treatment response, course and biologic indexes in first-episode schizophrenic patients. Am J Psychiatry 152:698–703, 1995
Thase ME, Reynolds CF, Frank E, et al: Do depressed men and women respond similarly to cognitive behavior therapy? Am J Psychiatry 151:500–505, 1994

Usall J, Araya S, Ochoa S, et al: Gender differences in a sample of schizophrenic outpatients. Compr Psychiatry 42:301–305, 2001

Usall J, Ochoa S, Araya S, et al: Gender differences and outcome in schizophrenia: a 2-year follow-up study in a large community sample. Eur Psychiatry 18:282–284, 2003

Williams JBW, Spitzer RL, Linzer M, et al: Gender differences in depression in primary care. Am J Obstet Gynecol 173:654–659, 1995

Wu L, Kouzis AC, Leaf PJ: Influence of comorbid alcohol and psychiatric disorders on utilization of mental health services in the National Comorbidity Survey. Am J Psychiatry 156:1230–1236, 1999

Young MA, Scheftner WA, Fawcett J, et al: Gender differences in the clinical features of unipolar major depressive disorder. J Nerv Ment Dis 178:200–203, 1990

10

GENDER AND DIAGNOSTIC CRITERIA

Thomas A. Widiger, Ph.D.
Michael B. First, M.D.

This chapter pertains directly to the heart of DSM: the diagnostic criteria themselves. A difficult issue that will need to be grappled with during the development of DSM-V is how much of an impact gender should have on the diagnosis of mental disorders. There are a number of options that range from virtually no impact to having separate diagnostic criteria for males and females. All of the options discussed here are included in DSM-IV-TR to varying degrees. Each is described briefly in turn, along with their potential advantages and disadvantages. An important agenda item during the development of DSM-V will be to more systematically consider which options are supported by the available data on gender differences and determining to which disorders these options should be applied.

Gender-Neutral Diagnostic Criteria

Gender-neutral diagnostic criteria use the same diagnostic criteria for both males and females, with the assumption that the diagnostic criteria are equally valid for both sexes. This option is used for all but a few of the diagnostic criteria sets in DSM-IV-TR (American Psychiatric Association 2000). An advantage of this approach is that differential sex prevalence rates are readily inferred from the valid application of these criteria sets within probability-based community samples, assuming that the criteria set applies equally well to, or is equally valid for, both males and females. Sex differences in the etiology, pathology, and course of a disorder are likewise readily inferred from the valid application of the criteria sets within unbiased samples of the population. Gender-biased diagnoses (e.g., the misapplication of the diagnosis to one sex more often than other) could be attributed to errors in the application of the criterion sets, biases in the instruments used in the assessment, or the impact of gender on symptom reporting, treatment seeking, or participant sampling, rather than reflecting gender biases in the diagnostic criteria themselves (Widiger and Spitzer 1991).

A difficulty with this option that arises for a number of disorders in DSM is that it is unclear how to develop gender-neutral diagnostic criteria that do in fact apply equally well to, or are equally valid for, males and females (Wakefield 1987; Widiger 1998). Consider, for example, somatization disorder. The DSM-III (American Psychiatric Association 1980) diagnostic criteria for somatization disorder included 37 somatic complaints organized into seven categories (e.g., gastrointestinal, pain, and so on), one of which was confined to "female reproductive symptoms" (p. 243), including painful menstruation, menstrual irregularity, excessive bleeding, and severe vomiting during pregnancy. These criteria could not be considered to be gender neutral, because they could be used only to diagnose somatization disorder in females. They certainly do not apply equally well to males, nor are they valid for diagnosing this disorder in males. Somatization disorder was said in DSM-III to be "rarely diagnosed in males" (p. 242), but this differential sex prevalence rate could be due in part to the absence of gender-neutral diagnostic criteria. Female-specific symptoms are still included as examples of symptoms in the diagnostic criteria for somatization disorder in DSM-IV (e.g., irregular menses, excessive menstrual bleeding, and vomiting throughout pregnancy; American Psychiatric Association 1994), but they are counterbalanced by male-specific examples (e.g., erectile or ejaculatory dysfunction) under the requirement for "one sexual symptom." It is still unclear, however, whether the addition of two examples of symptoms that are specific to males completely offsets, or compensates for, the three listed examples that are specific to women.

A somewhat less obvious example of a potentially gender-related diagnostic criterion is provided by conduct disorder. One of its diagnostic criteria is forcing someone into sexual activity (American Psychiatric Association 2000). Forcing someone into sexual activity is a behavior that is more likely to be done by males irrespective of its relationship to conduct disorder, and its inclusion as a diagnostic criterion for conduct disorder might then be contributing to an inaccurately higher prevalence of conduct disorder in males relative to females (Zoccolillo 1993; Zoccolillo and Rogers 1991). Robins (1986, 1991), one of the original authors of this criteria set for DSM-III, has suggested that changes made to the DSM-III-R (American Psychiatric Association 1987) criteria set for conduct disorder provided a major shift in the diagnosis of the disorder by replacing many nonaggressive acts (e.g., trouble in school, early sexual activity, and early substance use) with quite severe aggressive behaviors (e.g., cruelty to animals, physical cruelty to people, and sexual assault or rape) that are more likely to be male-related. This change was perhaps due in part to the fact that the research supporting these changes focused on data sets that primarily included males.

Similar concerns have been raised with respect to the diagnostic criteria for dependent personality disorder. Kaplan (1983) argued in her widely cited paper on sex biases in DSM-III that "DSM-III singles out for scrutiny and therefore diagnosis the ways in which women express dependency but not the ways in which men express dependency" (p. 789). Walker (1994) suggested that "men who rely on others to maintain their homes and take care of their children are...expressing personality-disordered dependency behaviors" (p. 25). Frances et al. (1995) stated similarly that "clinicians should be aware of a possible sex bias in their diagnoses [of dependent personality disorder]...so as not to miss stereotypically masculine forms of dependency expressed through domineering behavior, ordering others to help rather than demanding or pleading" (p. 377). Bornstein (1996, 1997) argued further that there might be as many males with dependent personality disorder as females, but the emphasis upon overt, explicit expressions of a need for others when making the diagnosis contributed to a failure to recognize and diagnose the disorder in males.

It might be difficult to develop gender-neutral diagnostic criteria for somatization disorder, conduct disorder, and dependent personality disorder if the gender-related symptoms are highly useful or important for its diagnosis, or if these disorders are themselves closely related to neurobiologically or socioculturally based gender differences that the diagnostic criteria accurately reflect (Widiger 1998; Zahn-Waxler 1993). For example, if irregular menses, excessive menstrual bleeding, and vomiting throughout pregnancy are clinically important and valid symptoms of somatization disorder in women, it could be problematic to remove them for the sake of "gender neutrality." There might in fact be few disorders that do not have a neurobiological or sociocultural relationship with gender that in some way meaningfully affects the disorder's symptoms or other clinical features (Hartung and Widiger 1998). If this is the case, then the provision of gender-neutral diagnostic criteria might be an unrealistic and undesirable goal. It might be preferable to have a single set of diagnostic criteria but accept that they may not in fact be gender neutral for disorders whose etiology or pathology are themselves gender related.

Gender Differences in Clinical Features or Symptoms Noted in the Text

One approach to acknowledging the impact of gender on the presentation of a disorder is to describe the variation across gender in the text discussion of the disorder rather than in the diagnostic criteria themselves. For example, the "Specific Culture, Age, and Gender Features" section of the DSM-IV-TR text notes that males with conduct disorder "frequently exhibit fighting, stealing, vandalism, and school discipline problems [whereas] females...are more likely to exhibit lying, truancy, running away, substance use, and prostitution" (p. 97). The text also notes that "women with schizophrenia tend to express more affective symptomatology, paranoid delusions, and hallucinations, whereas men tend to express more negative symptoms" (pp. 307–308). For histrionic personality disorder, the text states that "a man with this disorder may dress and behave in a manner often identified as 'macho' and may seek to be the center of attention by bragging about athletic skills, whereas a woman, for example, may choose very feminine clothes and talk about how much she impressed her dance instructor" (p. 712).

Information on how a disorder's presentation varies among men and women is descriptively informative, but a limitation of this approach is that it is unclear whether or how clinicians should use this information. One of the purposes of the DSM text is to facilitate the diagnosis of a respective disorder (American Psychiatric Association 2000; Frances et al. 1995), but it is not clear whether this information should have an impact on the application of the diagnostic criteria. For example, the features noted to be particularly typical of conduct disorder in males are included explicitly within the diagnostic criteria set (i.e., fighting, stealing, vandalism, and school discipline problems), whereas some of the features noted to be typical of the disorder in females are not included in the criteria set (e.g., prostitution) or are included only as an associated feature (e.g., substance use). Indicating in the text that prostitution and substance use are features that are common in or specific to females with the disorder might imply to some DSM users that these features should be used as diagnostic indicators for the presence of the disorder in females, particularly when the features noted to be common or specific to males are included in the diagnostic criteria. However, there is no indication or suggestion as to whether or how prostitution or substance use can be used as diagnostic criteria for conduct disorder in females. Most readers would probably understand the text information as being simply descriptive rather than diagnostic and would consider the diagnosis to be based primarily, if not solely, on the criteria set. However, in the case of conduct disorder, this would mean using diagnostic criteria for females that are said to be typical or specific to males with the disorder (e.g., forcing someone into a sexual activity) rather than features that are said to be more common in females.

Gender-Related Modifiers or Specifiers

The impact of gender-related variables on the presentation of a disorder can be so substantial that in some instances gender-related specifiers could be developed for males or females. For example, DSM-IV included for the first time a postpartum-onset specifier for major depressive disorder and bipolar disorder. The same diagnostic criteria are used for males and females, but a postpartum onset is provided only for women. In this instance, it was concluded that "the symptoms of the postpartum-onset...do not differ from the symptoms in nonpostpartum mood episodes" (American Psychiatric Association 2000, p. 422); therefore, separate diagnostic criteria or a separate diagnostic entity were not considered to be necessary (Purnine and Frank 1996). However, as noted elsewhere in this volume and in DSM-IV-TR, some symptoms (e.g., fluctuations in mood, mood lability, and preoccupation with infant well-being) might be more common with a postpartum onset than a nonpostpartum onset and, therefore, might warrant separate diagnostic criteria in the future.

Gender-Specific Thresholds for Diagnosis

A common procedure used in laboratory and psychological testing is to provide different cutoff points for gender, ethnic, cultural, and other demographic features. A rationale for doing so is to avoid or at least minimize the occurrence of possible gender biases within the instrument of assessment. If the indicators of the respective disorder are not considered to perform equally well for males and females, then the threshold for a diagnosis can be adjusted accordingly (Robins and Price 1991; Rutherford et al. 1995).

This procedure was used in DSM-III for the diagnosis of somatization disorder. Because it was recognized that the criteria set included symptoms that would be characteristic only of females (e.g., painful menstruation), the number of symptoms required for a diagnosis of somatization disorder was lower in males than in females (i.e., 12 of the 37 diagnostic criteria were required for males, compared with 14 for females). However, one difficulty with this approach is determining, in the absence of an unbiased gold standard, how much adjustment should be made to the diagnostic threshold to offset a possible gender bias in the criteria set. Cloninger et al. (1986) indicated, subsequent to the publication of DSM-III, that the diagnostic threshold would have to have been lowered to approximately 8 of 37 diagnostic criteria to result in an equal prevalence for males and females with DSM-III somatization disorder. However, it is unclear whether having a criteria set that results in an equal prevalence for males and females is valid for a disorder that perhaps does actually occur more often in females than in males (Widiger and Spitzer 1991). On the other hand, it is possible that the presence of female-only symptoms in the diagnostic criteria set for somatization disorder has itself lowered the threshold for the diagnosis in females because it provides females with ways in which they can meet the criteria that are not provided to males.

Gender-Specific Diagnostic Criteria

If adequate gender-neutral diagnostic criteria cannot be developed, or if it is apparent that gender-related diagnostic criteria perform better for a particular sex, then perhaps gender-specific diagnostic criteria should be used. DSM-IV-TR currently includes gender-specific diagnostic criteria for gender identity disorder because it was concluded that the optimal diagnostic indicators for the disorder are specific to each gender (e.g., in boys, aversion toward rough-and-tumble play and, in girls, marked aversion toward normative feminine clothing)—or at least that it was not possible to use the same diagnostic criteria for both males and females.

The inclusion of separate diagnostic criteria for males and females is analogous to the inclusion of separate diagnostic criteria for children and adults. Different diagnostic criteria are used for children and adults for the diagnosis of posttraumatic stress disorder, obsessive-compulsive disorder, major depressive disorder, gender identity disorder, social and specific phobia, and generalized anxiety disorder, because it is believed in each case that the disorder is largely the same across ages but that different diagnostic criteria are optimal for identifying the presence of the disorder across ages. A comparable rationale could guide the decision to develop different diagnostic criteria for males and females.

Zoccolillo (1993) recommended the development of separate diagnostic criteria for conduct disorder in girls to recognize that the disorder is expressed differently in boys and girls. His proposal places relatively more emphasis for the diagnosis in girls on rule violations at home and school, substance abuse, prostitution, chronic lying, running away, and poor school performance, and less emphasis on vandalism, fire setting, forcing someone to have sexual activity, burglary, use of a weapon, and stealing with confrontation of a victim. This option would essentially move the gender-related features described in the text into the diagnostic criteria sets so they would have an explicit impact on the diagnosis.

Zahn-Waxler (1993), however, argued that having different criteria for boys and girls would be problematic. The disorder may indeed be expressed differently in boys and girls, but alternative criteria sets might fail to provide the same threshold for the diagnosis in boys and girls (i.e., the risk of false positives might be different in the two sexes). Alternative criteria sets may instead define different disorders in boys and girls in terms of severity and level of behavioral dysfunction. For example, changing the criteria set for girls by placing less emphasis on confrontational, violent, and aggressive behavior in favor of more emphasis on nonaggressive behavior such as rule violations and deceitfulness could have the undesirable effect of labeling behavior that might be considered acceptable or normative in boys (e.g., aggressiveness) as mentally disordered, and potentially stigmatizing, in girls. Thus, boys would have to exhibit more severely dysfunctional behaviors than girls to receive the diagnosis of conduct disorder. Defining the disorder differently for boys and girls (i.e., providing criteria for girls that are inherently less severe than the criteria required for boys) could perhaps be even more problematically gender-biased than using a single diagnostic criteria set that is less applicable to girls.

Zahn-Waxler (1993) argued further that conduct disorder by its very nature involves aggressive, confrontational, and violent behavior, and that girls receive the diagnosis less often because they are less likely to engage in these behaviors. The behaviors are relatively more specific to boys because the sociocultural and neurobiological causes of these behaviors are themselves gender-related. Altering the criteria to include behaviors that are more evident in girls would be altering what is considered fundamental to the disorder's etiology and pathology. It may indeed be the case that girls who fall below the threshold for conduct disorder should receive a diagnosis of a mental disorder, but it would be a different disorder (e.g., oppositional defiant disorder) or at least a less severe disorder, that might also still occur more frequently in boys.

Phillips and Gunderson (1994) made a similar argument with respect to the diagnosis of dependent personality disorder. They suggested that dependent personality disorder has a differential sex prevalence rate because it is related to different sociocultural expectations and pressures that contribute to the disorder's etiology. If dependency on others is encouraged in females more than in males (or independence and autonomy are encouraged more in males), this would contribute to the differential sex prevalence (Bornstein 1999; Widiger 1998). The diagnostic criteria are perhaps then female related because the disorder itself is gender related in its etiology.

Gender-Specific Disorders

Some of the diagnoses in DSM-IV-TR include not only different diagnostic criteria but also different titles and code numbers for males and females. For example, DSM-IV-TR includes "female orgasmic disorder" (302.73) and "male orgasmic disorder" (302.74), and "female sexual arousal disorder" (302.72) and "male erectile disorder" (302.72). There are even disorders that are specific to only one sex, such as premature ejaculation and vaginismus. A diagnosis included in a research appendix to DSM-IV-TR is also confined to just one sex, premenstrual dysphoric disorder.

The gender-specific diagnoses are defined according to different criteria sets. For example, the diagnostic criteria for female orgasmic disorder state that "the diagnosis…should be based on the clinician's judgment that the woman's orgasmic capacity is less than would be reasonable for her age, sexual experience, and the adequacy of sexual stimulation she receives" (American Psychiatric Association 2000, p. 549). However, in contrast, there is no recommendation to consider sexual experience in making the diagnosis of male orgasmic disorder. In a manner analogous to Zahn-Waxler's (1993) critique of the provision of separate diagnostic criteria for boys and girls with conduct disorder, Wakefield (1987) suggested that these alternative criteria sets for males and females with sexual dysfunction disorders are problematic.

Wakefield's (1987) suggestion was in response to an argument by Kaplan (1983) of a gender bias in DSM-III in the diagnosis of inhibited orgasm and inhibited sexual desire in women. Wakefield argued that the DSM-III criteria for inhibited orgasm were at least less sex biased than, for example, the Masters and Johnson (1982) criteria. Masters and Johnson diagnosed inhibited orgasm in females if they had no history of attempting to achieve orgasms (e.g., no history of sexual intercourse or masturbation), whereas males were diagnosed only if they attempted and failed to achieve orgasm. In addition, females could be diagnosed with inhibited orgasm whether or not they were sexually aroused, whereas in males the diagnosis could only be made if there was no orgasm despite being fully sexually aroused. In other words, it was much easier to make the diagnosis in females than in males, because there was no requirement that the anorgasmia occur in the presence of full sexual arousal. Wakefield suggested that the DSM-III criteria for inhibited orgasm were in fact less biased than the Masters and Johnson criteria because the DSM-III criteria were relatively more consistent across males and females. The only inconsistency in DSM-III was the requirement for females that the clinician determine whether the sexual activity leading to orgasm was "adequate in focus, intensity, and duration" (American Psychiatric Association 1980, p. 280). "The fact that the female criterion specifies these additional conditions means that, at least in theory, [the criteria are] biased toward greater diagnosis of males" (Wakefield 1987, p. 470), yet the disorder was said in DSM-III to occur more often in females.

DSM-IV-TR continues to provide somewhat different criteria for males and females with an orgasmic disorder. For females, the diagnosis must consider whether her orgasmic capacity is less than would be reasonable for her sexual experience, and it is noted that females "exhibit wide variability in the type or intensity of stimulation that triggers orgasm" (p. 549). No such qualifications are made for the diagnosis in males. Wakefield (1987) suggested that any difference in the criteria across males and females could contribute to a biased diagnosis. "Although there is a certain sense to the asymmetry, it is still on balance unwarranted and should be eliminated" (Wakefield 1987, p. 470). The different criteria in DSM-IV-TR for males and females reflect presumably real differences in physiology and the importance of prior sexual experiences. However, if there are different sociocultural experiences or differences in physiology that result in a different liability for, or predisposition toward, the development of a disorder, then perhaps the criteria sets should not be adjusted so as to make the prevalence rates more comparable. Potential differences in physiology and sociocultural experiences might contribute to the etiology of the disorder in a manner that is gender related and thereby contributes to the differential sex prevalence for the disorder. In this case, it does not seem warranted for the diagnostic criteria to minimize or eliminate a real, and clinically relevant, gender difference.

How Might These Issues Be Resolved?

The impact and role of gender on the diagnosis of mental disorders has been among the most controversial and discussed topics in the development of the recent editions of DSM (Ross et al. 1995). Most of the DSM-IV criteria sets are intended to be used with both males and females. However, it is unclear whether these criteria sets are always equally valid for males and females. This concern is particularly evident for disorders that have substantially different sex prevalence rates or for which there are gender differences in the disorder's neurobiological or sociocultural etiology. Given the likely impact of gender on the etiology and expression of most mental disorders, the development of gender-neutral diagnostic criteria sets can be quite problematic. However, the nature and extent to which gender differences should impact diagnostic criteria sets is unclear. Gender-specific diagnostic criteria can be potentially more problematic than gender-neutral diagnostic criteria because they can provide an explicit but potentially invalid distinction between the sexes with respect to diagnostic thresholds and descriptions.

How best to resolve these complex, yet clearly important, questions is not entirely clear.

1. At the very least, as discussed throughout the first part of this volume, there is a need for more research concerned specifically with how each of the disorders is manifested in males and females. Increased understanding of phenomenology and whether symptom expression differs in males and females is needed to inform the development of valid diagnostic criteria. Of course, this is an iterative process, because research on phenomenology is usually based on the DSM criteria sets and vice versa.
2. Research is needed on how the diagnostic criteria sets perform for males and females. There is surprisingly little such research on these issues (Hartung and Widiger 1998). In fact, in many instances much of the diagnostic criteria research is confined largely to just one sex (e.g., somatization disorder and conduct disorder).
3. In the absence of an independent, objective gold standard for the valid diagnosis of a respective mental disorder, it is not clear how gender differences in etiology, pathology, and symptomatology should impact diagnostic criteria sets. Nevertheless, in the absence of a perfect gold standard, studies could compare across males and females the relationship of criteria sets to external validators (e.g., course, level of impairment, treatment responsivity, and family history). As disorders' etiopathology is increasingly elucidated, criteria sets could be examined in relationship to various etiopathological variables.
4. Item response theory analyses can also be useful in determining whether males and females at comparable levels of a disorder respond differentially to individual diagnostic criteria (e.g., Santor et al. 1994).
5. More studies are needed that are concerned specifically with the potential existence and precise nature of gender-biased diagnoses.

References

American Psychiatric Association: Diagnostic and Statistical Manual of Mental Disorders, 3rd Edition. Washington, DC, American Psychiatric Association, 1980

American Psychiatric Association: Diagnostic and Statistical Manual of Mental Disorders, 3rd Edition, Revised. Washington, DC, American Psychiatric Association, 1987

American Psychiatric Association: Diagnostic and Statistical Manual of Mental Disorders, 4th Edition. Washington, DC, American Psychiatric Association, 1994

American Psychiatric Association: Diagnostic and Statistical Manual of Mental Disorders, 4th Edition, Text Revision. Washington, DC, American Psychiatric Association, 2000

Bornstein RF: Sex differences in dependent personality disorder prevalence rates. Clinical Psychology: Science and Practice 3:1–12, 1996

Bornstein RF: Dependent personality disorder in the DSM-IV and beyond. Clinical Psychology: Science and Practice 4:175–187, 1997

Bornstein RF: Dependent and histrionic personality disorders, in Oxford Textbook of Psychopathology. Edited by Millon T, Blaney PH, Davis RD. New York, Oxford University Press, 1999, pp 535–554

Cloninger CR, Martin RL, Guze SB, et al: A prospective follow-up and family study of somatization in men and women. Am J Psychiatry 143:873–878, 1986

Frances AJ, First MB, Pincus HA: DSM-IV Guidebook. Washington, DC, American Psychiatric Press, 1995

Hartung C, Widiger TA: Gender differences in the diagnosis of mental disorders: conclusions and controversies of DSM-IV. Psychol Bull 123:260–278, 1998

Kaplan M: A woman's view of DSM-III. Am Psychol 38:786–792, 1983

Masters WH, Johnson VE: Human Sexuality. Boston, MA, Little, Brown, 1982

Phillips KA, Gunderson JG: Personality disorders, in Textbook of Psychiatry, 2nd Edition. Edited by Hales RE, Yudofsky SC, Talbott JA. Washington, DC, American Psychiatric Press, 1994, pp 701–728

Purnine D, Frank E: Should postpartum mood disorders be given a more prominent or distinct place in DSM-IV?, in DSM-IV Sourcebook, Vol 2. Edited by Widiger TA, Frances AJ, Pincus HA, et al. Washington, DC, American Psychiatric Association, 1996, pp 261–279

Robins LN: The consequences of conduct disorder in girls, in The Development of Antisocial and Prosocial Behavior. Edited by Olweus D, Yarrow MR, Block J. New York, Academic Press, 1986, pp 385–414

Robins LN: Conduct disorder. J Child Psychol Psychiatry 32:193–212, 1991

Robins LN, Price RK: Adult disorders predicted by childhood conduct disorder problems: results from NIMH Epidemiologic Catchment Area project. Psychiatry 54:116–132, 1991

Ross R, Frances AJ, Widiger TA: Gender issues in DSM-IV, in Review of Psychiatry, Vol 14. Edited by Oldham JM, Riba MB. Washington, DC, American Psychiatric Press, 1995, pp 205–226

Rutherford MJ, Alterman AI, Cacciola JS, et al: Gender differences in diagnosing antisocial personality disorder in methadone patients. Am J Psychiatry 152:1309–1316, 1995

Santor DA, Ramsay JO, Zuroff DC: Nonparametric item analyses of the Beck Depression Inventory: evaluating gender item bias and response option weights. Psychol Assess 6:255–270, 1994

Wakefield JC: Sex bias in the diagnosis of primary orgasmic dysfunction. Am Psychol 42:464–471, 1987

Walker LEA: Are personality disorders gender biased?, in Controversial Issues in Mental Health. Edited by Kirk SA, Einbinder SD. New York, Allyn and Bacon, 1994, pp 22–29

Widiger TA: Sex biases in the diagnosis of personality disorders. J Personal Disord 12:95–118, 1998

Widiger TA, Spitzer RL: Sex bias in the diagnosis of personality disorders: conceptual and methodological issues. Clin Psychol Rev 11:1–22, 1991

Zahn-Waxler C: Warriors and worriers: gender and psychopathology. Dev Psychopathol 5:79–89, 1993

Zoccolillo M: Gender and the development of conduct disorder. Dev Psychopathol 5:65–78, 1993

Zoccolillo M, Rogers K: Characteristics and outcome of hospitalized adolescent girls with conduct disorder. J Am Acad Child Adolesc Psychiatry 30:973–981, 1991

11

CONCLUDING THOUGHTS

Katharine A. Phillips, M.D.
Michael B. First, M.D.

As the chapters in the first part of this book clearly indicate, gender is a critically important aspect of psychopathology. Although the quantity of research on gender has dramatically increased in recent years, the field is still young, and much additional research is needed—especially on the causes of gender differences. Many of the intriguing findings presented in this part of this book, while illustrating advances in our understanding, raise more questions than answers. For example, why is unipolar depression about twice as common in women as in men, whereas alcohol and drug use disorders are more common in men? How does childhood adversity affect neurobiological functioning differently in men versus women? Why do a variety of "female-typical" psychopathologies, such as unipolar depression and eating disorders, so often arise during adolescence (Rutter et al. 2003)?

Increasing our understanding of gender will have profound implications for DSM. As discussed in Chapter 10 ("Gender and Diagnostic Criteria"), for example, gender considerations have immediate implications for the DSM-V revision process, given their impact on the validity and applicability of the diagnostic criteria sets. Although gender issues were given greater visibility in the DSM-IV (American Psychiatric Association 1994) text with the inclusion of a new text section on "Specific Culture, Age, and Gender-Related Features," the actual amount of information pertaining specifically to gender was disappointingly small, reflecting the limited empirical base on gender issues in psychopathology. We hope that the explosion of research on gender over the past decade and in the near future will allow the inclusion of much more detailed and clinically useful information in the DSM-V text.

Furthermore, as discussed throughout the first part of this volume, gender has profound implications for our understanding of the etiology and pathophysiology of mental disorders. If we can answer questions such as *why* some disorders are more common in women and others in men, *why* differences in gender ratio for some disorders change during puberty and at menopause, and *why* men and women with the same disorder may experience different symptoms, we can begin to understand what causes and maintains these disorders. Classification systems in psychiatry may someday be based on pathoetiology rather than a description of clinical features. This transition has largely already occurred in nonpsychiatric medicine, where systems based on pathogenesis (e.g., infectious organisms) have largely replaced syndrome-based classification (Kendell 1991). Without a doubt, classifications based on the structural or functional abnormalities underlying the syndrome are likely to be more useful and valid (Kendell 1989). Adopting an etiopathologically based approach to classification is expected to greatly improve our ability to identify, treat, and prevent disorders (Hyman 2003; Phillips et al. 2003). A challenge for our field, however, is that the DSM-V revision process is coming at an awkward time: we do not know enough about the underlying neurobiological or environmental bases of mental disorders to reflect this understanding in the structure of the classification. The transition from a syndrome-based classification system to one based on pathogenesis will inevitably be gradual and sputtering, because research will progress at different rates for different disorders. Additional gender research, such as that recommended by the Institute of Medicine, will contribute substantially to this paradigm shift.

As noted in Chapter 1 ("Introduction"), the Institute of Medicine recommended expanding research on sex differences in brain organization and function, monitoring sex differences and similarities for all human diseases that affect both sexes, supporting and conducting additional research on sex differences, and encouraging and supporting interdisciplinary research on sex differences. The National Institute of Mental Health (NIMH; 2003) has taken concrete steps to foster such research in mental health by issuing a Program Announcement in 2003 on "Women's Mental Health and Sex/Gender Differences Research" that "seeks to increase understanding of the significance of sex/gender differences in mental health outcomes and to assess their significance for mental health prevention, treatment, and services." It identified three major areas for research emphasis: 1) basic and clinical neuroscience (e.g., research on sex differences in brain processes contributing to behavior as determined by brain imaging; gene regulatory and gene–environment interactions contributing to mental disorders; and the development of models to examine the impact of hormonal transitions across the life span on brain function); 2) epidemiology and risk factors (e.g., research on disparities in prevalence of mental illness, disability, and access to care among females of different ethnic and socioeconomic backgrounds; and childhood risk and protective factors related to gender disparities in the incidence and course of mental disorders); and 3) intervention and services research (e.g., research on sex/gender differences in acute and maintenance treatment outcomes; taxonomies of functional outcomes and disabilities in women and girls with mental disorders; and preventive interventions for mental disorders with female-specific risk factors [e.g., stressors in caregiver roles]). It is hoped that important efforts such as this will translate into increased research on women's mental health as well as gender more broadly.

In the rush to discover the etiology and pathophysiology of mental disorders, as well as prevent such disorders, we should not forget the fundamental importance of research on disorders' clinical features. This is important for several reasons. First, the reality is that disorders in our diagnostic system will continue to be defined in terms of their clinical features for the foreseeable future. Thus, research on gender-related similarities and differences using the current definitions of disorders will remain of crucial importance. Second, valid data on pathogenesis can be obtained only by using well-defined clinical phenotypes. Studies of pathogenesis that are not based on clearly defined and well-described phenotypes will be of limited usefulness. As long ago as 1942, Brown noted, "The part played by heredity in the development of the psychoneuroses is one of the fundamental unsolved problems in psychiatry.... But the chief difficulty is to define the condition the heredity of which one is attempting to trace." More recently, Smoller and Tsuang (1998) similarly noted: "With recent advances in molecular genetics, the rate-limiting step in identifying susceptibility genes for psychiatric disorders has become phenotype definition." Of course, this is an iterative process—more valid phenotype definitions will enhance research on etiopathology, and increased understanding of etiopathology will gradually elucidate more valid phenotypes. It is also worth noting that the dimensional approach to classification is potentially powerful, and it is important that gender be incorporated into studies of potentially useful and valid dimensions (e.g., personality dimensions).

Gender must be more than an afterthought in ongoing and future research, both basic science and clinical research. Too often, gender is considered a "nuisance" variable that researchers feel obligated to control for in their statistical analyses but otherwise disregard. Often, it is neglected altogether. However, some studies do not yield much of interest or meaning until gender is considered. We need to take a fresh look at gender. Both males and females should be included in all studies unless there is a highly compelling reason to do otherwise. NIMH-funded clinical trials require examination of outcome by gender, even if statistical power to do so is limited. Such analyses should substantially advance understanding of whether men and women respond to treatment differently. In fact, studies of all topics should test for sex differences, and all gender-related findings—both differences and lack of differences—should be reported (Institute of Medicine 2001).

New gender-focused studies are certainly critically important to increasing our understanding of gender. However, studies that do not focus primarily on gender can also shed valuable light on gender similarities and differences. For example, questions pertaining to gender can be investigated using existing databases. In addition, studies (such as treatment studies) that are not focused primarily on gender should examine, or reexamine, treatment outcomes in terms of differential effects in men versus women—perhaps when analyzed in this way, new insights can be gleaned about treatment efficacy. It can be very (i.e., prohibitively) expensive for such studies to have adequate statistical power for such analyses; nonetheless, gender can be examined and effect sizes (in addition to statistical significance) can be reported to estimate the magnitude of the effect. Conversely, secondary gender-related analyses may be subject to type I error. If secondary or post-hoc analyses are done to examine gender, such analyses should be identified as such, and potential implications for both type I and type II error should be considered. Rutter et al. (2003) usefully and eloquently discuss some additional methodological considerations when conducting gender research—for example, the importance of studying representative population samples, of adequate measurement and significance testing, and of adequate attention to the complexity of causes of sex differences in psychopathology.

This is a very exciting time for our field, and gender deserves to be at the forefront of our efforts to increase understanding of psychopathology. This increased understanding will undoubtedly improve the validity of future editions of DSM. The Institute of Medicine (2001) report stated it well: "Until the question of sex is routinely asked and the results—positive or negative—are routinely reported, many opportunities to obtain a better understanding of the pathogenesis of disease and to advance human health will surely be missed."

References

American Psychiatric Association: Diagnostic and Statistical Manual of Mental Disorders, 4th Edition. Washington, DC, American Psychiatric Association, 1994

Brown F: Heredity in the psychoneuroses. Proc R Soc Med 35:785–790, 1942

Hyman S: Foreword, in Advancing DSM: Dilemmas in Psychiatric Diagnosis. Edited by Phillips KA, First MB, Pincus HA. Washington, DC, American Psychiatric Association, 2003, pp xi–xxi

Institute of Medicine: Exploring the Biological Contributions to Human Health: Does Sex Matter? Washington, DC, National Academy Press, 2001

Kendell RE: Clinical validity, in The Validity of Psychiatric Diagnosis. Edited by Robins LE, Barrett JE. New York, Raven Press, 1989

Kendell RE: Relationship between DSM-IV and ICD-10. J Abnorm Psychol 100:297–301, 1991

National Institute of Mental Health: Women's mental health and sex/gender differences research (PA number PA-03-143). Bethesda, MD, National Institutes of Health, June 20, 2003. Available online at http://grants2.nih.gov/grants/guide/pa-files/PA-03-143.html.

Phillips KA, Price LH, Greenberg BD, et al: Should DSM's diagnostic groupings be changed?, in Advancing DSM: Dilemmas in Psychiatric Diagnosis. Edited by Phillips KA, First MB, Pincus HA. Washington, DC, American Psychiatric Publishing, 2003, pp 57–84

Rutter M, Caspi A, Moffitt TE: Using sex differences in psychopathology to study causal mechanisms: unifying issues and research strategies. J Child Psychol Psychiatry 44:1092–1115, 2003

Smoller JW, Tsuang MT: Panic and phobic anxiety: defining phenotypes for genetic studies. Am J Psychiatry 155:1152–1162, 1998

PART II

EARLY CHILDHOOD

12

DIAGNOSIS OF PSYCHOPATHOLOGY IN INFANTS, TODDLERS, AND PRESCHOOL CHILDREN

Irene Chatoor, M.D.
Daniel S. Pine, M.D.
William E. Narrow, M.D., M.P.H.

The need for a valid nosology for psychiatric diagnosis in early childhood represents one of the most pressing issues in psychiatric classification. To address the need for such standards, the American Psychiatric Association established a work group to take stock of progress in this area and delineate a research agenda. This group included a broad range of child psychiatrists and clinical psychologists conducting leading-edge research across the spectrum of childhood disorders and developmental measurement. Over the course of a year, the Infant and Young Child Diagnostic Work Group communicated through more than a dozen conference calls. In the spring of 2005, the group met in Washington, D.C., to discuss general issues relevant to this area.

To summarize the conclusions emerging through this process, the group produced nine white papers, individually represented as chapters in this volume, that focused on specific issues in nosology. This introduction defines general issues pertinent to nosology in this age group, with the goal of delineating areas of consensus as well as specific challenges that confront clinicians and researchers working in this area. This discussion revolves around two sets of issues: those that occur in nosology at all ages but create relatively novel problems in infants, toddlers, and preschoolers, and those that are unique to this age period. In both areas, the Infant and Young Child Diagnostic Work Group was able to reach considerable consensus during the 2005 conference.

Core Challenges That Occur at All Ages

A standard nosology must address two core challenges: delineating boundaries between health and illness and determining the boundaries separating the various specific disorders. Although the boundaries between "normal" and "pathological" behavior can be difficult to discern in all age groups, drawing a firm line in the first years of life can be particularly difficult, particularly in the first 2 years of life. This difficulty arises in part from the rapid changes in behavior that accompany the initial acquisition of emotion and behavior regulation skills during the early developmental periods. Periods of developmental transition can pose particular difficulties for clinicians who must distinguish extremes of "normal" behavior in such areas as sleep, attachment, and physical activity from clear-cut instances of psychopathology that may indicate sleep disorders, separation anxiety disorder, social phobia, oppositional defiant disorder, attention-deficit/hyperactivity disorder (ADHD), and so on. The centrality of the parent–child relationship as the social context of early childhood can further increase the complexity of the evaluation by requiring a disentangling of problems in parenting from disordered behavior in the child.

As a general guide for identifying pathology, the work group reached consensus on criteria that can help to distinguish between normal behavioral variations and psychopathology in infants, toddlers, and preschoolers. This determination rests on the quality and pervasiveness of the behaviors in question and the extent to which the behaviors are experienced as distressing or interfere with functioning. These principles are consistent with criteria for established DSM mental disorders as applied to older children, adolescents, and adults, although the unique social context of young children must be taken into consideration. Most importantly, behaviors of the young child exhibit distinctive and intricate relationships with behavior of the parents. Thus, in infants, toddlers, and preschoolers, the group reached consensus, as a general principle, that a mental disorder can be diagnosed in an infant, toddler, or young child in the absence of distress or functional impairment in the child, if the disorder causes significant distress or functional impairment in a parent or the family.

Despite the emergence of this consensus, many questions remain concerning application of the principle. In some clinical circumstances, a relatively strong case can be made for applications of this principle. For example, in the case of nocturnal sleep problems, an infant's difficulties may disrupt sleep only at night, and the infant might compensate for such difficulties by sleeping during the day. The group agreed that "impairment," in this situation, could emerge entirely through effects on a parent, who must go to work in a state of relative sleep deprivation. In other clinical circumstances, however, it can be more difficult to classify behavior as "normal" or "abnormal" based merely on the extent to which the behavior is impairing for the parent. For example, in the case of behavior problems, the very same behaviors in the child may produce widely varying levels of family disruption, depending on the parent's skillfulness, tolerance for behavior, or own psychiatric status (e.g., depression). Firm rules do not exist for deciding when such situations call for classification of a disorder in the infant, in the parent, or in both. Some members of the group suggested an additional axis that would address the parent–child relationship. However, at the present time, there are virtually no empirical data to guide diagnostic decisions under such circumstances. However, to clarify this principle, further research is needed on the contributions of parental psychopathology and parenting skills to distress and impairment in the child and in other family members. Furthermore, more research is needed to fully characterize how young children experience and manifest distress and impairment individually, beyond the effects on family members. Some instruments, such as the Preschool Age Psychiatric Assessment (PAPA) recently developed by Egger and Angold (Egger et al. 1999), begin to provide relevant guidelines for determining impairment for children 2–5 years of age. There is no psychometrically validated instrument for measuring impairment in infants or toddlers younger than 2 years of age. Considerably more work is needed in this area.

Beyond the major challenge of establishing clear definitions of disorders, a second challenge in this age group concerns standards for distinguishing among individual psychiatric disorders in children presenting with a range of impairing symptoms. The lack of such standards can contribute to disagreements over comorbidity. Empirically testing whether existing nosological constructs are distinct categories, as opposed to minor variations of a core underlying syndrome, will require systematic efforts applying diverse research approaches. Drawing on prior work among older children, adolescents, and adults, in particular the well-known conceptualization of Robins and Guze, the group recognized four criteria that clearly can be used for classifying a disorder as distinct. Specifically, to be considered a "distinct" condition, a symptom constellation should 1) manifest as a systematic, reliably observed collection of typically co-occurring features that each occur less frequently in other classes of disorder; 2) show a selective association with specific familial and genetic factors, distinguishing the syndrome both from states of health and other classes of disorder; 3) exhibit a longitudinal course that also distinguishes the syndrome from health and other classes of disorder; and 4) exhibit unique neurobiological correlates. The group also debated the utility of differential responses to treatment as a validating criterion, and while recognizing its current value for some conditions, could not reach consensus for this fifth criterion. It should be noted that for virtually all psychiatric disorders in DSM-IV (American Psychiatric Association 1994), these criteria have not yet been fully met. Relative to most disorders in DSM-IV, the conditions discussed by the work group have been the focus of even less research on validation. This fact should be kept in mind by the DSM-V Task Force and Work Groups when guidelines for the addition of potential new disorders are discussed and decided upon.

Problems Unique to This Age Period

A nosology of infants, toddlers, and preschoolers must also address problems that are relatively unique to this age period. Much like problems in defining the presence of a disorder or of specific syndromes, these problems also arise from the complex and rapid pace of development in the first years of life, coupled with the unusual degree of dependency in this age period. The group focused on four sets of general problems unique to this age period.

First, the group recognized the need to clearly demarcate distinct age periods, due to the rapid changes in development during the first years of life. This is truly a unique aspect of approaches to classification with this age group, because the magnitude of change during infancy is unparalleled during any other developmental period. Because such rapid changes, demarcations of distinct age-related periods involve a much finer level of resolution than for other ages. To serve as an approximate guide for future studies, the group demarcated three discrete developmental periods: infancy (0–11 months), toddlerhood (12–35 months), and preschool (36–60 months). In considering various forms of psychopathology, the group agreed to conceptualize psychiatric syndromes as they display common or discontinuous manifestations across these three developmental periods.

Second, the group recognized the challenges involved in relating symptoms in infants, toddlers, and preschoolers to symptoms manifest in older children, adolescents, and adults. Describing symptoms in young children may involve the need to translate *existing* nosology into terms that are suitable for young children, or it may emphasize the need to define relatively *novel* symptoms in young children that more precisely capture clinical manifestations during this age period. Ideally, a broad nosology should be developed that is applicable across the life span while characterizing unique manifestations and/or criteria for specific developmental periods. In accord with this, several studies have examined whether symptoms from DSM-IV for depressive disorders, anxiety disorders, and posttraumatic stress disorder can be applied to young children. These studies have found that many items assessing psychiatric symptoms can be applied to young children; others require modification of the wording without altering the intent of the item; and still others may need to be omitted and diagnostic algorithms may have to be changed to capture relevant psychopathology. However, as in virtually all aspects of work with psychopathology in young children, research in this area is only beginning. In addition, considerable research is needed on heterotypic continuity—that is, the varying manifestations of a latent behavioral construct that change across developmental periods. An example of such research would be the relationship of feeding problems during the early years of life and eating disorders during the adolescent and young adult years.

Third, existing duration and pervasiveness criteria in DSM-IV may not be appropriate in infants, toddlers, and young children because of the rapid developmental changes and strong context dependency of behavior in young children. For example, given the rapid pace of development, it may be inappropriate to adopt the currently employed 6-month duration criteria for disorders such as ADHD, oppositional defiant disorder, or generalized anxiety disorder. Similarly, the pervasiveness criterion for some disorders, such as ADHD Criterion C, requires special attention in this age group. Many young children spend virtually all of their time in a single social setting—the home—with parents serving as the only source of information concerning the child's behavior. As such, the "pervasiveness" of the child's behaviors cannot reasonably be judged across multiple social settings. Further research is necessary to specify criteria for the duration and pervasiveness of symptoms in young children.

Fourth, advances are needed in assessment techniques for this age period. Unique complexities arise in this area because of the relative inability of young children to report on their own symptoms, coupled with the restricted range of social settings to which young children are exposed. These complications limit opportunities for collecting information directly from children and from parallel informants, such as teachers. Therefore, the issue of multimethod diagnostic procedures takes on special importance for this young age group. As pointed out by Angold, Egger, and Carter (see Chapter 15, "Measurement of Psychopathology in Children Under the Age of Six," this volume), during recent years a number of validated instruments, interviews, and questionnaires have become available for the diagnosis of young children, although there continues to be a lack of standardized interviews and measures of impairment for infants and toddlers younger than 2 years of age.

In addition to the parent interview and questionnaires, direct observation in the laboratory has become an important part of the assessment for some disorders in infants and young children, particularly for the pervasive developmental disorders. These methods should be further developed as a diagnostic tool for other disorders as well. As a component of some observation tools, prior experience suggests the benefits of using techniques that "press" for clinically salient behaviors characteristic of particular disorders and rate the behaviors using a standardized coding system. By developing clinically relevant "presses" for other syndromes, similar advances in the observational assessment technology may emerge for a broader range of syndromes. For example, in the area of behavior disorders, this approach is exemplified by the Disruptive Behavior Diagnostic Observation Schedule developed by Wakschlag, Leventhal, and colleagues (Wakschlag et al. 2005).

Work over the past decade, as summarized in this volume, clearly establishes the fact that broad categories of psychopathology delineated in DSM-IV exist and are clinically meaningful in young children. Considerable progress has been made in the development of assessment tools for young children and the definition of psychiatric disorders in this young age group. Consensus has emerged on key principles and on future directions. However, as outlined here and described in the chapters in this part of the book, this promise must serve as the foundation for rigorous research that can characterize the nature of psychiatric manifestations in young children in a developmentally informed manner for DSM-V. Such work will enable early identification, inform applications of treatment, and substantially advance etiological research on the origins of psychopathology. Ultimately, this work will benefit the infants and young children who would not receive treatment unless their symptomatology is defined within the framework of DSM.

References

American Psychiatric Association: Diagnostic and Statistical Manual of Mental Disorders, 4th Edition. Washington, DC, American Psychiatric Association, 1994

Egger H, Ascher BH, Angold A: The Preschool Age Psychiatric Assessment (PAPA). Durham, NC, 1999

Wakschlag LS, Leventhal BL, Briggs-Gowan MJ, et al: Defining the "disruptive" in preschool behavior: what diagnostic observation can teach us. Clin Child Fam Psychol Rev 8(3):183–201, 2005

13

A RESEARCH AGENDA FOR POSTTRAUMATIC STRESS DISORDER IN INFANTS, TODDLERS, AND PRESCHOOL CHILDREN

Michael S. Scheeringa, M.D., M.P.H.

Current State of the Science

When the DSM-IV (American Psychiatric Association 1994) nosology for PTSD was published in 1994, there had been no studies of infants or preschool children that examined posttraumatic symptomatology. Little more than a decade later, in contrast, six systematic group studies have examined PTSD criteria in 193 children younger than 7 years of age (Ghosh-Ippen et al. 2004; Levendosky et al. 2002; Ohmi et al. 2002; Scheeringa et al. 1995, 2001, 2003). Two other studies have examined posttraumatic symptomatology in 230 children, but these did not focus on diagnostic criteria (Laor et al. 1996, 1997).

PTSD is one of the disorders in this volume that affects individuals of all ages, in contrast to predominantly childhood disorders (e.g., oppositional defiant disorder, reactive attachment disorder, feeding disorders). In this context, it is worth noting that there are benefits of consistency in a nosology for PTSD across ages whenever possible and useful. Consistency makes communication among professionals, and comparison across studies, more feasible.

EVIDENCE THAT DSM-IV NOSOLOGY CAN BE APPLIED TO PRESCHOOLERS WITH RELATIVELY MINOR MODIFICATIONS

In a programmatic series of research studies (Scheeringa et al. 1995, 2001, 2003), we began by asking disarmingly straightforward questions: Does PTSD exist in very young children? If so, in what ways is it similar to PTSD in older children and adults, and in what ways is it different? These are important questions for several reasons. First, despite contentions of various social critics (Summerfield 2001), PTSD is a well-validated disorder that is enormously useful for clinical treatment and clinical research. The conceptualization of PTSD in DSM-III (American Psychiatric Association 1980) fostered the blossoming of treatment efficacy research and neuroscientific investigations encompassing psychophysiological and functional brain imaging studies. Second, critics' assertions that PTSD is an inappropriate diagnosis for children because children show many forms of non-PTSD symptomatology after traumatic events miss the point of what is useful about diagnosis. Third, the most rapid period of postnatal brain development occurs in young children, in whom important cognitive and language capacities are emerging; whether PTSD shows downward continuity into this age group despite this period of development is a logical empirical question.

In our series of studies cited earlier, we initially examined individual signs and symptoms in detail, an approach that had been applied rarely to early childhood disorders. In systematically listing all signs and symptoms that real cases of traumatized young children had demonstrated (Scheeringa et al. 1995), this approach extended well beyond DSM-IV symptomatology. Findings clearly revealed two telling challenges to the diagnostic assessment of young children. First, symptomatology that *depends on verbalizations* from the individual are difficult to detect in preverbal or barely verbal children. For example, detection of the item "avoidance of thoughts, feelings, or conversations associated with the traumatic event" requires children to verbalize that they experienced these phenomena. Although this item may be detected partially through behavioral observations of avoidance, an adult's presence is required to observe, infer, and report on the child's behavioral reactions. Second, symptoms that are experienced *internally* are difficult or impossible to detect, even with the presence of an adult. This holds true even for young children who have developed narrative language capacities but in whom a capacity to self-report on any internalized symptomatology is still a nascent skill.

Reviewing signs and symptoms of these highly symptomatic, traumatized young children showed that they could not meet the algorithm for the DSM-IV diagnosis of PTSD (Scheeringa et al. 1995), principally because of the requirement for three avoidance and numbing (criterion C) items. The seven "avoidance and numbing" items are also the most internal of the 17 possible PTSD criteria. Our research demonstrated that if the requirement for the numbing and avoidance items was reduced to one item, a reasonable proportion of young children could qualify for the diagnosis (Scheeringa et al. 1995, 2001, 2003).

On the basis of these data, we proposed a set of alternative criteria (Scheeringa et al. 1995) that were modified in subsequent studies (Scheeringa et al. 2001, 2003). These criteria were used as the basis for traumatic stress disorder in *Diagnostic Classification: 0–3* (Zero to Three 1994). Current recommendations for these alternative criteria are similar to the DSM-IV, albeit with the following six modifications.

1. Do not require the A2 item that the child's response at the time of the traumatic event involved helplessness, fear, or horror. This transient reaction cannot be known if children are preverbal or adults were not present to witness the children's reactions.
2. For the item "recurrent and intrusive distressing recollections of the event," include a note that the distress may not be obvious. We have found empirically that some young children spontaneously talk about or play out their intrusive traumatic recollections but do not appear obviously distressed. The reason for this is unclear.

The next three modifications are minor wording changes that enhance the face validity of the items for young children, but do not alter the intent of the original DSM-IV items. The rationale for these modifications is that when asking about young children, it may help to ask about the phenomenology in developmentally appropriate terms.

3. For the item "markedly diminished interest or participation in significant activities," it makes relatively more sense to ask about "significant activities" in terms of play, social interactions, and daily routines.
4. Inquire about the item "feeling of detachment or estrangement from others" (a highly internal phenomenon) in more behavioral terms, as social withdrawal from loved ones.
5. When asking about the item "irritability or outbursts of anger," include inquiry about extreme temper tantrums.
6. Lower the threshold for the avoidance and numbing criterion from three items to one item, as mentioned previously. Lowering the threshold for criterion C has also been proposed for adults (Kilpatrick and Resnick 1993).

Using this alternative algorithm and criteria sets that were similar to the wording changes recommended here, five studies now have calculated rates of PTSD in head-to-head comparisons with the DSM-IV rules (Table 13–1). The last column of Table 13–1 reports the mean number of PTSD symptoms for three of the studies. The rates of PTSD in young children identified by using DSM-IV are considerably lower than those identified with the alternative rules. This finding, coupled with the observation that children diagnosed by the alternative rules were highly symptomatic (6.1 symptoms in nonclinical cohorts and 9.9 symptoms in a clinical

TABLE 13–1. Rates of posttraumatic stress disorder (PTSD) by DSM-IV criteria compared with the alternative criteria in five studies of preschool children

Study	Rate of PTSD by DSM-IV criteria	Rate of PTSD by alternative criteria	Mean number of PTSD symptoms
Scheeringa et al. 1995, *N*=12, clinic	13%	69%	Not reported
Scheeringa et al. 2001, *N*=15, clinic	20%	60%	9.9
Ohmi et al. 2002, *N*=32, non-clinic	0%	25%	6.1
Scheeringa et al. 2003, *N*=62, non-clinic	0%	26%	6.1
Ghosh-Ippen et al. 2004, *N*=156, clinic	2% (0–3 years) 1% (4–6 years)	47% (0–3 years) 39% (4–6 years)	Not reported

Note. "Clinic"=Parents of children were seeking help in clinics; "Non-clinic"=Parents were not all help-seeking and were recruited in the community.

sample), suggests that DSM-IV criteria require some modification for use in young children.

Our research also identified four items of symptomatology that were commonly shown by young children but were not present in DSM-IV: 1) regression in skills (e.g., verbal skills, dressing skills, and toileting); 2) new separation anxiety; 3) new aggression; and 4) new fears of things not related to the trauma (e.g., going to the bathroom alone, the dark). We attempted to include these in the alternative criteria but found that they did not increase the diagnostic sensitivity (Scheeringa et al. 2003). These items may have other uses, however, such as constituents of dimensional symptom checklists or treatment outcome measures.

We conclude that with the developmental modifications in the alternative criteria and algorithm, PTSD can be reliably detected in young children. We emphasize that PTSD does not capture every manifestation of possible posttraumatic symptomatology, but if one looks systematically for PTSD in young children, one can reliably and validly identify it.

LIMITATIONS OF EXISTING METHODOLOGY

Measurement of PTSD symptomatology in young children is almost entirely dependent on parent report. We have documented that a systematic procedure of observational assessments, including examiner-directed trauma-related play, provided only limited diagnostic information above and beyond caregiver report (Scheeringa et al. 2001). Furthermore, children younger than 7 years do not possess the cognitive capacities to self-report validly about psychiatric symptoms. Because caregivers cannot be aware of all of the internalized symptomatology of their children, measurement of PTSD symptoms in young children will almost always be an underestimate. In a study of a cohort of traumatized children ages 0–18 years, we determined that the extent of PTSD symptomatology in infant and preschool children was underestimated by 8.9-fold compared with that of older children for whom both child- and caregiver-report were available (Scheeringa et al. 2006).

PHENOMENOLOGY

We prospectively followed a cohort of 62 young children who had been assessed for PTSD following trauma (Scheeringa et al. 2003) 1 year (n=47) and 2 years later (n=35). Two findings are particularly noteworthy from that follow-up (Scheeringa et al. 2005). First, when the group who had been diagnosed with PTSD based on the alternative criteria at the first evaluation (Initial PTSD, n=16) was compared over time with the group that was diagnosed as not having PTSD (Initial No PTSD, n=46), the Initial PTSD group continued to show significantly more PTSD symptoms 1 year and 2 years later than the Initial No PTSD group (Figure 13–1). These data support the predictive validity of the alternative method for diagnosing PTSD—that is, requiring one rather than three numbing and avoidance items is not too low a threshold. In contrast to the remainder of the cohort, children who were diagnosed at this threshold initially continued to be significantly more symptomatic at high levels (i.e., a mean of more than five signs and symptoms after 2 years).

A second unexpected—and disturbing—finding was that the entire group showed no significant reduction in PTSD symptomatology over 2 years (Figure 13–1), nor was there any treatment effect over time for a subset of 19 subjects who received traditional treatment in the community during the course of the study. Despite evidence that PTSD can be a chronic illness in approximately 50% of patients (Davidson and Fairbank 1993), the vast majority of longitudinal studies in adults have demonstrated significant reductions in mean symptoms over time, even if the signs and symptoms do not completely disappear. Nevertheless, a pattern of unremitting signs and symptoms has been demonstrated previously in older, traumatized children (McFarlane 1987; Stuber et al. 1991).

Laor et al. (1997) conducted the only other known prospective, longitudinal study of traumatized preschool children. Their study of 3- through 5-year-old children was not confined to diagnostic items of PTSD. The more severely stressed subgroup decreased their symptomatology after 30 months, but the less stressed subgroup did not.

We conclude that these early findings show predictive validity for using alternative criteria for diagnosing PTSD in young children, in contrast to the DSM-IV criteria, which identify relatively few cases. Also, these early prospective findings

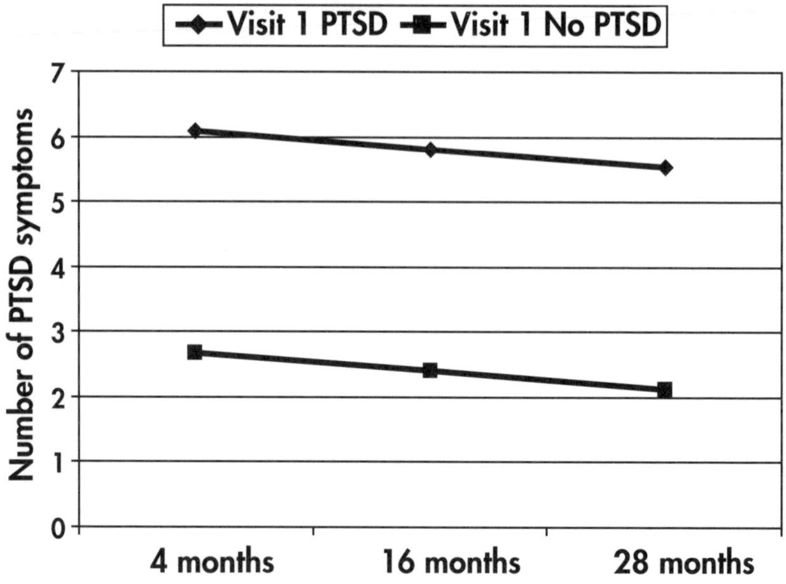

FIGURE 13–1. Number of posttraumatic stress disorder (PTSD) symptoms over time from a mixed models analysis equation adjusted for time from trauma.

Visit 1 in this study is approximated by 4 months posttrauma, Visit 2 by 16 months posttrauma, and Visit 3 by 28 months posttrauma.

Source. Reprinted from Scheeringa M, Zeanah C, Myers L, et al.: "Predictive Validity in a Prospective Follow-up of PTSD in Preschool Children." *Journal of American Academy of Child and Adolescent Psychiatry* 44:899–906, 2005. Copyright 2005, Lippincott Williams & Wilkins. Used with permission.

raise concerns about the chronicity of PTSD symptomatology in young children, lending some support to suggestions that trauma experienced in the preschool period may have more lasting and pernicious effects relative to older populations.

This raises a question: Why might trauma in the toddler/preschool period predict a worse prognosis? Two plausible explanations are the vulnerability of the rapidly developing and immature central nervous system (Schore 2002), and the unique dependence of young children on the caregiving context, subjects to be explored in a subsequent section.

Advances in Developmental Neuroscience

Two recent studies with preschool children provide preliminary evidence for the usefulness of neuroscientific approaches to understanding the manifestations of

PTSD symptomatology. The first study (Scheeringa et al. 2004) examined heart rate reactivity and variability in response to non-trauma- and trauma-related memory recall. It has been reliably shown in adult populations that when individuals with PTSD (Trauma/PTSD) are exposed to trauma-related stimuli, their heart rate increases significantly more than that of trauma-exposed participants who do not have PTSD (Trauma/No PTSD) (Keane et al. 1998).

In attempting replicate this finding for the first time in young children, we included an approach from developmental psychopathology and added a measure of the parasympathetic component of cardiac control. Heart rate is controlled by a combination of the two branches of the autonomic nervous system, the sympathetic and the parasympathetic branches. The parasympathetic component can be estimated as a subset of heart period variability, called *respiratory sinus arrhythmia* (RSA), and baseline measures are more commonly referred to in the child development literature as *vagal tone* (Porges 1995). Because the sympathetic and parasympathetic branches are separate neural networks, measuring the parasympathetic contribution ought to illuminate the neural mechanisms underlying PTSD. It is easiest perhaps to think of RSA (parasympathetic function) as a measure of an organism's adaptability, or flexibility, to respond to stress. The greater the flexibility (higher RSA), the better for the organism to adapt to stress. Studies of at-risk children have shown consistently that higher levels of RSA were associated with better psychosocial outcomes. We hypothesized that the Trauma/PTSD group would show either decreased RSA or relatively less increased RSA compared with the Trauma/No PTSD group during the trauma stimulus period.

For heart period, we partially replicated the adult studies by finding the same pattern of results. The Trauma/PTSD group increased their heart rate (decreased heart period 6.3 ms) more than the Trauma/No PTSD group (decreased heart period 1.4 ms), as expected, but this was not statistically significant. We found that, as hypothesized, the Trauma/PTSD group decreased RSA during the trauma stimulus period compared with baseline (–2.3 ms), whereas the Trauma/No PTSD group increased RSA (3.7 ms). Although the difference between groups was not statistically significant, when a measure of the parents' level of positive discipline during a cleanup episode in the laboratory was added to the analyses, this produced significant interaction effects. Specifically, children who had the "double whammy" of high levels of PTSD symptomatology (High PTSD) plus low levels of positive parental discipline (Low PD) were the subset that followed our hypotheses (increased heart rate and decreased RSA during the trauma stimulus period).

Figure 13–2 shows the fuller pattern of results for this interaction for the RSA data. Interestingly, the figure depicts different trajectories for the Low PTSD and High PTSD subgroups. The two lines for the two Low PTSD subgroups in Figure 13–2 are relatively flat, meaning that there was no real difference in RSA response between the Pleasant Memory and Trauma Memory. However, the two lines for the two High PTSD subgroups slope sharply and in opposite directions from each other.

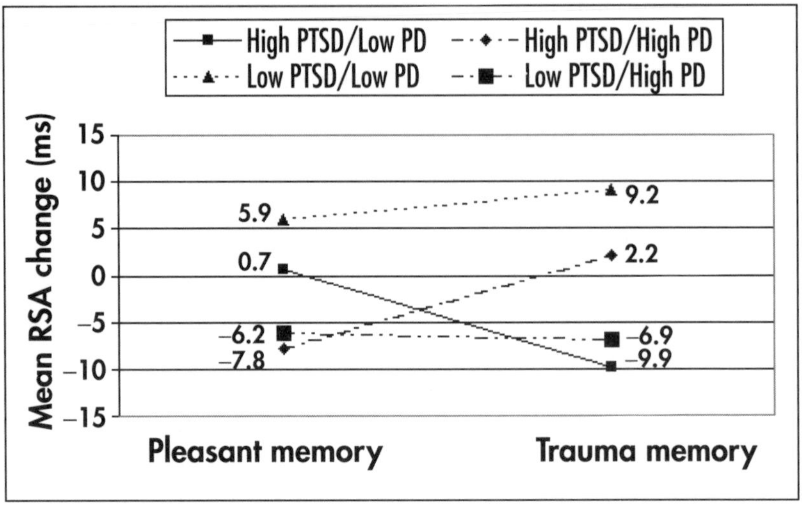

FIGURE 13–2. Change in mean respiratory sinus arrhythmia (RSA) for the subgroups with High Posttraumatic Stress Disorder (PTSD)/Low Parental Positive Discipline (PD) (*n*=13), High PTSD/High PD (*n*=12), Low PTSD/Low PD (*n*=23), and Low PTSD/High PD (*n*=7) during each memory condition.

Source. Reprinted from Scheeringa MS, Zeanah CH, Myers L, et al.: "Heart Period and Variability Findings in Preschool Children With Posttraumatic Stress Symptoms." *Biological Psychiatry* 55:685–691, 2004. Copyright 2004, with permission from the Society of Biological Psychiatry.

The High PTSD/High PD group is sloping upward, indicating that these children increased RSA when stressed by the Trauma Memory compared with the Pleasant Memory. The High PTSD/Low PD subgroup (the "double whammy" group) slopes downward, indicating that these children decreased RSA (lost flexibility) when stressed by the Trauma Memory compared with the Pleasant Memory.

It is tempting at this point to speculate that the Low PTSD subgroup represents a more "resilient" population of children. For reasons that are not known, they are not "vulnerable" to the effects of their parenting. Whether their parents had low positive discipline or high positive discipline styles, these children responded the same physiologically in both stimulus periods (flat lines in Figure 13–2). Likewise, it is also tempting to speculate that the High PTSD subgroup represented a more "vulnerable" population of children. When these children had parents with high positive discipline, they were able to adapt better and increase RSA. However, when they had parents with low positive discipline, they were not able to adapt as well and decreased RSA. It is not clear what makes one child "resilient" and another "vulnerable" in this context, but these psychophysiological data suggest a distinction.

What do these findings tell us about a nosology for PTSD? Bearing in mind the preliminary nature of these findings, they may suggest two things. First, evidence of resilient and vulnerable subgroups logically leads to speculation about genetically driven traits that confer resilience and/or vulnerability to stress. Second, parenting may influence children's psychophysiology and therefore may also influence the manifestation of symptomatology in parallel or linear fashions. Overall, these findings suggest the existence of subtypes and possible etiological insights.

Scheeringa et al. (2006) were the first to examine a cohort that spanned from 0–18 years of age who had all experienced a similar type of trauma. Within this cohort, children began to manifest more criterion C items (avoidance and numbing items) at around 7 years of age compared with younger children. The difference in the number of criterion C items between the 0- to 6-years group reached statistical significance when compared with the 12- to 18-years group. The shift at age 7 converges neatly with existing models of normal development that describe cognitive shifts around 7 years with the emergence of concrete operations (Piaget 1929) and more advanced executive functions (Pascualvaca and Morote 2000). Also, normative electroencephalographic studies have shown alterations in normal hemispheric coherence development between 5 and 8 years and again between 10 and 14 years (Hanlon et al. 1999) and a progression from undifferentiated to differentiated brain processing from 6 to 12 years, possibly due to the selective atrophy of unused neural circuits (Koenig et al. 2002). This convergence of biobehavioral data implies that the natural maturation of neural networks drives the differential manifestation of criterion C pathology, but this has yet to be integrated into a mechanism-driven theory.

Generating a Developmentally Informed Phenotype: Research Agenda for Validation

How much evidence is enough to declare that the existing diagnostic criteria need to be modified in DSM-V for young children? This is likely to be a controversial topic. Modifications are probably best made as consensus judgments that take into account the complexity and uniqueness of each issue, including research needs and practical clinical needs, on an individual basis. Waiting for more scientific proof, and opting not to modify the PTSD criteria for the next iteration of DSM, make it certain that three to four times fewer young children will be diagnosed with PTSD. From a clinical perspective, those children will not be referred for treatment, and even if treatment is recommended, payors may deny coverage for subsyndromal symptomatology. Limited access to treatment is a major challenge at present; even when young children are referred for treatment, it often is enormously difficult for parents to find competent clinicians. If lowering the threshold results in more children who are symptomatic and impaired being referred to treatment, this might exceed the treatment capacity of communities, but it is not a "disadvantage" for those individual children. On the other hand, if the criteria are modified (with a lower threshold), the potential disadvantages seem relatively greater for research than for clinical purposes. For research studies, overinclusion of "cases" would potentially cloud studies of assessment and treatment response.

If the extant evidence is insufficient to trigger modifications, what else is needed? A research agenda for gathering more evidence should include 1) more studies; 2) more sites, including independent investigative teams; and 3) studies of homogeneous types of traumas (abuse vs. natural disaster vs. accidents vs. witnessing domestic violence vs. witnessing community violence, etc.; single-blow vs. repeated/chronic) that focus on the issues reviewed in this chapter.

In summary, the empirical evidence that has emerged makes a compelling case for the existence of PTSD in young children. Less clear are the exact modifications in criteria that should be applied to preschool children. Few precedents exist for modifying criteria in a disorder that was defined for adults in order to make them more applicable to young children. What is clear, however, is that the DSM-IV criteria and algorithm would benefit from minor modifications. Fortunately, there is now a growing evidence base. The ongoing DSM-V planning process has made an historic step in formally beginning the debate about PTSD in infants and young children.

Commentary: Fred Volkmar, M.D.

As Scheeringa notes in his review, understanding the expression of PTSD as it might manifest in infants and young children is a particularly complex issue. In important ways, this and related conditions offer models for understanding the complicated interaction of stressful life events and developmental, social, and neurobiological factors in the expression of stress-related disorders. Although interest in the effects of stress on children can be traced to the studies of Freud and Burlingham on the responses of children in London to air raids during World War II, it was only in 1987 that DSM-III-R (American Psychiatric Association 1987) permitted the diagnosis of PTSD to be made explicitly in children. The concept, as it is applied to older children, has evolved, and, as Scheeringa emphasizes, it has become possible to consider how the disorder might manifest itself in very young children.

The potential importance of developmental factors is particularly critical here because the perception of the stress relates both to the social factors (e.g., parental distress and availability to the child) and the cognitive ones (appreciation of the stress and ability to manifest characteristic symptoms as presently defined). Although the minor modifications to current DSM-IV criteria that Scheeringa recommends may be sufficient, other, more basic issues also need to be considered, for example, regression as a manifestation of stress response and new manifestations of anxiety not always simply related to the trauma. Issues of measurement and assessment will be particularly critical, and longitudinal studies are sorely needed. Clarification of these issues will provide important insights into the experience of stress in infants and young children and help us better understand sources of continuity and discontinuity of the disorder over the life span.

References

American Psychiatric Association: Diagnostic and Statistical Manual of Mental Disorders, 3rd Edition. Washington, DC, American Psychiatric Association, 1980

American Psychiatric Association: Diagnostic and Statistical Manual of Mental Disorders, 3rd Edition Revised. Washington, DC, American Psychiatric Association, 1987

American Psychiatric Association: Diagnostic and Statistical Manual of Mental Disorders, 4th Edition. Washington, DC, American Psychiatric Association, 1994

Davidson J, Fairbank J: The epidemiology of posttraumatic stress disorder, in Posttraumatic Stress Disorder: DSM-IV and Beyond. Edited by Davidson J, Foa E. Washington, DC, American Psychiatric Press, 1993, pp 147–169

Ghosh-Ippen C, Briscoe-Smith A, Lieberman A: PTSD symptomatology in young children. Paper presented at the annual meeting of the International Society for Traumatic Stress Studies, New Orleans, LA, November 2004

Hanlon H, Thatcher R, Cline M: Gender differences in the development of EEG coherence in normal children. Dev Neuropsychol 16:479–506, 1999

Keane T, Kolb L, Kaloupek D, et al: Utility of psychophysiological measurement in the diagnosis of posttraumatic stress disorder: results from a Department of Veterans Affairs Cooperative Study. J Consult Clin Psychol 66:914–923, 1998

Kilpatrick K, Resnick H: Posttraumatic stress disorder associated with exposure to criminal victimization in clinical and community populations, in Posttraumatic Stress Disorder: DSM-IV and Beyond. Edited by Davidson J, Foa E. Washington, DC, American Psychiatric Press, 1993, pp 113–143

Koenig T, Prichep L, Lehmann D, et al: Millisecond by millisecond, year by year: normative EEG microstates and developmental stages. Neuroimage 16:41–48, 2002

Laor N, Wolmer L, Mayes L, et al: Israeli preschoolers under Scud missile attacks. Arch Gen Psychiatry 53:416–423, 1996

Laor N, Wolmer L, Mayes L, et al: Israeli preschool children under scuds: a 30-month follow-up. J Am Acad Child Adolesc Psychiatry 36:349–356, 1997

Levendosky A, Huth-Bocks A, Semel M, et al: Trauma symptoms in preschool-age children exposed to domestic violence. J Interpers Violence 17:150–164, 2002

McFarlane A: Posttraumatic phenomena in a longitudinal study of children following a natural disaster. J Am Acad Child Adolesc Psychiatry 26:764–769, 1987

Ohmi H, Kojima S, Awai Y, et al: Post-traumatic stress disorder in pre-school aged children after a gas explosion. Eur J Pediatr 161:643–648, 2002

Pascualvaca D, Morote G: Cognitive development from a neuropsychologic perspective, in Functional Neuroimaging in Child Psychiatry. Edited by Ernst M, Rumsey J. Cambridge, United Kingdom, Cambridge University Press, 2000, pp 137–154

Piaget J: The Child's Conception of the World. New York, Harcourt, Brace, 1929

Porges S: Orienting in a defensive world: mammalian modifications of our evolutionary heritage: A Polyvagal Theory. Psychophysiology 32:301–318, 1995

Scheeringa M, Zeanah C, Drell M, et al: Two approaches to the diagnosis of posttraumatic stress disorder in infancy and early childhood. J Am Acad Child Adolesc Psychiatry 34:191–200, 1995

Scheeringa M, Peebles C, Cook C, et al: Toward establishing procedural, criterion, and discriminant validity for PTSD in early childhood. J Am Acad Child Adolesc Psychiatry 40:52–60, 2001

Scheeringa M, Zeanah C, Myers L, et al: New findings on alternative criteria for PTSD in preschool children. J Am Acad Child Adolesc Psychiatry 42:561–570, 2003

Scheeringa MS, Zeanah CH, Myers L, et al: Heart period and variability findings in preschool children with posttraumatic stress symptoms. Biol Psychiatry 55:685–691, 2004

Scheeringa M, Zeanah C, Myers L, et al: Predictive validity in a prospective follow-up of PTSD in preschool children. J Am Acad Child Adolesc Psychiatry 44:899–906, 2005

Scheeringa M, Wright M, Hunt J, et al: Factors affecting the diagnosis and prediction of PTSD symptomatology in children and adolescents. Am J Psychiatry 163:644–651, 2006

Schore A: Dysregulation of the right brain: a fundamental mechanism of traumatic attachment and the psychogenesis of posttraumatic stress disorder. Aust N Z J Psychiatry 36:9–30, 2002

Stuber M, Nader K, Yasuda P: Stress responses after pediatric bone marrow transplantation: preliminary results of a prospective longitudinal study. J Am Acad Child Adolesc Psychiatry 30:952–957, 1991

Summerfield D: The invention of posttraumatic stress disorder and the social usefulness of a psychiatric category. Br Med J 322:95–98, 2001

Zero to Three: Diagnostic Classification: 0–3. Washington, DC, Zero to Three: National Center for Infants, Toddlers, and Families, 1994

14

REACTIVE ATTACHMENT DISORDER

Charles H. Zeanah Jr., M.D.

Current State of the Science

Reactive attachment disorder (RAD) appeared in psychiatric nosologies for the first time in DSM-III (American Psychiatric Association 1980), and the criteria were revised for DSM-III-R (American Psychiatric Association 1987) and again for DSM-IV (American Psychiatric Association 1994). Nevertheless, these revisions were made largely in the absence of any pertinent research, because the first study directly addressing the validity of the criteria did not appear until 1998 (Boris et al. 1998).

With regard to defining attachment disorders, DSM-IV and its text update, DSM-IV-TR (American Psychiatric Association 2000), define RAD as a markedly disturbed and developmentally inappropriate social relatedness in most contexts, beginning before age 5 years, as evidenced by either emotionally withdrawn/inhibited behavior or by indiscriminately social/disinhibited behavior. Neither developmental delay nor autism/pervasive developmental disorder (PDD) is supposed to account for the abnormal social relatedness. In addition, evidence of "pathogenic care," such as occurs in institutionalization, emotional or physical neglect, or multiple changes in primary caregivers, may explain the aberrant social behavior. Furthermore, RAD comprises two types of attachment disorder: an indiscriminately social or "disinhibited" type and an emotionally withdrawn or "inhibited" type (O'Connor and Zeanah 2003). These types appear to have been derived from earlier studies of children in institutions (Tizard and Rees 1975; Wolkind 1974) and from the social behavior of maltreated children (Main and George 1985). Finally, consistent with the notion of disorder, both DSM-IV-TR and ICD-10 (World Health Organization 1992) require that the disturbance be evident across situations and across relationships.

Despite limited attention to validation, attachment disorders do appear to define symptom patterns not captured by criteria of other disorders. In fact, recent evidence indicates that attachment disorder behavior is unassociated or only moderately associated with traditional forms of behavioral/emotional problems in young children (O'Connor and Rutter 2000; Smyke et al. 2002). Insecure and disorganized attachments, on the other hand, are more clearly risk factors for internalizing and externalizing behavior problems (Green and Goldwyn 2002; Greenberg 1999).

Case reports (e.g., Hinshaw et al. 1999; Richters and Volkmar 1994; Zeanah et al. 1993), studies using continuous measures of RAD (Chisholm 1998; Chisholm et al. 1995; O'Connor and Rutter 2000; O'Connor et al. 1999, 2003; Smyke et al. 2002; Zeanah et al. 2003), and studies using categorical measures of RAD (Boris et al. 2005; Zeanah et al. 2004) all have affirmed that these two types of RAD are reliably identified in maltreated, institutionalized, and formerly institutionalized children. Research on international adoptees has focused on the disinhibited type, but studies of children being reared in institutions and maltreated children have included the inhibited type as well. In all, about a dozen studies have contributed to an evaluation of the criteria for RAD in young children. Collectively, these studies have supported the construct validity of RAD, but several important questions have arisen regarding how the disorder is defined.

Advances in Developmental Psychopathology of Reactive Attachment Disorder

Although it has been described formally in the psychiatric nosologies for nearly 25 years, RAD has been studied systematically only recently. There are fewer than a dozen studies, involving only seven samples of young children, that have assessed signs of RAD or applied diagnostic criteria: two samples of internationally adopted children (Chisholm 1998; Chisholm et al. 1995; O'Connor and Rutter 2000; O'Connor et al. 1999, 2003); two samples of children currently institutionalized (Smyke et al. 2002; Zeanah et al. 2002, 2003, 2004); one sample of maltreated toddlers (Zeanah et al. 2004); one sample of maltreated, homeless, and young children attending Head Start (Boris et al. 2004); and one sample of clinic-referred toddlers (Boris et al. 1998).

STUDIES OF MALTREATED CHILDREN

Three studies of young, maltreated children, which assessed the presence or absence of categorical diagnosis of RAD, all indicated that RAD can be reliably diagnosed in young children (see Boris et al. 1998, 2004; Zeanah et al. 2004). These are the first studies that examined formally the reliability and validity of DSM criteria for RAD.

Boris et al. (1998) were the first to examine the reliability of alternative versus DSM-IV diagnostic criteria. They used a retrospective chart review of 48 consecutive clinical cases (mean age, 24 months; range, 9–36 months) referred to an infant psychiatry clinic. The clinic was a primary referral source for the state child protective services (accounting for 79% of cases in this study); the remainder had been referred by private pediatricians or community clinics or had been self-referred. The authors found substantially greater interrater agreement on emotionally withdrawn/inhibited RAD (kappa of 0.70 vs. 0.46) and indiscriminately social/disinhibited RAD (kappa of 0.81 vs. 0.36) using alternative criteria compared with DSM-IV criteria. In addition, using the Parent–Infant Relationship Global Assessment Scale (Zero to Three 1994, 2005), they demonstrated more severe parent–child relationship impairments in children with RAD compared with children with other clinical problems, providing preliminary construct validity for RAD.

In another study, Zeanah et al. (2004) interviewed clinicians treating young children in foster care, using a structured interview designed to assess signs of attachment disorder. Three raters applied diagnostic criteria for RAD to the interview responses in order to determine which children met criteria. There was more than adequate interrater agreement for DSM-IV criteria for RAD (kappa = 0.76–0.80) in that study.

In another recent study, Boris et al. (2004) used structured interviews and a structured clinic observation to diagnose attachment disorders. They compared DSM, ICD, and alternative criteria for attachment disorders in three groups of young children: those in foster care, those in a homeless shelter, and those in Head Start. As expected, the children in foster care were far more often diagnosed with serious disturbances of attachment than those in the other two groups, but only 1 of 69 children in the sample met DSM-IV criteria for RAD, and only 4 met ICD-10 criteria.

STUDIES OF INSTITUTIONALIZED AND POST-INSTITUTIONALIZED CHILDREN

Studies of attachment disorder measured continuously have included studies of institutionalized young children in Romania (O'Connor et al. 1999; Smyke et al. 2002; Zeanah et al. 2002, 2005a) and children adopted out of institutions in Romania into Canada (Chisholm 1998; Chisholm et al. 1995) and into the United Kingdom (O'Connor and Rutter 2000; O'Connor et al. 2003).

Studies of children currently institutionalized have demonstrated expected differences in signs of both types of RAD in different caregiving environments. For example, a study comparing a typical unit in a large institution for young children, in which a large number of caregivers (usually about 17) were involved in the course of a week, with a unit in which the number of caregivers was reduced to 4 found significantly fewer signs of both types of attachment disorder in the unit with fewer caregivers. Significantly fewer signs of RAD also were found among children living at home with their parents and attending child care (Smyke et al. 2002).

In another study of institutionalized children, Zeanah et al. (2005a) found caregiving quality was associated with presence or absence of signs of RAD among institutionalized children. We also found that transferring placement of children from institutions to foster care led to complete disappearance of signs of emotionally withdrawn/inhibited RAD and to diminution but not elimination of signs of indiscriminate/disinhibited RAD (Zeanah et al. 2004). At all points in time, signs of both types of RAD were higher in institutionalized than in community children.

Studies of internationally adopted children have found little evidence of emotionally withdrawn/inhibited RAD in their samples but have found a substantial minority of children who are indiscriminately social/disinhibited (Chisholm 1998). These studies have demonstrated that signs of indiscriminate behavior are linearly related to length of time in institutional care (O'Connor and Rutter 2000). They have also found some association (comorbidity) between indiscriminate/disinhibited behavior and inattention/overactivity, both measured continuously (Kreppner et al. 2001).

Taken together, results of these studies indicate that both categorical and continuous approaches can be used to reliably identify RAD in young children. Furthermore, as expected, signs of RAD and prevalence of RAD are greater in young children who have experienced more severe deprivation (Boris et al. 2004; Chisholm 1998; O'Connor et al. 2003; Smyke et al. 2002; Zeanah et al. 2004, 2005a).

CONSTRUCT VALIDITY

As noted, signs of RAD are clearly more common among children expected to be at greater risk—namely, maltreated and institutionalized children—than among nonmaltreated and noninstitutionalized children (Boris et al. 2004; O'Connor and Rutter 2000; Zeanah et al. 2003). Given that the criteria of RAD specify pathogenic care as the cause of the disorder, it is important to examine caregiving quality in relation to signs of RAD. All institutionalized children share prenatal risk factors and postnatal social deprivation, and yet not all young children raised in institutions develop RAD. In fact, among institutionalized children in Romania, Zeanah et al. (2005a) have shown that individual differences in quality of caregiving are related to individual differences in signs of the emotionally withdrawn/inhibited type of RAD, even after other child and environmental characteristics were controlled for.

With regard to convergent validity, Zeanah et al. (2002) demonstrated convergence of four different measures of indiscriminate behavior that ranged from 0.64

to 0.97, indicating substantial convergence in what these four scales measure. Recent data have demonstrated substantial levels of agreement (kappa = 0.65) between an interview measure of indiscriminate/disinhibited RAD and an observational procedure designed to assess a young child's willingness to "go off" with a stranger (Zeanah et al. 2005b). With regard to the emotionally withdrawn/inhibited type, Zeanah et al. (2005a) also demonstrated moderate convergence ($r = 0.44$) between the degree of attachment development rated from behavior in the Strange Situation Procedure and an interview measure. Thus, interview measures of RAD have been validated preliminarily with observational procedures.

Discriminant validity, on the other hand, has been less well examined. Although it is clear that there are only modest associations between RAD and internalizing and externalizing behavior problems (O'Connor et al. 2003; Smyke et al. 2002; Zeanah et al. 2003), there have been limited attempts to assess discriminant validity with regard to other disorders. Comorbidity has hardly been explored at all.

ATTACHMENT DISORDER IN SCHOOL-AGE CHILDREN

Despite considerable interest, there are few reliable indicators of attachment-disordered behavior in school-age children. In fact, there are no well-validated means of measuring attachment in this group. Current approaches include coding separation reunion behavior (Main and Cassidy 1988), as with younger children; use of family drawings; and story stem completion of narratives (e.g., MacArthur Story Stem Battery [Page and Bretherton 2001], the Separation Anxiety Test [Wright et al. 1995] and Manchester Child Attachment Story Test [Goldwyn et al. 2000; Green et al. 2000]).

Emotionally withdrawn/inhibited attachment disorder has not been described in school-age children. Indiscriminate behavior, on the other hand, has been described in the Tizard longitudinal study (Tizard and Hodges 1978) as well as in some case reports. On the other hand, DSM-IV and ICD-10 criteria for indiscriminant/disinhibited attachment disorder were written to describe the behavior of young children rather than school-aged children, and the reliability and validity of these criteria have not been assessed in the latter group. In fact, it is unlikely that they could be applied without some modification.

Generating a Developmentally Informed Phenotype

Unlike most other disorders in this volume, RAD is an early childhood disorder rather than a disorder well described in older children and adolescents that is being adapted for early childhood. The difficulty of defining RAD is the problem of delineating disorder from more normative behavior.

The reason for this challenge is the very ubiquity of attachment in young children. Under species-typical rearing conditions, virtually all children form selected attachments to their caregivers. A substantial body of evidence indicates that individual differences in quality of attachment relationships, measurable as early as 12 months of age, are predictable from infant–caregiver interactive patterns and predict subsequent psychosocial adaptations. Secure, insecure, and disorganized attachments may be measured both continuously (e.g., Waters and Deane 1985) and categorically (Ainsworth et al. 1978; Main and Hesse 1990) and may be assessed as risk and protective factors in early childhood. In children with clinical disturbances of a variety of types, attachment may be compromised. Thus the question is when the disturbed attachment is the primary problem—in which case it would constitute an attachment disorder—and when attachment is merely one of a number of developmental domains that is compromised.

CRITIQUE OF THE DSM-IV DEFINITION OF REACTIVE ATTACHMENT DISORDER

Despite broad agreement about the two distinctive subtypes of RAD, a number of criticisms of the DSM-IV conceptualization of RAD have been enumerated. Highlighting these areas of controversy begins to form the basis of a research agenda for illuminating this disorder.

The RAD criteria are focused more on abnormalities of social behavior than on disturbed attachment behaviors per se. This approach has led to broader and less well-defined descriptions of social abnormalities rather than to a focus on the disordered attachment behaviors themselves (Zeanah 1996). Studies have been mixed about interrater reliability of DSM-IV criteria for RAD (see Boris et al. 1998, 2004; Zeanah et al. 2004), and questions remain about the diffuseness of the criteria (O'Connor and Zeanah 2003).

Core behavioral features of indiscriminate/disinhibited attachment disorder in young children include inappropriate approach of unfamiliar adults and lack of wariness of strangers as well as a willingness to wander off with strangers. There is also a lack of appropriate physical boundaries, so children may interact with strangers at close distance (that is felt by the stranger as being intrusive) and may even seek out physical contact (O'Connor and Zeanah 2003). These behaviors are reported in many studies and may constitute a coherent set of objectively defined "symptoms." The same kinds of behaviors are implied by DSM-IV, but the language used (e.g., "indiscriminate sociability with marked inability to exhibit appropriate selective attachments") is less specific and somewhat vague. Perhaps for this reason, 8% of 3-year-old children met criteria for RAD in a pediatric clinic sample (H. Egger, personal communication, September 27, 2000), if one ignored the pathogenic care criterion.

"Pathogenic care" has been criticized both for precluding the possibility of intrinsic abnormalities being important etiological contributors and for being unnecessarily vague. Although severe neglect does seem a necessary factor for emotionally withdrawn/inhibited attachment disorder to develop, it is clearly not sufficient. A minority of children who are abused and neglected develop attachment disorders, and even among institutionalized children, most probably do not develop attachment disorders (Zeanah et al. 2003, 2005a). In addition, pathogenic care is not always disclosed or identified in clinical assessments or evaluations. The diagnostic criteria preclude the diagnosis of RAD in children whose maltreatment is not known to the clinician.

On the other hand, indiscriminate behavior has been described in Williams syndrome (Dykens 2003) and in fetal alcohol syndrome (Streissguth et al. 1997), for example, although it is unclear to date whether it is distinguishable from the indiscriminate behavior in RAD. The presence of indiscriminate behavior in children with known biological abnormalities and no evidence of neglect suggests that maintaining the pathogenic care criterion may be justifiable, although more specific indicators of environmental contributors to the disorder would be useful.

Presence of PDD is considered an exclusionary condition for diagnosing RAD, and it may be that these two disorders cannot co-occur. The exclusionary criterion is designed to distinguish between aberrant social behavior induced by severe neglect and deprivation versus that induced by intrinsic central nervous system abnormalities such as autistic spectrum disorders (Zeanah 1996). On the other hand, this criterion may pose a problem, because PDD or "quasi-autistic" behavior seems to be induced at times by institutional rearing. Rutter et al. (1999) reported on a small number of children who met criteria for autism soon after placement in adoptive homes but improved over the 2 subsequent years and no longer met the criteria thereafter. The implication is that it may not be necessary to exclude a diagnosis of attachment disorder among children who exhibit PDD-like behavior immediately following institutional deprivation. This issue clearly needs further study (O'Connor and Zeanah 2003).

Socially aberrant behaviors in attachment disorders are not supposed to be due "solely to developmental delay." This is problematic in that social behaviors in young children who have only developmental delays *by definition* should be delayed rather than deviant. Furthermore, the same conditions that give rise to attachment disorders—that is, social deprivation—are quite likely to give rise to cognitive delays. Indeed, it is somewhat difficult to imagine conditions that might cause RAD without also causing cognitive delays. Thus, given that cognitive delays and attachment disorders will often if not always co-occur, it is unclear why this criterion is included (O'Connor and Zeanah 2003; Zeanah 1996). In a recent sample of institutionalized children in Romania, the convergence of cognitive delays and signs of RAD was modest, in the range of 0.20 and 0.25, suggesting that they are distinguishable issues (Smyke et al. 2007).

The more important issue, in my view, is ensuring that cognitive age be considered with regard to presence or absence of attachment behaviors. This is not a diagnosis that should be made before the child is developmentally expected to have formed selected attachments (i.e., 7–9 months). Thus, a minimum cognitive age for making the diagnosis should be included.

In keeping with the DSM-IV's view of psychopathology within the individual, RAD is not conceptualized as a disorder of the attachment relationship, but rather it is a disorder of social relatedness within the child. Considerable developmental research has determined that attachment may be different between the child and different caregivers. Reactive attachment disorder, in current diagnostic systems, is a disorder of social relatedness within the child rather than a characteristic of that child's relationship with a specific caregiver. As RAD is currently defined (essentially as a disorder of nonattachment), this is not a problem, but if RAD were broadened to cover dyadic, relationship-specific disturbances, it would be a serious limitation in the diagnostic process (Zeanah 1996). Lieberman and Zeanah (1995) and Zeanah and Boris (2000) have described secure base distortions—that is, pathological attachment relationship patterns that are relatively relationship specific rather than traits within the child—but these have not been validated. This challenge to the DSM-IV conceptualization has not been addressed with sufficient data to recommend any modifications in criteria at present.

In summary, although the criteria established by diagnostic systems reflect the history of existing research and clinical reports, they are not always as clear and reliable as they might be. We should hope to be more precise in defining the symptoms of the disorder than are the current diagnostic systems (O'Connor and Zeanah 2003), particularly as new research clarifies many of the issues described herein.

Areas for Future Research

For RAD, assessment of discriminant validity and comorbidity of the disorder are especially pressing concerns, because studies addressing these issues have not yet been conducted. For emotionally withdrawn/inhibited RAD the autistic spectrum disorders, depressive disorders, and posttraumatic stress disorder need to be examined, and for indiscriminate/disinhibited RAD, attention-deficit/hyperactivity disorder needs to be examined.

As noted in this review, RAD has been assessed in research conducted to date both categorically and continuously. A continuous approach, of course, complicates the issue of distinguishing normal variants from "true" psychopathology and complicates assessment of "caseness," whereas a categorical approach may miss clinically significant subsyndromal psychopathology. At this point, from the perspective of a research agenda, there is value in maintaining this dual approach rather than prematurely concluding that one is always preferable.

Unexplained to date is why the two subtypes of RAD, which are phenomenologically so distinct, arise in similar conditions of risk. Correlates of the two subtypes have not been delineated. Whether temperamental disposition, or some aspect of experience, leads to such different clinical pictures is unclear. To date, the major feature that differentiates the two beyond their behavioral manifestations is differential response to improvements in the caregiving environment. Specifically, emotionally withdrawn/inhibited RAD responds much more readily to improved caregiving than indiscriminately social/disinhibited (Zeanah et al. 2005b).

Despite the convergence of extant measures of indiscriminate behavior, clinical experience and observations from extant research suggest that it is a far more heterogeneous condition than has been recognized in the literature (O'Connor and Zeanah 2003). Some young children actively avoid their attachment figures when threatened and seek proximity from strangers selectively rather than indiscriminately. Others are quite aggressive in their interactions with unfamiliar adults—hitting them, throwing objects at them, and so on. Still others are intrusive in their violations of social boundaries—for example, on first meeting hugging (often too tightly) the unfamiliar person, touching/grabbing the stranger's hair, or grabbing the stranger's glasses. The distinctiveness (and stability) of these subtypes is unknown because they have not been described with sufficient precision nor assessed systematically. If these observations are substantiated, however, the approach to studying indiscriminate behavior needs to be more comprehensive. Furthermore, its links to inhibitory control more generally need to be explored. There is some evidence, for example, from amygdala-lesioned Rhesus monkeys that both social and nonsocial impulsivity are intensified in these animals after ablation of the amygdala (Emery and Amaral 2000). Therefore, it should be determined whether young children who lack reticence in approaching unfamiliar people are also more impulsive about approaching novel objects.

Determining impairment related to RAD represents a major challenge, especially for the indiscriminate type of RAD. Evidence to date implicates disturbances in peer relations and possible abnormalities in social cognition rather than more tangible behavior problems. These preliminary findings are compatible with impairment in social relationships, although this issue needs to be explored formally.

Studies of children placed in foster care after serious neglect and those of children raised in institutions offer opportunities to study the effects of timing of intervention on outcomes. Findings to date indicate that attachment begins to form within weeks of placement in an adequate environment (Stovall and Dozier 2000) and that some signs of RAD begin to disappear within months (Zeanah et al. 2005b).

Among the more interesting and challenging questions in developmental neuroscience concern issues of *plasticity*—that is, critical and sensitive periods and the capacity to recover from abnormal states. Plasticity is a salient issue for attachment disorders because the most important question about treatment is the degree to which healthy, robust, and secure attachments can be formed by children who had early experiences characterized by severe neglect and deprivation and who developed attachment disorders as a result. The limited data to date suggest that some recovery occurs, but lasting adverse effects are also evident (O'Connor et al. 2003). Real progress in understanding attachment disorders is likely to be limited until we have a better appreciation of the neural circuitry involved in these behaviors as well as that involved in normative attachment. This represents a major challenge to the field. Phenomenological similarities between RAD indiscriminate/disinhibited and the hypersociability characteristic of Williams syndrome suggest possible similarities in brain functioning. A recent functional magnetic resonance imaging study (Meyer-Lindenberg et al. 2005) demonstrated that individuals with Williams syndrome demonstrated a number of abnormalities while shown frightening pictures. In response to angry or scary faces, individuals with Williams syndrome demonstrated hypoactivation of the amygdala, but when viewing pictures of threatening scenes, such as plane crashes, their amygdalar response was overactive. Three key areas of the prefrontal cortex—the dorsolateral area, involved in establishing and maintaining social goals governing interactions; the medial area, associated with empathy and regulating negative emotions; and the orbitofrontal region, involved in assigning emotional valence to experiences—all were hypoactive in the Williams syndrome participants during stimulus presentation.

Conclusions

Preliminary progress has been made in delineating the features of attachment disorders, which have been reliably demonstrated in young children reared in conditions of neglect and severe deprivation. Preliminary research also has demonstrated responsiveness of these disorders to enhanced caregiving. Much research is needed to more completely explore neurobiological correlates, course, prevalence, and pathogenesis of these disorders of early childhood.

Commentary: Joan L. Luby, M.D.

This comprehensive and cogent review of the nosological history and more recent empirical database on RAD clarifies the history and diagnostic features of this disorder, which is unique in part for its specificity to early childhood.

Several issues seem to make this important, highly disabling and potentially preventable condition elusive to clinicians and researchers. One is the clear and critical importance of the caregiver and caregiving environment to the etiology of the disorder. Related to this is the issue of whether the disorder can be most accurately understood as an internal feature of the individual child or as a disorder of the caregiver–child relationship. It also supports to some degree the unusual use of "pathogenic care" as a criterion for the diagnosis, a rare distinction within established diagnostic nosologies.

Zeanah points out the numerous critical questions that have yet to be addressed to clarify the issue of convergent validity of attachment disorders. This list comprises the need to understand the presence of associated developmental delay in other domains, the need to understand the presence of comorbidity, and, perhaps most importantly, the need to focus more specifically on attachment behaviors, per se, and distinguish them from related but less specific social delays. Populations of institutionalized and adopted children provide compelling opportunities to understand these processes more clearly, and investigations in such populations are ongoing as described.

Two areas of major importance, in my view, are mentioned but not fully developed in this review. One is the issue of the distinction between the inhibited and the disinhibited subtypes. Zeanah outlines the potential lack of specificity of disinhibited behavior and also notes its enduring quality even after other signs of lack of attachment resolve. This is a particularly important issue for mental health clinics, where the disinhibited subtype is far more commonly observed than the inhibited type and therefore can be more easily confused with other disorders.

Another area that is mentioned but not fully elaborated on is the issue of neuroplasticity and critical periods. Although this complex area of brain development is surely beyond the scope of this review, it seems that even in the absence of an elaboration of the details and the gaps in our data on brain development, key facts about the trajectory of the development of attachment are well understood at this point. It seems that these facts could—and should—inform public policy on prevention of attachment disorders based on principles of early placement. Unfortunately, these developmental data have not fully impacted these policies. This represents a clear way that the data to date should affect the lives of young children at risk despite the great need for further study.

References

Ainsworth MDS, Blehar MS, Waters E, et al: Patterns of Attachment: A Psychological Study of the Strange Situation. Hillsdale, NJ, Erlbaum, 1978

American Psychiatric Association: Diagnostic and Statistical Manual of Mental Disorders, 3rd Edition. Washington, DC, American Psychiatric Association, 1980

American Psychiatric Association: Diagnostic and Statistical Manual of Mental Disorders, 3rd Edition Revised. Washington, DC, American Psychiatric Association, 1987

American Psychiatric Association: Diagnostic and Statistical Manual of Mental Disorders, 4th Edition. Washington, DC, American Psychiatric Association, 1994

American Psychiatric Association: Diagnostic and Statistical Manual of Mental Disorders, 4th Edition, Text Revision. Washington, DC, American Psychiatric Association, 2000

Boris NW, Zeanah CH, Larrieu JA, et al: Attachment disorders in infancy and early childhood: a preliminary investigation of diagnostic criteria. Am J Psychiatry 155:295–297, 1998

Boris NW, Hinshaw-Fuselier SS, Smyke AT, et al: Comparing criteria for attachment disorders: establishing reliability and validity in high-risk samples. J Am Acad Child Adolesc Psychiatry 43:568–577, 2004

Boris NW, Zeanah CH, Work Group on Quality Issues: Practice parameters for the assessment and treatment of children and adolescents with reactive attachment disorder of infancy and early childhood. J Am Acad Child Adolesc Psychiatry 44:1206–1219, 2005

Chisholm K: A three year follow-up of attachment and indiscriminate friendliness in children adopted from Romanian orphanages. Child Dev 69:1092–1106, 1998

Chisholm K, Carter MC, Ames EW, et al: Attachment security and indiscriminately friendly behavior in children adopted from Romanian orphanages. Dev Psychopathol 7:283–294, 1995

Dykens EM: Anxiety, fears, and phobias in persons with Williams syndrome. Dev Neuropsychol 23:291–316, 2003

Emery NJ, Amaral DG: The role of the amygdala in primate social cognition, in Cognitive Neuroscience of Emotions. Edited by Lane RD, Nadel L. New York, Oxford University Press, 2000, pp 156–191

Goldwyn R, Stanley C, Smith, V, et al: The Manchester child attachment story task: relationship with parental AAI, SAT and child behavior. Attach Hum Dev 2:71–74, 2000

Green J, Goldwyn R: Attachment disorganization and psychopathology: new findings in attachment research and their potential implications for developmental psychopathology in childhood. J Child Psychol Psychiatry 43:835–846, 2002

Green J, Stanley C, Smith V, et al: A new method of evaluating attachment representations in young school-age children: the Manchester Child Attachment Story Task. Attach Hum Dev 2:48–70, 2000

Greenberg MT: Attachment and psychopathology in childhood, in Handbook of Attachment. Edited by Cassidy J, Shaver P. New York, Guilford, 1999, pp 469–496

Hinshaw-Fuselier S, Boris NW, Zeanah CH: Reactive attachment disorder in maltreated twins. Infant Ment Health J 20:42–59, 1999

Kreppner JM, O'Connor TG, Rutter ML: Can inattention/hyperactivity be an institutional deprivation syndrome? J Abnorm Child Psychol 29:513–528, 2001

Lieberman A, Zeanah CH: Disorders of attachment in infancy. Child Adolesc Psychiatr Clin N Am 4:539–554, 1995

Main M, Cassidy J: Categories of response to reunion with the parent at age 6: predictable from infant attachment classifications and stable over a 1-month period. Dev Psychol 24:1–12, 1988

Main M, George C: Responses of abused and disadvantaged toddlers to distress in age mates: a study in the daycare setting. Dev Psychol 21:407–412, 1985

Main M, Hesse E: Parents' unresolved traumatic experiences are related to infant disorganized status: is frightened and/or frightening parental behavior the linking mechanism? in Attachment in the Preschool Years: Theory, Research and Intervention. Edited by Greenberg M, Cicchetti D, Cummings E. Chicago, IL, University of Chicago Press, 1990

Meyer-Lindenberg RA, Hariri AR, Munoz KE, et al: Neural correlates of genetically abnormal social cognition in Williams Syndrome. Nat Neurosci 8:991–993, 2005

O'Connor TG, Rutter M: Attachment disorder behavior following early severe deprivation: extension and longitudinal follow-up. J Am Acad Child Adolesc Psychiatry 39:703–712, 2000

O'Connor TG, Zeanah CH: Assessment strategies and treatment approaches. Attach Hum Dev 5:223–244, 2003

O'Connor TG, Bredenkamp D, Rutter M: Attachment disturbances and disorders in children exposed to early severe deprivation. Infant Ment Health J 20:10–29, 1999

O'Connor TG, Marvin RS, Rutter M, et al: Child–parent attachment following early institutional deprivation. Dev Psychopathol 15:19–38, 2003

Page T, Bretherton I: Mother– and father–child attachment themes in the story completions of preschoolers from post-divorce families: do they predict relationships with peers and teachers? Attach Hum Dev 3:1–29, 2001

Richters MM, Volkmar F: Reactive attachment disorder of infancy and early childhood. J Am Acad Child Adolesc Psychiatry 33:328–332, 1994

Rutter M, Anderson-Wood L, Beckett C, et al: Quasi-autistic patterns following severe early global privation. J Child Psychol Psychiatry 40:537–549, 1999

Smyke AT, Dumitrescu A, Zeanah CH: Disturbances of attachment in young children, I: the continuum of caretaking casualty. J Am Acad Child Adolesc Psychiatry 41:972–982, 2002

Smyke AT, Koga SF, Johnson DE, et al: The caregiving context in institution-reared and family-reared infants and toddlers in Romania. J Child Psychol Psychiatry 48:210–218, 2007

Stovall KC, Dozier M: The development of attachment in new relationships: single subject analyses for ten foster infants. Dev Psychopathol 12:133–156, 2000

Streissguth A, Barr H, Kogan J, et al: Primary and secondary disabilities in fetal alcohol syndrome, in The Challenge of Fetal Alcohol Syndrome: Overcoming Disabilities. Edited by Streissguth A, Kanter J. Seattle, WA, University of Washington Press, 1997

Tizard B, Hodges J: The effect of early institutional rearing on the development of eight year old children. J Child Psychol Psychiatry 19:99–118, 1978

Tizard B, Rees J: The effect of early institutional learning on the behavior problems and affectional relationships of four-year-old children. J Child Psychol Psychiatry 16:61–73, 1975

Waters E, Deane K: Defining and assessing individual differences in attachment relationships: Q-methodology and the organization of behavior in infancy and early childhood, in Growing Points in Attachment Theory and Research (Monographs of the Society for Research in Child Development 50, Ser No. 209). Edited by Bretherton I, Waters E. Chicago, IL, University of Chicago Press, 1985, pp 41–65

Wolkind SN: The components of "affectionless psychopathy" in institutionalized children. J Child Psychol Psychiatry 15:215–220, 1974

World Health Organization: The ICD-10 Classification of Mental and Behavioral Disorders: Clinical Descriptions and Diagnostic Guidelines. Geneva, Switzerland, World Health Organization, 1992

Wright JC, Binney V, Smith PK: Security of attachment in 8–12-year-olds: a revised version of the Separation Anxiety Test, its psychometric properties and clinical interpretation. J Child Psychol Psychiatry 36:757–774, 1995

Zeanah CH: Beyond insecurity: a reconceptualization of attachment disorders of infancy. J Consult Clin Psychol 64:42–52, 1996

Zeanah CH, Boris NW: Disturbances and disorders of attachment in early childhood, in Handbook of Infant Mental Health, 2nd Edition. Edited by Zeanah CH. New York, Guilford, 2000, pp 353–368

Zeanah CH, Mammen O, Lieberman A: Disorders of attachment, in Handbook of Infant Mental Health. Edited by Zeanah CH. New York, Guilford, 1993, pp 332–349

Zeanah CH, Smyke AT, Dumitrescu A: Disturbances of attachment in young children, II: indiscriminate behavior and institutional care. J Am Acad Child Adolesc Psychiatry 41:983–989, 2002

Zeanah CH, Nelson CA, Fox NA, et al: Studying the effects of institutionalization on brain and behavioral development: the Bucharest early intervention project. Dev Psychopathol 15:885–907, 2003

Zeanah CH, Scheeringa MS, Boris NW, et al: Reactive attachment disorder in maltreated toddlers. Child Abuse Negl 28:877–888, 2004

Zeanah CH, Smyke AT, Koga S, et al: Attachment in institutionalized and community children in Romania. Child Dev 76:1015–1028, 2005a

Zeanah CH, Smyke AT, Koga S: Attachment in institutionalized and non-institutionalized Romanian children. Paper presented at the biennial meeting of the Society for Research in Child Development, Atlanta, GA, April 2005b

Zero to Three: Diagnostic Classification: 0–3R. Washington, DC, Zero to Three: National Center for Infants, Toddlers, and Families, 2005

15

MEASUREMENT OF PSYCHOPATHOLOGY IN CHILDREN UNDER THE AGE OF SIX

Adrian Angold, M.B., MRCPsych
Helen Link Egger, M.D.
Alice Carter, Ph.D.

It is a notable feature of the history of psychiatric research over the past half century that assessment approaches developed originally for adults have proved applicable to ever younger populations. This has resulted in the realization that the onsets of many disorders occur much earlier than was once thought, and that, in turn, has resulted in a substantial expansion of psychiatric research on children and adolescents. However, each step in this "down-aging" process has been accompanied in its early stages by opposition to the idea that younger people can or should be "diagnosed" using the algorithmic approach that began life in the 1970s with the Present State Examination and its accompanying CATEGO diagnostic system (Wing et al. 1981), and the Research Diagnostic Criteria and (Spitzer et al. 1978); continued through the various DSMs; and was incorporated into DSM-IV (American Psychiatric Association 1994) and ICD-10 (World Health Organization 1992). In this chapter, we review the status of the assessment of *preschool* psychopathology. Carter et al. (2004) recently completed a wide-ranging review of measures of psychopathology in young children, so here we focus only on conceptual issues. We recommend, however, that this paper be read in conjunction with that review.

Lack of Self-Reports of Symptoms

The key assessment approach for adult diagnosis—the structured diagnostic interview—works as reliably by *self*-report with children as young as age 9 as it does with adults (Angold and Fisher 1999; Shaffer et al. 1999). It is now generally agreed that diagnoses based on such interviews are as appropriate in children down to this age as they are in adults. There is also agreement that information from interviews conducted with parents about their children and symptom reports from teachers provide reliable (and necessary) clinical information. Standardized assessments are available for all of these informants, and methods for combining information from them into a single diagnostic statement are in routine use with older children.

Unfortunately, research on children younger than 9 years has been unnecessarily limited by uncertainties about whether, or how, to incorporate information reported directly by the child or obtained by observation. The older child assessment literature shows clearly that the absence of one source of information (in this case information derived directly from the child) reduces the *sensitivity* of the diagnostic process (i.e., some children with disorders are missed), but the absence of information directly from the child does not reduce the *validity* of diagnoses made on the basis of information obtained from the remaining informants (i.e., those diagnosed on the basis of other informants' reports really do have disorders) (Angold 2002). The key task is to collect the best possible information from the available informants. After all, most adult research is conducted on the basis of information collected from only a single informant (the patient or study participant). Adult reports about preschool children should, therefore, be seen as being an adequate (if, perhaps, less than perfect) basis for diagnosis.

Lack of a Standard Out-of-Home Setting

Similar considerations apply to the fact that children younger than school age are not expected to be involved in any particular out-of-home activity. Reports from schoolteachers are commonly collected in diagnostic studies of school-age children, but no "standard" equivalent to the teacher is available before the school years. Some children attend preschool, others are in day care, and still others experience no out-of-home care whatsoever. In the last case, no other reporter about the child's behavior except the parent may be available. From a methodological point of view, it is comforting to have information from equivalent informants in each case, but it is appropriate to use the only informants available and to recognize that if a child does not spend time in an out-of-home setting, then they cannot have problems in such a setting. The fact that younger children may be exposed to only a limited range of environments could present a problem in assessing diagnoses such as attention-deficit/hyperactivity disorder (ADHD) that require *impairment* in more than one setting. Whether that will be a problem in practice remains to be seen, but we return to the measurement of impairment later.

Potential Objections to DSM-Style Diagnoses in Younger Children

When it comes to preschoolers, a number of additional objections to DSM-style diagnosis are often raised (reviewed in Emde et al. 1993), and again, we note that similar objections were once raised against childhood diagnosis in general:

1. It has been suggested a) that the boundaries between different types of preschool emotions and behaviors are not as differentiated as they are in older children or adults, and b) that putative psychiatric symptoms and syndromes are inherently unstable and transient in young children. These considerations lead to the conclusion that it is not possible to identify discrete diagnostic categories of disorders. However, a substantial parent/teacher questionnaire literature suggests that preschool psychopathology shows a factor structure rather similar to that seen in older children in both content and complexity (e.g., Achenbach and Rescorla 2000; Koot et al. 1997; Rescorla 1986; Richman et al. 1982; van den Oord et al. 1995). Moreover, there is no evidence that preschool symptoms and syndromes are any less stable than those of older individuals. Indeed, many studies have indicated that preschool externalizing and internalizing problems are a) predictors of negative outcomes years later, and b) often quite stable (e.g., Campbell and Ewing 1990; Fischer et al. 1984; Ialongo et al. 1995; Keenan et al. 1998; Kellam et al. 1998; Lavigne et al. 1998; McGee et al. 1991; Richman et al. 1982). We conclude, therefore, that attempts to diagnose preschool psychiatric disorders are not limited, *a priori*, by syndrome undifferentiation or instability.
2. It is said that current diagnostic systems take little account of the fact that early childhood is a period of rapid development. This may be true, but the more important question is "given that we need a classification of some sort, where should we start?" If the aim is to develop a helpfully developmental scheme that identifies underlying psychopathological consistencies across developmentally varying presentations, it makes sense to start with what we know about older children. The DSM system has been justly criticized for giving only the faintest nods to developmental issues, but that has often been because insufficient data were available to support modification of adult-based diagnostic criteria. On the other hand, the application of adult criteria to older children and adolescents has sometimes led to the surprising conclusion that they worked much better than expected, as in the case of depression (Angold 1988). Investigating the properties of a *non*-developmental set of criteria is, in fact, a good strategy for identifying ways in which those criteria need to be modified to take account of developmental phenomena.

3. There is no doubt that there are developmental changes in the prevalences of specific behaviors that are referred to in standard psychiatric nosologies (attentional abilities, levels of aggression, and separation responses are three obvious examples). The fear is that the application of such nosologies to younger children will result in entirely normative behaviors being labeled as "psychopathology." It is fair to note, however, that DSM often reminds us that symptomatic behaviors should be inappropriate for the child's developmental stage. This issue is an empirical one of determining what the appropriate norms of behavior are. This is true at any age, and the problem is that little information exists about the relevant behavioral norms in younger children. There is great need for such information, and as discussed later, measures are now available for collecting it. This objection is therefore not a problem, in principle, for DSM but rather an indication of work that needs to be done to improve diagnostic validity for younger children.
4. Concern is expressed that the categorical approach to diagnosis locates the pathology "in the child" rather than "in the child's relationships" and so ignores the importance of the relational contexts of a young child's behaviors. For many reasons it has proved useful to regard certain phenomena as being characteristics of individuals, but that does not deny the importance of social context as cause, mediator, and moderator of those phenomena. Furthermore, we already know that some forms of childhood psychopathology (e.g., autism) certainly are better regarded as being characteristics of the child, and old formulations of them in terms of caregiver interaction style have been abandoned. There is also plenty of evidence that

    a. Certain relatively stable behavioral and physiological reaction patterns are associated with current and future psychopathology—see, for example, the many studies of infant temperament and its interactions with physiological measures and social contextual factors (e.g., Bates et al. 1985; Calkins and Fox 1992; Carey et al. 1977; Earls and Jung 1987; Emde et al. 1992; Gersten 1986; Gunnar et al. 1995; Hay and O'Brien 1984; Jansen et al. 1995; Kagan 1994; Maziade et al. 1990; Rothbart and Mauro 1990; Tubman and Windle 1995; Wertlieb et al. 1987); and
    b. There are genetic components involved in preschool behavioral variation and psychopathology (Kagan 1994; van den Oord et al. 1996). The issue is not whether psychopathology "resides in" the child or the child's social context, but how the characteristics of the child and of the social context work to produce psychopathology.

5. There has been a great deal more work on infant and early childhood *temperament* than there has been on psychopathology, and some would argue that what DSM might call "psychopathology" is better regarded as being extremes of temperament. However, as Lahey (2004) has pointed out:

> Before one can relate temperament to psychopathology, one must define these terms in independent ways. This is more difficult than it first appears, largely because there is no inherent distinction between temperament and psychopathology in nature. Rather, we theorists have *imposed* a distinction in which some aspects of behavior are classified as temperament and some are classified as psychopathology. (p. 88)

Indeed, at the level of questionnaire measures of temperament and psychopathology, there is enormous item overlap. For instance, by our count, the 94-item Children's Behavior Questionnaire (a temperament measure; Rothbart et al. 2001) contains 24 items that are identical to, or the inverse of, items found in the 108-item Child Behavior Checklist, 1½–5 Years (Achenbach and Rescorla 2000). Examination of the rest of the items in these two measures reveals even greater conceptual overlap. However, there are great differences between the conceptualization of temperament and that of psychopathology. Although there is no generally agreed-on formal definition of psychiatric disorders, it is probably uncontroversial to state that, as implemented by DSM-IV and ICD-10, psychiatric disorders are characteristic clusterings of behavioral, emotional, and psychological phenomena, or extremes of behavioral/emotional/psychological dimensions, that lead to distress, disability, or negative outcomes over time. There is also no generally agreed-on definition of temperament (Frick 2004), but Rothbart's oft-quoted definition—"constitutionally based, individual differences in reactivity and self-regulation" (Rothbart et al. 2001)—will serve here to show that psychiatric disorders and temperamental extremes are conceptually different things. Certainly some "extremes of temperament" could qualify as psychiatric disorders, but extremity on a temperament dimension is neither a necessary nor a sufficient condition for the identification of a psychiatric disorder. It is also important to recognize that psychiatric disorders encompass many symptoms that are not included in any temperament assessment. This is particularly true at the severe end of the spectrum, and so, from a measurement perspective, the temperamental approach fails to cover what is clinically often the most important material. The point here is not that there is anything wrong with the measurement of temperament, but that temperament does not provide a viable conceptual or practical framework for psychopathology as a whole.

6. Some worry that the assignment of psychiatric diagnoses to young children carries a risk of labeling the child, who might then be defined or stigmatized in ways that might adversely affect his or her future development (Campbell 1990). This argument was raised long ago against the use of psychiatric diagnosis for children and adolescents in general. It has largely fallen by the wayside as the utility of specific treatments for specific diagnoses has been established (as with stimulants in the treatment of ADHD; Goldman et al. 1998), and it seems likely to continue thus as we learn more about preschool psychopathology.

There are also many circumstances in which a diagnosis *has* to be made. For instance, the decision to provide treatment services must be based upon a categorical (yes/no) decision about whether there is "something that needs treatment." "Something that needs treatment" is a crude form of diagnosis. When continuous measures derived from questionnaires are used to measure psychopathology, cutpoints are still applied to define "clinical ranges." Being in the "clinical range" or "above a certain t-score on a subscale" are both forms of diagnosis. The descriptive, prescriptive nosologies embodied in DSM-IV-TR and the Diagnostic Classification: 0–3 (Zero to Three 1994) are in many ways no different from these examples, except that they rely upon specific categories derived from clinical experience. We should also be aware that DSM-IV-TR diagnoses are mandated for the receipt of federal block grant funds to states for the provision of services for seriously emotionally disturbed children (U.S. Government 1993).

In summary, we conclude that DSM-style approaches to the diagnosis of preschoolers are as appropriate as such approaches to diagnosis at other ages.

Available Measures

As we mentioned earlier, Carter et al. (2004) recently reviewed the literature on this topic, and their key finding is that we have in place the basic toolset for the assessment of psychopathology in young children, down to the age of 2 years at least. For instance, "the assessment methodology currently exists to routinely screen very young children for social-emotional and behavior problems as well as delays in the acquisition of competencies in pediatric settings as well as in early intervention programs." (p. 128). There are also parent and teacher/caregiver questionnaire assessments (like the Infant-Toddler Social and Emotional Assessment [Carter et al. 2003] or the Child Behavior Checklist, 1½–5 Years [Achenbach and Rescorla 2000]) available to assess general levels of psychopathology. However, measures of this sort do not provide the detailed symptom coverage required to make full DSM diagnostic assessments.

Until recently, no standardized diagnostic interviews were available for use with parents of preschoolers, and "diagnostic" assessments had relied upon questionnaires plus unstructured clinical interviews (e.g., Lavigne et al. 1993, 1996) or DSM-IV-referenced rating scales (Gadow and Sprafkin 1997, 2000; Gadow et al. 2001; Sprafkin and Gadow 1996). More recently, several groups have modified sections of preexisting diagnostic interviews like the Diagnostic Interview Schedule for Children–DSM-IV version or the Kiddie Schedule for Affective Disorders and Schizophrenia for diagnostic purposes (e.g., Keenan and Wakschlag 2000; Keenan et al. 1997; Luby and Morgan 1997; Luby et al. 2003) or developed semistructured interviews for particular diagnoses (e.g., Scheeringa et al. 2003). These appear to have worked as expected in practice, but their test-retest reliabilities have not been established.

The Preschool Age Psychiatric Assessment (PAPA) is a parent-report interview that covers a wide range of diagnoses (but not learning disorders or pervasive developmental disorders), and it has recently been found to have test-retest reliabilities comparable with those achieved with interviews for older children and adults (Egger et al. 2006). The structure of the PAPA makes it possible to compare the reliability and validity of unmodified DSM-IV-TR or ICD-10 criteria with proposed alternative criteria for preschoolers, as well as to determine the normative ranges of potentially pathological behaviors (Egger and Angold 2004).

It appears, therefore, that the diagnostic interview approach is likely to work just as well with preschoolers down to age 2 as it does at later ages. In the literature on older children, the specifics of interview format (e.g., respondent- vs. interviewer-based) seem to have made little difference to reliability, and there is no reason to suppose that variations in interview format will have much effect on the reliability of parent interviews about their younger children.

In the area of the pervasive developmental disorders, the Autism Diagnostic Interview–Revised (Lord et al. 1994), and the Autism Diagnostic Observation Schedule–Generic (Lord et al. 1989) have undergone extensive development aimed at making them suitable for use with children as young as 2 years (Volkmar et al. 2004).

However, for non–autism-spectrum diagnoses, the questions of whether and how to incorporate observational measures, or material elicited directly from the child, have not been settled. A variety of measures have been developed that focus on the free responses of children to story stems, puppet interactions (Measelle et al. 1998; Warren et al. 2000), and simple picture-based questionnaire responses (Ialongo et al. 1995; Martini et al. 1990). Wakschlag et al. (2002) developed an observational assessment modeled conceptually on the Autism Diagnostic Observation Schedule for eliciting and assessing behaviors relevant to the diagnosis of the disruptive behavior disorders in preschool children.

The Problem of Impairment

How can we measure psychosocial impairment in very young children? The problem is that younger children are not expected to be able to do very much in the way of taking responsibility for self-care, having stable friendships, performing well at school, or engaging in extracurricular activities. So the sorts of measures of psychosocial impairment and disability that have become a standard part of the assessment of psychopathology in older children do not appear to be immediately applicable to younger children. Here again, the issue of there not being a single non-home type of setting in which all children under school age are engaged is relevant. All younger children are not enrolled in a relatively standardized range of childcare or preschool activities the way school-age children are, so each child's "test" for impairment is subject to greater stimulus variation than is the case at later ages. In part, there is nothing that can be done about this—if one is not engaged in certain activities, one simply cannot be impaired in them, unless the nonengagement is clearly generated by psychopathology. If a child has not been exposed to a particular setting, then we simply will not be able to tell whether he or she would have been impaired in it. Work is currently under way to produce robustly usable measures of impairment for younger children.

However, a way around this limitation suggests itself if we are willing to allow negative effects on the lives of others to stand in for impairment in the child's own functioning. The idea here is that the younger child is intimately bound to his or her caretaker's social functioning (Carter et al. 2004). It therefore makes sense to see negative effects of the child's psychopathology on parents' and caretakers' social lives and activities as being equivalent to impairment in the child's functioning. We refer here to what has usually been called parental or caretaker "burden" or "impact" (Messer et al. 1996). Measures of burden or impact have proven to be quite straightforwardly applicable to toddlers and preschoolers, and such a measure is included in the PAPA.

Conclusions

At the symptom level, a broad range of assessment tools is now available for children between ages 2 and 5 years. A lack of measures can no longer be seen as a reason for not pursuing research in this age group. A priority here is to use the detailed symptom ratings available from the newer structured interviews to establish norms and symptomatic cutoffs for behaviors that have been seen as being "characteristic" of younger children, such as disobedience or short attention span.

More work is needed in relation to impairment and the incorporation of child self-report and observational materials into the production of the final diagnosis, but the present parlous lack of information about psychiatric disorders in younger children can no longer be put down to deficiencies in the available assessment tools. Rather the fault now is in the lack of resources committed to deploying the excellent tools we have.

Commentary: Lauren S. Wakschlag, Ph.D., and Bennett L. Leventhal, M.D.

By examining the issue of measurement in the diagnosis of early childhood psychopathology within historical context, Drs. Angold, Egger, and Carter provide an excellent framework with which to analyze the current state of the science. There are none better suited to frame this issue, because their own work is at the leading edge of the "measurement revolution" in assessing clinical problems in young children.

These authors suggest that we should not hold ourselves to a higher standard than has been accepted for diagnosis of older children and adults. They make a cogent argument that the standard of "good enough" has been achieved in relation to preschool psychopathology: substantial empirical evidence indicates that DSM-IV-TR criteria can be meaningfully applied to the assessment of preschool children.

Meeting this standard of "good enough" has freed us from the recurrent question about the basic existence of psychopathology in young children, but it obligates us to thoughtfully characterize the actual expression of clinical phenomena during this developmental period. Achieving this will require careful integration of developmental and clinical science. Once completed, this will at last afford clinical scientists the opportunity to equip DSM-V with a truly developmentally informed nosology. After careful consideration, one may even conclude that the dynamic tension around the validity of diagnosis in young children has already served as the catalyst for the creation of an unparalleled set of developmentally specific diagnostic instruments. For the first time, such instruments may enable the establishment of clinical criteria firmly anchored within a developmental framework. We can then test whether this level of developmental specificity has incremental utility for the identification and treatment of clinical disorders.

Rapid advances in the basic sciences since the development of DSM-IV suggest that in the not-too-distant future, nosology may be substantially informed by etiological mechanisms. This will require precise phenotypic characterization. Such precision will be especially important for the description of clinically relevant behaviors during early childhood, when the emergence of early signs and symptoms of many disorders is first evident.

With developmentally validated clinical assessment tools in hand, early childhood psychopathology has firmly earned its place in the ranks of clinical disorders, but there are "miles to go before we sleep."

References

Achenbach TM, Rescorla LA: Manual for the ASEBA Preschool Forms and Profiles: An Integrated System of Multi-Informant Assessment. Burlington, VT, University of Vermont Department of Psychiatry, 2000

American Psychiatric Association: Diagnostic and Statistical Manual of Mental Disorders, 4th Edition. Washington, DC, American Psychiatric Association, 1994

American Psychiatric Association: Diagnostic and Statistical Manual of Mental Disorders, 4th Edition, Text Revision. Washington, DC, American Psychiatric Association, 2000

Angold A: Childhood and adolescent depression, II: research in clinical populations. Br J Psychiatry 153:476–492, 1988

Angold A: Diagnostic interviews with parents and children, in Child and Adolescent Psychiatry: Modern Approaches, 4th Edition. Edited by Rutter M, Taylor E. Oxford, United Kingdom, Blackwell Scientific Publications, 2002, pp 32–51

Angold A, Fisher PW: Interviewer-based interviews, in Diagnostic Assessment in Child and Adolescent Psychopathology. Edited by Shaffer D, Lucas C, Richters J. New York, Guilford, 1999, pp 34–64

Bates JE, Maslin CA, Frankel KA: Attachment security, mother–child interaction, and temperament as predictors of behavior-problem ratings at age three years. Growing Points in Attachment Theory and Research. Monographs of the Society for Research in Child Development 50:167–193, 1985

Calkins SD, Fox NA: The relations among infant temperament, security of attachment, and behavioral inhibitions at twenty-four months. Child Dev 63:1456–1472, 1992

Campbell SB: Behavior Problems in Preschool Children: Developmental and Clinical Issues. New York, Guilford, 1990

Campbell SB, Ewing LJ: Follow-up of hard-to-manage preschoolers: adjustment at age 9 and predictors of continuing symptoms. J Child Psychol Psychiatry 6:871–889, 1990

Carey WB, Fox M, McDevitt SC: Temperament as a factor in early school adjustment. Pediatrics 60:621–624, 1977

Carter AS, Briggs-Gowan MJ, Jones SM, et al: The Infant-Toddler Social and Emotional Assessment (ITSEA): factor structure, reliability, and validity. J Abnorm Child Psychol 31:495–514, 2003

Carter AS, Briggs-Gowan MJ, Davis NO: Assessment of young children's social-emotional development and psychopathology: recent advances and recommendations for practice. J Child Psychol Psychiatry 45:109–134, 2004

Earls F, Jung KG: Temperament and home environment characteristics as causal factors in the early development of childhood psychopathology. J Am Acad Child Adolesc Psychiatry 26:491–498, 1987

Egger HL, Angold A: The Preschool Age Psychiatric Assessment (PAPA): a structured parent interview for diagnosing psychiatric disorders in preschool children, in Handbook of Infant, Toddler, and Preschool Mental Assessment. Edited by DelCarmen-Wiggins R, Carter A. New York, Oxford University Press, 2004, pp 223–243

Egger HL, Erkanli A, Keeler G, et al: The test-retest reliability of the Preschool Age Psychiatric Assessment. J Am Acad Child Adolesc Psychiatry 45:538–549, 2006

Emde RN, Plomin R, Robinson J, et al: Temperament, emotion, and cognition at fourteen months: the MacArthur longitudinal twin study. Child Dev 63:1437–1455, 1992

Emde RN, Bingham RD, Harmon RJ: Classification and the diagnostic process in infancy, in Handbook of Infant Mental Health. Edited by Zeanah CH Jr. New York, Guilford, 1993, pp 225–235

Fischer M, Rolf JE, Hasazi JE, et al: Follow-up of a preschool epidemiological sample: cross-age continuities and predictions of later adjustment with internalizing and externalizing dimensions of behavior. Child Dev 55:137–150, 1984

Frick P: Integrating research on temperament and childhood psychopathology: its pitfalls and promise. J Clin Child Adolesc Psychol 33:2–7, 2004

Gadow KD, Sprafkin J: Early Childhood Symptom Inventory–4 Norms Manual. Stony Brook, NY, Checkmate Plus, 1997

Gadow KD, Sprafkin J: Early Childhood Symptom Inventory–4 Screening Manual. Stony Brook, NY, Checkmate Plus, 2000

Gadow KD, Sprafkin J, Nolan EE: DSM-IV symptoms in community and clinic preschool children. J Am Acad Child Adolesc Psychiatry 40:1383–1392, 2001

Gersten M: The contribution of temperament to behavior in natural contexts. PhD diss., Harvard University Graduate School of Education, Cambridge, MA, 1986

Goldman LS, Genel M, Bezman RJ, et al: Diagnosis and treatment of attention-deficit/hyperactivity disorder in children and adolescents. JAMA 279:1100–1107, 1998

Gunnar MR, Porter FL, Wolf CM, et al: Neonatal stress reactivity: predictions to later emotional temperament. Child Dev 66:1–13, 1995

Hay DA, O'Brien PJ: The role of parental attitudes in the development of temperament in twins at home, school, and in test situations. Acta Genet Med Gemellol (Roma) 36:239–248, 1984

Ialongo N, Edelsohn G, Werthamer-Larsson L, et al: The significance of self-reported anxious symptoms in first grade children: prediction to anxious symptoms and adaptive functioning in fifth grade. J Child Psychol Psychiatry 36:427–437, 1995

Jansen RE, Fitzgerald HE, Ham HP, et al: Pathways into risk: temperament and behavior problems in three- to five-year-old sons of alcoholics. Alcohol Clin Exp Res 19:501–509, 1995

Kagan J: Galen's Prophecy: Temperament in Human Nature. New York, Basic Books, 1994

Keenan K, Wakschlag LS: More than the terrible twos: the nature and severity of behavior problems in clinic-referred preschool children. J Abnorm Child Psychol, 28:33–46, 2000

Keenan K, Shaw DS, Walsh B, et al: DSM-III-R disorders in preschool children from low-income families. J Am Acad Child Adolesc Psychiatry 36:620–627, 1997

Keenan K, Shaw D, Delliquadri E, et al: Evidence for the continuity of early problem behaviors: application of a developmental model. J Abnorm Child Psychiatry 26:441–452, 1998

Kellam S, Ling X, Merisca R, et al: The effect of the level of aggression in the first grade classroom on the course and malleability of aggressive behavior into middle school. Dev Psychopathol 10:165–185, 1998

Koot HM, van den Oord EJCG, Verhulst FC, et al: Behavioral and emotional problems in young preschoolers: cross-cultural testing of the validity of the Child Behavior Checklist/2–3. J Abnorm Child Psychol 25:183–196, 1997

Lahey B: Commentary: role of temperament in developmental models of psychopathology. J Clin Child Adolesc Psychol 33:88–93, 2004

Lavigne JV, Binns HJ, Christoffel KK, et al: Behavioral and emotional problems among preschool children in pediatric primary care: prevalence and pediatricians' recognition. Pediatrics 91:649–655, 1993

Lavigne JV, Gibbons RD, Christoffel KK, et al: Prevalence rates and correlates of psychiatric disorders among preschool children. J Am Acad Child Adolesc Psychiatry 35:204–214, 1996

Lavigne JV, Arend R, Rosenbaum D, et al: Psychiatric disorders with onset in the preschool years, I: stability of diagnoses. J Am Acad Child Adolesc Psychiatry 37:1246–1254, 1998

Lord C, Rutter M, Goode S, et al: Autism Diagnostic Observation Schedule: a standardized observation of communicative and social behavior. J Autism Dev Disord 19:185–212, 1989

Lord C, Rutter M, LeCouteur A: Autism Diagnostic Interview—Revised: a revised version of a diagnostic interview for caregivers of individuals with possible pervasive developmental disorders. J Autism Dev Disord 24:659–685, 1994

Luby JL, Morgan K: Characteristics of an infant/preschool psychiatric clinic sample: implications for clinical assessment and nosology. Infant Ment Health J 18:209–220, 1997

Luby J, Heffelfinger A, Mrakotsky C, et al: The clinical picture of depression in preschool children. J Am Acad Child Adolesc Psychiatry 42:340–348, 2003
Martini DR, Strayhorn JM, Puig-Antich J: A symptom self-report measure for preschool children. J Am Acad Child Adolesc Psychiatry 29:594–600, 1990
Maziade M, Caron C, Côté R, et al: Extreme temperament and diagnosis. Arch Gen Psychiatry 47:477–484, 1990
McGee R, Partridge F, Williams S, et al: A twelve-year follow-up of preschool hyperactive children. J Am Acad Child Adolesc Psychiatry 30:224–232, 1991
Measelle JR, Ablow JC, Cowan PA, et al: Assessing young children's views of their academic, social, and emotional lives: an evaluation of the self-perception scales of the Berkeley Puppet Interview. Child Dev 69:1556–1576, 1998
Messer SC, Angold A, Costello EJ, et al: The Child and Adolescent Burden Assessment (CABA): measuring the family impact of emotional and behavioral problems. Int J Methods Psychiatr Res 6:261–284, 1996
Rescorla LA: Preschool psychiatric disorders: diagnostic classification and symptom patterns. J Am Acad Child Psychiatry 25:162–169, 1986
Richman N, Stevenson J, Graham P: Preschool to School: A Behavioural Study. London, England, Academic Press, 1982
Rothbart MK, Derryberry DE: A psychobiological approach to the development of temperament, in Temperament: Individual Differences at the Interface of Biology and Behavior, 2nd Edition. Edited by Bates JE, Wachs TD. Washington, DC, American Psychological Association, 1994, pp 83–116
Rothbart MK, Mauro JA: Temperament, behavioral inhibition, and shyness in childhood, in Handbook of Social and Evaluation Anxiety. Edited by Leitenberg H. New York, Plenum, 1990, pp 139–160
Rothbart M, Ahadi S, Hersey K, et al: Investigations of temperament at three to seven years: The Children's Behavior Questionnaire. Child Dev 72:1394–1408, 2001
Scheeringa MS, Zeanah C, Myers L, et al: New findings on alternative criteria for PTSD in preschool children. J Am Acad Child Adolesc Psychiatry 42:561–571, 2003
Shaffer D, Fisher PW, Lucas CP: Respondent-based interviews, in Diagnostic Assessment in Child and Adolescent Psychopathology. Edited by Shaffer D, Lucas CP, Richters JE. New York, Guilford, 1999, pp 3–33
Spitzer RL, Endicott J, Robins E: Research diagnostic criteria: rationale and reliability. Arch Gen Psychiatry 35:773–782, 1978
Sprafkin J, Gadow KD: Early Childhood Inventories Manual. Stony Brook, NY, Checkmate Plus, 1996
Tubman JG, Windle M: Continuity of difficult temperament in adolescence: relations with depression, life events, family support, and substance use across a one-year period. J Youth Adolesc 24:133–153, 1995
U.S. Government: Federal Register 58, 29425, 1993
van den Oord EJCG, Koot HM, Boomsma DI, et al: A twin-singleton comparison of problem behaviour in 2–3 year-olds. J Child Psychol Psychiatry 36:449–458, 1995
van den Oord EJCG, Verhulst FC, Boomsma DI: A genetic study of maternal and paternal ratings of problem behaviors in 3 year-old twins. J Abnorm Psychol 105:349–357, 1996

Volkmar FR, Lord C, Bailey A: Autism and pervasive developmental disorders. J Child Psychol Psychiatry 45:135–170, 2004

Wakschlag LS, Leventhal BL, Danis B, et al: Manual for Disruptive Behavior Diagnostic Observational Schedule. Chicago, IL, University of Chicago, 2002

Warren SL, Emde RN, Sroufe A: Internal representations: predicting anxiety from children's play narratives. J Am Acad Child Adolesc Psychiatry 39:100–107, 2000

Wertlieb D, Weigel C, Springer T, et al: Temperament as a moderator of children's stressful experiences. Am J Orthopsychiatry 57:234–245, 1987

Wing JK, Bebbington P, Robins LN: What Is a Case? London, England, Grant McIntyre, Ltd, 1981

World Health Organization: International Statistical Classification of Diseases and Related Health Problems, 10th Revision. Geneva, Switzerland, World Health Organization, 1992

Zero to Three: Diagnostic Classification: 0–3. Washington, DC, Zero to Three: National Center for Infants, Toddlers, and Families, 1994

16

NOSOLOGY OF MOOD DISORDERS IN PRESCHOOL CHILDREN

State of Knowledge and Future Directions

Joan L. Luby, M.D.

Depression

A long history of skepticism among developmental theorists and clinicians about the possibility that young children could experience many of the key emotions inherent to mood disorders has, until recently, thwarted serious consideration of clinical mood symptoms among young children. The concept of mood disorders arising in preschoolers is one that often meets resistance, perhaps because it is both disturbing and counterintuitive to imagine a young child having a serious mood disturbance. In light of the unfortunate social stigma that continues to surround mental disorders, it is important to avoid prematurely or incorrectly diagnosing young children with mood disorders. At the same time, the potential for more effective intervention earlier in life makes it equally important to identify clinical mood disturbances at the earliest possible developmental point.

HISTORY OF RECOGNITION OF DEPRESSIVE MANIFESTATIONS IN EARLY CHILDHOOD

In the 1940s, the first reports of the altered behaviors and emotional expressions of infants with a presumed depressive syndrome were provided by Rene Spitz. His remarkable descriptions of the behaviors of institutionalized infants experiencing relative emotional neglect represent the first published reports of depressed mood in human infants (Spitz 1949). Despite how robust and remarkable these observations were, they had relatively little clinical or developmental impact, or application, until high-risk studies of the infants of depressed mothers, initiated in the early 1980s, renewed interest and attention to alterations in infant affect. These high-risk studies demonstrated observable changes in infant affect expression during mother–infant interactions—which were also detected in other interpersonal interactions and suggested generalization—and set the stage for later clinical investigations of clinical depression in preschoolers (Field et al. 1998).

VALIDATION OF AGE-ADJUSTED CRITERIA FOR DEPRESSION

Explorations of clinical depression arising in young children gained momentum in the early 1980s, at which time case studies and controlled investigations in small samples were conducted. Despite the fact that these studies were hampered by lack of developmentally sensitive measures and use of restrictive DSM-III (American Psychiatric Association 1980) criteria, they suggested that a depressive syndrome might be identifiable in preschool children (e.g., Kashani 1982; Kashani and Carlson 1985; Kashani and Ray 1983; Kashani et al. 1984, 1986; Poznanski and Zrull 1970). Kashani et al. (1986) studied DSM-III symptoms of depression in community samples of preschoolers and identified "concerning symptoms," but because few children met formal criteria for major depressive disorder (MDD), the authors suggested the possible need for developmental modifications to the criteria for depression for preschoolers.

Building on this work more recently, my colleagues and I conducted a larger investigation focusing on validation of age-adjusted criteria for preschool depression utilizing newly developed age-appropriate assessment tools. A sample of 174 children between the ages of 3.0 and 5.6 years recruited from community pediatric and specialty mental health clinics was assessed using a now-validated screening checklist (Luby et al. 2004a). A group of children with two or more putative depressive symptoms as well as those with symptoms of attention-deficit/hyperactivity disorder (ADHD)/oppositional defiant disorder (ODD) and those with no symptoms were included for study. Children with major medical or neurological disorders, serious developmental delays, or autistic spectrum disorder were excluded. Preschoolers and their caregivers underwent a comprehensive mental health and developmental assessment that had both dyadic and individual components, utilizing a multimodal age-appropriate assessment strategy (e.g., observational assessments, puppet interviews, parent interviews). Salivary cortisol was collected both before and after mildly stressful events to explore whether alterations in hypothalamic-pituitary-adrenal axis activity could be identified similar to those known in depressed adults.

Phenomenology of Depression

Findings from this investigation demonstrated that the "typical" symptoms of MDD could be identified in preschool children when symptom states were "translated" to describe age-appropriate manifestations of DSM-IV (American Psychiatric Association 1994) MDD constructs (Luby et al. 2003b, 2003c). Developmental modification of symptom manifestations included that *anhedonia* was described as the "inability to enjoy activities and play" and that *negative themes in play* were considered as an adjusted manifestation of a depressive symptom in lieu of (or in addition to) direct expression of sadness, guilt, negative thoughts, or other related depressive symptoms.

Biological Correlates of Depression

We found a unique pattern of cortisol reactivity in response to psychosocial stress characterized by persistently increasing cortisol levels in the depressed group in contrast to a U-shaped curve in comparison groups (Luby et al. 2003a). This finding, which bears similarity to those established in depressed adults and animal models, suggests that biological changes are already occurring in very early onset depressive states. Biological correlates of depression in preschool children confer additional validity according to the schema developed by Robins and Guze (1970). Adding to validity in a similar fashion, neuropsychological impairments and differences in emotion labeling also have been detected in the depressed group (Mrakotsky 2001).

Continuity of Established Nosology in Young Children

Taken together, our findings have supported the basic integrity of the core depressive constructs (the adult manifestation of which are described in DSM-IV-TR) for application as early as age 3 years. Some earlier investigators had suggested that young children would manifest "masked" symptoms of depression instead of depressed affect. Instead, as in investigations of this issue in older depressed children, we found that although masked symptoms of depression appeared in young children, they occurred much less frequently than "typical" symptoms such as sadness, irritability, or vegetative signs (e.g., changes in activity, sleep and appetite) (Carlson and Cantwell 1980; Luby et al. 2003a, 2003b, 2003c).

Depressive Subtypes

Notably, the inability to enjoy activities and play known as "anhedonia" emerged as a highly specific symptom of depression among preschool children in this investigation. This symptom was reported only by the parents of depressed preschoolers and was never reported by any parent in either comparison group. Depressed preschoolers whose parents reported that they displayed anhedonia were more severely depressed than those without anhedonia and met criteria for a melancholic depression as described in the DSM-IV-TR (Luby et al. 2004b). Furthermore, anhedonia also emerged as a highly specific symptom of depression because it was not observed in any child in the psychiatric or healthy comparison groups. Therefore, this subgroup is of interest as a potentially more severe, biologically based, "endogenous" depressive subtype, and it has been targeted for ongoing investigations of structural neurobiological changes (e.g., structural neuroimaging).

The notion that an inability to experience pleasure and joy from activities and play would be a clinical symptom in a preschooler and a marker of serious psychopathology is consistent with the concept that young children are inherently joyful and pleasure seeking. Therefore, impairments in the young child's ability to experience joy and pleasure could be a marker of a clinical problem. In keeping with this concept, preschoolers were more likely to appear and to describe themselves as "less happy" rather than as overtly "sad" than same-age nondepressed peers (Luby et al. 2003a, 2003b).

Familial Aggregation and Impairment

Higher familial aggregation of affective disorders was also found in the first- and second-degree relatives of the depressed group in our investigation (Luby et al. 2002). Familial continuity of disorders, whether genetic or psychosocial, is another feature of a valid psychiatric disorder according to the schema proposed by Robins and Guze (1970).

The conclusion that these children were "impaired" and therefore in need of clinical attention was supported by the finding of significantly lower scores (more than two standard deviations below the normative mean) on the social scale of the Vineland Adaptive Behavior Scales compared with those of preschoolers without a psychiatric disorder. The requirement for impairment is also a feature of DSM criteria for clinical caseness.

Convergent Validity

Notably, the symptom of anhedonia, which appeared as a robust marker of depression when reported by the parent, was also evident when objective observational measures of the child's behavior during dyadic interactions were used (Belden and Luby 2006; Luby et al. 2006). Anhedonically depressed preschoolers were observed as less enthusiastic than preschoolers without psychiatric disorders during a dyadic task with their mothers. This finding provides some support for the validity of parent report measures, which is important because of the concern that parent reports of depressive symptoms in the child are merely the distorted perception of mood-disordered parents. Depressed preschoolers in general (anhedonic and nonanhedonic subgroups) were also observed to display numerous other differences in behavior along expected lines, providing objective observational evidence of more negative and fewer positive behaviors and emotions among depressed preschoolers. Similar observational findings have also been provided by Mol Lous et al. (2002), who reported alterations in play behavior among preschool children who received a clinical diagnosis of depression (finding delayed and impoverished play) compared with well control subjects.

Questions About Episode Duration

It remains unclear whether young children with the valid depressive symptoms experienced symptoms in a sustained fashion over a 2-week duration as required by DSM-IV. Although parents of "depressed" preschoolers endorsed that the child had symptoms "for a long time each day," "most of the day," and "almost every day," the majority of this group did not endorse that the symptoms occurred for "2 weeks in a row" on the Diagnostic Interview Schedule for Children–IV–Young Child (Lucas et al. 1998). The question of the time course of symptoms within an episode is a current focus of study, because it is not clear that it was captured in a sufficiently detailed fashion by the structured psychiatric interview.

Limitations of Available Data and Ongoing Data Collection

Limitations of this first preliminary investigation were that the sample was predominantly Caucasian, was only moderate in size, and was not population based and therefore is not representative. Related to this, the sample was followed for only 6 months after baseline. Our ongoing study in the St. Louis, Missouri, metropolitan area has ascertained a larger, more ethnically and socioeconomically diverse community-based sample (N=305) and will follow the cohort for 2 years after baseline. More detailed information about symptom onset, durations, and course will be obtained. Furthermore, more sensitive measures of the child's internal emotional state (e.g., using narrative techniques) are also being used. In addition, we are including a more detailed assessment of the parent's observation of the child's behaviors and emotions as well as their onset and durations in the mood domain using expanded versions of the Preschool Age Psychiatric Assessment (PAPA; Egger et al. 1999) MDD and Mania sections. A multimodal assessment of impairment has also been included in this study design to address the distinction between clinical thresholds and high-risk states.

Next Steps for Validating Depressive Disorders in Early Childhood

Replication of the findings from a single study as described earlier is needed from independent investigative teams and epidemiologically derived samples. To date, Egger et al. (1999) have identified a depressed group using the PAPA in their community-based sample (N>300) of preschool children, using the Child Behavior Checklist as a screening tool. Although some studies suggest that dysthymia is rare in young children, further investigation of whether the distinction between other depressive subtypes known in older children and adults (e.g., dysthymic disorder, MDD) also can be detected in young children is needed (Kashani et al. 1997; Masi et al. 2001). Longitudinal outcome of depressed preschoolers at school age and later in life is key to determining whether there is continuity of this disorder to the later-life form when it arises in early childhood. Imaging studies (both structural and functional) of depressed preschoolers are needed to investigate the neurobiological correlates of this early onset disorder and to determine whether brain changes that are evident later in development can also be detected at these early stages. Investigation of the disorder across cultures is also needed and is ongoing. Larger sample sizes also will allow exploration of age and other developmental variations in the disorder's manifestations across early childhood. More detailed studies of family history using direct interview of family members are also warranted. Twin studies in samples of young children that address gene–environment interactions would also be of value.

Mania and Bipolar Disorder

The questions of whether mania can arise in the preschool period and, if so, how it manifests are currently insufficiently tested. Numerous case studies have been done, as well as a few studies of small sample size limited by the use of unstructured clinician diagnoses or psychiatric interviews designed for older children. These studies have suggested that bipolar disorder can arise in the preschool period and that it is characterized by irritable mood, elation, decreased need for sleep, and impaired functioning. Nevertheless, the distinction between these features and normative and developmentally transient emotional extremes has not been established. Despite the lack of validity data, a few small-scale treatment studies have suggested efficacy of various mood-stabilizing agents in overall mood regulation (Wozniak 2005).

AVAILABLE CASE DESCRIPTIONS AND INVESTIGATIONS

To date, eight studies of preschool mania have been published. Three of these are single case studies that describe mania-like behavior in individual patients (Pavulari et al. 2003; Poznanski et al. 1984; Tuzun 2002). Another is a sample of 44 preschool children who were assessed with the Schedule for Affective Disorders and Schizophrenia, Epidemiological version (designed for older children). The report identified similar patterns of comorbidity in preschool and school-age "bipolar" samples (Wilens et al. 2003). Another study in which 6 (17%) of 32 inpatient preschoolers received a clinical diagnosis of bipolar disorder found that all children had family histories of bipolar disorder and previous diagnoses of ADHD (Tumuluru et al. 2003). Investigators who studied nine cases of preschoolers who were given clinical diagnoses of bipolar disorder reported that validators included family history, worsening on stimulants, and good response to mood stabilizers (Mota-Castillo et al. 2001). Despite these highly suggestive findings, there are no studies of sufficient sample size using age-appropriate measures and careful consideration of appropriate developmental norms.

MEASUREMENT DEVELOPMENT

On the basis of limited extant data, we are currently assessing for the presence of mania symptoms (based on the PAPA expanded mania section) in our ongoing study of preschool mood disorders. To conduct this study, we developed an expanded mania module of the PAPA. The module assesses for the presence of age-appropriate manifestations of elation, grandiosity, flight of ideas, and all DSM-IV-TR mania symptoms as they could manifest in a preschool child. This module has demonstrated high test-retest reliability that is comparable to that established in other PAPA modules (Luby and Belden 2006). In addition, the age-adjusted DSM-IV-TR core mania symptoms on the module clustered together in a factor analysis.

To tap the child informant, we also developed a mania module of the Berkeley Puppet Interview (Ablow and Measelle 1993) and determined test-retest reliability. However, reliability was in general modest to low. Further measurement development for the assessment of mania symptoms in young children is now needed (using multiple modalities such as narrative and observational approaches).

KEY DEVELOPMENTAL ISSUES

In addressing the question of whether mania can arise during the preschool period, it is necessary to consider two broad developmental issues. One is whether it is developmentally possible for cardinal symptoms of mania to manifest at this early stage of development. For example, we need to have an understanding of the normative trajectory of the development of self-concept to consider whether it is possible for a preschool child to be truly "grandiose." This question is particularly salient because preschoolers are well known for making bold and fanciful statements, but it is not clear that such expression from a preschool child represents fixed and false beliefs with the same significance as such claims would have in an older child or adult. Related to this developmental issue is the question of how normative expressions of broad mood and ideation can be distinguished from clinically significant phenomena. For example, the distinction between joyful, silly, and giddy mood that is normative and true clinical elations must be made clear. Along these lines, the distinction between the known greater fluctuations in mood state from clinical mood cycling must also be clarified. These distinctions are key to determining whether a valid mania syndrome can occur in preschool children.

PRELIMINARY FINDINGS AND ONGOING INVESTIGATIONS

An exploratory investigation of mania symptoms within our preschool sample has demonstrated a group of preschoolers who meet all DSM-IV symptom criteria for bipolar disorder I. Notably, several symptoms emerged as highly specific for this syndrome. For example, the symptom of elation had a very high odds ratio, demonstrating a very clear and robust distinction between clinical elation and normative joyful mood in the preschool period (Luby and Belden 2006). Also of clinical importance, preschoolers who met symptom criteria for bipolar disorder I had very high levels of impairment, even higher than levels found in groups of preschoolers with other Axis I psychiatric disorders. Longitudinal follow-up of this group will be informative to further clarify the clinical significance of this early-onset syndrome.

One research group is currently investigating the behaviors of high-risk preschoolers of bipolar parents. Another study looking at preschool children of bipolar parents is also being conducted, and a treatment study of preschool bipolar disorder is ongoing using inclusion criteria based on those established in older children and not yet validated for preschoolers.

Commentary: Michael S. Scheeringa, M.D., M.P.H., and Charles H. Zeanah Jr., M.D.

As noted by Luby, the extant evidence for mood disorders in preschool children has addressed the major guidelines for diagnostic validity put forth by Robins and Guze (1970). Recent research has more convincingly demonstrated that depressive disorders are identifiable in young children, sharing both strong similarities with depressive disorders in older children and some important differences. It is worth highlighting that the key change in Luby's group's method for diagnosing young children is loosening the requirement for sustained mood change (i.e., all day, every day) for 2 weeks. They used the slightly lower threshold of "most of the day" or "almost every day" but still had a minimum 2 week's duration. Their ongoing study ought to shed light on the issue of whether depressed children show sadness all day, every day and, if so, whether they are a more severe subtype from those who show sadness most of the day. However, it is also fair to reverse the question and ask whether research with adults actually demonstrates individuals who experience depressed mood (as observed by others) "all day, every day."

Luby notes that bipolar disorder is considerably less substantiated in the preschool years, and the limited research to date has not been developmentally sensitive. However, the controversy about bipolar disorder is not limited to the preschool period. Luby frames the conundrum in terms of developmental norms, which is an important issue, but it also may involve our emerging understanding of nonbipolar emotional dysregulation in children of all ages. The extant studies have not included appropriate subgroups that can answer this question of discriminant validity.

Three final points suggest directions for future research. First, like most other disorders of early childhood, mood disorders have not been subjected to extensive tests of discriminant validity, particularly against anxiety disorders. Investigations of biological correlates may reflect nonspecific disturbances associated with negative affect rather than specific links to depression. Large-scale population-based studies using omnibus measures of psychopathology will be important in this regard. Second, it is unclear whether any of the findings about depression in these children hold for children younger than 3 years of age, particularly in light of Field's pioneering work with infants of depressed mothers (as cited by Luby). That research demonstrated relationship specificity of the signs of depression in these infants as they interacted with their depressed mothers versus their nondepressed fathers and childcare providers. Third, longitudinal data are desperately needed for virtually all putative disorders of early childhood. Such data are vital for considering the question of the degree to which disorders of early childhood represent early expressions of the phenotype, discrete disorders lacking continuity with later disorders, or disorders characterized by varying degrees of heterotypic continuity.

References

Ablow JC, Measelle JR: The Berkeley Puppet Interview. Berkeley, University of California, 1993

American Psychiatric Association: Diagnostic and Statistical Manual of Mental Disorders, 3rd Edition. Washington, DC, American Psychiatric Association, 1980

American Psychiatric Association: Diagnostic and Statistical Manual of Mental Disorders, 4th Edition. Washington, DC, American Psychiatric Association, 1994

Belden AC, Luby JL: Preschoolers' depression severity and behaviors during dyadic interactions: mediating role of parental support. J Am Acad Child Adolesc Psychiatry 45:213–222, 2006

Carlson GA, Cantwell DP: Unmasking masked depression from childhood through adulthood: analysis of three studies. Am J Psychiatry 145:1222–1225, 1980

Egger HL, Ascher BH, Angold A: Preschool Age Psychiatric Assessment. Durham, NC, Duke University Medical Center, 1999

Field T, Pickens J, Fox NA, et al: Facial expression and EEG responses to happy and sad faces/voices by 3-month-old infants of depressed mothers. Br J Dev Psychol 16:485–494, 1998

Kashani JH: Depression in the preschool child. Journal of Children in Contemporary Society 15:11–17, 1982

Kashani JH, Carlson GA: Major depressive disorder in a preschooler. J Am Acad Child Adolesc Psychiatry 24:490–494, 1985

Kashani JH, Ray JS: Depressive related symptoms among preschool-age children. Child Psychiatry Hum Dev 13:233–238, 1983

Kashani JH, Ray JS, Carlson GA: Depression and depressive-like states in preschool-age children in a child development unit. Am J Psychiatry 141:1397–1402, 1984

Kashani JH, Holcomb, WR, Orvaschel H: Depression and depressive symptoms in preschool children from the general population. Am J Psychiatry 143:1138–1143, 1986

Kashani JH, Allan WD, Beck NC, et al: Dysthymic disorder in clinically referred preschool children. J Am Acad Child Adolesc Psychiatry 36:1426–1433, 1997

Luby JL, Belden AC: Defining and validating bipolar disorder in the preschool period. Dev Psychopathol 18:971–988, 2006

Luby JL, Heffelfinger A, Mrakotsky C, et al: Preschool major depressive disorder: preliminary validation for developmentally modified DSM-IV criteria. J Am Acad Child Adolesc Psychiatry 41:928–937, 2002

Luby JL, Heffelfinger A, Mrakotsky C, et al: Alterations in stress cortisol reactivity in depressed preschoolers relative to psychiatric and no-disorder comparison groups. Arch Gen Psychiatry 60:1248–1255, 2003a

Luby JL, Heffelfinger AK, Mrakotsky C, et al: The clinical picture of depression in preschool children. J Am Acad Child Adolesc Psychiatry 42:340–348, 2003b

Luby JL, Mrakotsky C, Heffelfinger A, et al: Modification of DSM-IV criteria for depressed preschool children. Am J Psychiatry 160:1169–1172, 2003c

Luby JL, Heffelfinger A, Koenig-McNaught A, et al: The preschool feelings checklist: a brief and sensitive screening measure for depression in young children. J Am Acad Child Adolesc Psychiatry 43:708–717, 2004a

Luby JL, Mrakotsky C, Heffelfinger A, et al: Characteristics of depressed preschoolers with and without anhedonia: evidence for a melancholic depressive subtype in young children. Am J Psychiatry 161:1998–2004, 2004b

Luby JL, Sullivan J, Belden AC, et al: An observational analysis of behavior in depressed preschoolers: further validation of early onset depression. J Am Acad Child Adolesc Psychiatry 45:203–212, 2006

Lucas CP, Fisher P, Luby J: Young-Child DISC-IV Research Draft: Diagnostic Interview Schedule for Children. New York, Joy and William Ruane Center to Identify and Treat Mood Disorders, 1998

Masi G, Favilla L, Mucci M, et al: Depressive symptoms in children and adolescents with dysthymic disorder. Psychopathology 34:29–35, 2001

Mol Lous AM, deWit CAM, deBruyn EJ, et al: Depression markers in young children's play: a comparison between depressed and nondepressed 3- to 6-year-olds in various play situations. J Child Psychol Psychiatry 43:1029–1038, 2002

Mota-Castillo M, Torruella A, Engels B, et al: Valproate in very young children: an open case series with a brief follow-up. J Affect Disord 67:193–197, 2001

Mrakotsky C: Visual perception, spatial cognition and affect recognition in preschool depressive syndromes. PhD diss., University of Vienna/Washington University School of Medicine, Vienna, Austria, Austrian National Library, 2001

Pavuluri MN, Janicak PG, Naylor MW, et al: Early recognition and differentiation of pediatric schizophrenia and bipolar disorder, in Adolescent Psychiatry: Developmental and Clinical Studies, Vol 27. Edited by Flaherty LT. Hillsdale, NJ, Analytic Press, 2003, pp 117–134

Poznanski E, Zrull JP: Childhood depression: clinical characteristics of overtly depressed children. Arch Gen Psychiatry 23:8–15, 1970

Poznanski EO, Grossman JA, Buchsbaum Y, et al: Preliminary studies of the reliability and validity of the children's depression rating scale. J Am Acad Child Adolesc Psychiatry 23:191–197, 1984

Robins E, Guze SB: Establishment of diagnostic validity in psychiatric illness: its application to schizophrenia. Am J Psychiatry 126:983–986, 1970

Spitz R: Motherless infants. Child Dev 20:145–155, 1949

Tumuluru RV, Weller EB, Fristad MA, et al: Mania in six preschool children. J Child Adolesc Psychopharmacol 13:489–494, 2003

Tuzun U, Zoroglu SS, Savas HA: A 5-year-old boy with recurrent mania successfully treated with carbamazepine. Psychiatry Clin Neurosci 56:589–591, 2002

Wilens TE, Biederman J, Forkner P, et al: Patterns of comorbidity and dysfunction in clinically referred preschool and school-age children with bipolar disorder. J Child Adolesc Psychopharmacol 13:495–505, 2003

Wozniak J: Recognizing and managing bipolar disorder in children. J Clin Psychiatry 66 (suppl):18–23, 2005

17

DIAGNOSIS OF ANXIETY DISORDERS IN INFANTS, TODDLERS, AND PRESCHOOL CHILDREN

Susan L. Warren, M.D.

Current State of the Science

Despite the fact that anxiety disorders are prevalent and disabling conditions (Cantwell and Baker 1989; Hettema et al. 2001; Ost and Treffers 2001; Woodward and Fergusson 2001), little research has been conducted thus far concerning anxiety disorders in infants and young children. Part of this omission might result from the fact that fears and anxiety-related behaviors in young children are common and are thought therefore to be innocuous, and it has been difficult to differentiate anxiety disorders from typical developmental processes. Moreover, young children frequently lack verbal skills necessary to meet criteria for anxiety disorders as specified by DSM-IV-TR (American Psychiatric Association 2000). The tendency has thus been to delay the diagnosis of anxiety disorders in some cases until children are older (Rapoport and Ismond 1996). However, clinicians have reported cases of young children showing anxiety-related suffering and impairment (Warren 2004; Wright et al. 2002). In addition, some recent studies have begun to examine DSM-IV-TR anxiety disorders in young children (Angold et al. submitted) as well as investigate possible modifications to the criteria (Warren et al. 2006).

Several different types of anxiety disorders have been previously described in older children and adults: separation anxiety disorder (anxiety in response to separation from caregivers), social phobia (anxiety in response to social situations), generalized anxiety disorder (GAD; persistent and excessive anxiety concerning a number of events or activities), and specific phobia (anxiety in response to a specific feared object or situation) (American Psychiatric Association 2000). Obsessive-compulsive disorder, posttraumatic stress disorder, panic disorder, and agoraphobia have also been classified as anxiety disorders, but these are not addressed in this chapter.

Table 17–1 outlines the studies that have reported anxiety disorders in children younger than 5 years of age. For each study, the table lists the sample size, ages studied, type of sample, diagnostic procedures used, and rates of disorders if reported. One major difficulty for reviewing this research is that the authors have generally used instruments developed for older children. While implementing or applying the instruments and diagnostic criteria to the younger children, the authors might have found it necessary to make modifications to the instruments and to the diagnostic criteria that were not clearly specified. Another problem is that investigators have employed different versions of DSM, and few studies have used DSM-IV (American Psychiatric Association 1994). An additional issue is that although the table reports rates of disorders—because few of the studies used probability-based sampling designed to be statistically representative of the population—the rates generally do not represent prevalence rates in the population. Notable research that has appropriately addressed these issues was conducted by Angold et al. (submitted), who used the Preschool Age Psychiatric Assessment (PAPA; Egger et al. 1999), an interview about preschoolers that was based on the Child and Adolescent Psychiatric Assessment (Angold and Costello 2000). This research used probability-based sampling, DSM-IV, and clearly specified symptom-based criteria for making the diagnoses. The PAPA diagnostic algorithms that were used to make the diagnoses were reviewed with H. Egger (personal communication, July 22, 2005). In order to implement the diagnostic criteria with the younger children, decisions were made that resulted in modifications to the criteria in some cases. The specific implementation modifications are described more fully later, within the separate discussions for each anxiety disorder.

According to DSM-IV-TR, the diagnosis of separation anxiety disorder requires that a child show three out of eight symptoms related to separation anxiety disorder. Four of these symptoms require good verbal skills (worrying, complaints, and reports of nightmares), which could make it difficult for a young child to meet the criteria. The additional symptom of reluctance or refusal to go to school or elsewhere could also be difficult to meet, because at young ages, most children are generally not required to leave their parents. In addition, the manual warns clinicians not to diagnose developmentally appropriate levels of separation anxiety (American Psychiatric Association 2000). Thus, some clinicians have been reluctant to diagnose separation anxiety disorder in young children (Rapoport and Ismond 1996). Yet some toddlers seem to meet criteria and have experienced significant distress

TABLE 17–1. Studies investigating anxiety disorders in children less than five years of age

Study	Sample size	Age	Type of sample	Diagnostic procedure[a]	Type of anxiety disorder studied/Prevalence (%) if obtained						
					ANX	SAD	AVD	SOC	OAD	GAD	SP
Angold et al. submitted	307	2–5 yr	Pediatric clinic[b]	PAPA:DSM-IV		2.4[c,d]		2.2[c,d]		6.5[d]	2.3[c]
Beitchman et al. 1987	98	2.5–6 yr	Psychiatric preschool	DSM-III			4		11		
Briggs-Gowan et al. 2000	1060	4–9 yr	Pediatric practices[b]	DISC-R:DSM-III-R	6.1	3.6			0.5		3.9[e]
Cantwell and Baker 1987	600	1.7–15.9 yr	Speech clinic	DICA:DSM-III	10	3.2	4.8		2		0.2
Cordeiro et al. 2003	343	0–48 mo	Infant mental health clinic	DC:0–3	8[f]						
Dunitz et al. 1996	82	9 days–24 mo	Pediatric psycho-therapy clinic	DC:0–3 and DSM-IV	6[f]	7					
Earls 1982	100	3 yr	Island population[b]	DSM-III		5	2				
Frankel et al. 2004	177	0–58 mo	Mental health clinic	DC:0–3 and DSM-IV; chart review	3[f], 4						

TABLE 17–1. Studies investigating anxiety disorders in children less than five years of age *(continued)*

Study	Sample size	Age	Type of sample	Diagnostic procedure[a]	Type of anxiety disorder studied/Prevalence (%) if obtained						
					ANX	SAD	AVD	SOC	OAD	GAD	SP
Guédeney et al. 2003	85	0–3 yr	Mental health centers	DC:0–3	10.6[f]						
Hooks et al. 1988	193	0–5 yr	Mental health clinic	DSM-III; chart review		3			4.7	0.05	
Keenan et al. 1997	104	4.6–5.8 yr	WIC program	K-SADS:DSM-III-R		2.3		4.6	1.1		11.5
Lavigne et al. 1996	510	2–5 yr	Pediatricians[b]	DSM-III-R		0.5	0.7		0.7		0.6
Lee 1987	129	1–6 yr	Mental health clinic	DSM-III; chart review		2					
Luby and Morgan 1997	120	9–70 mo	Mental health clinic	DSM-III-R	10						
Maldonado-Durán et al. 2003	167	0–3 yr	Infant mental health clinic	DC:0–3	6.5[f]						
Minde and Tidmarsh 1997	57	15–48 mo	Disruptive behavior disorders	DC:0–3 and DSM-IV	5[f]	7					

TABLE 17–1. Studies investigating anxiety disorders in children less than five years of age *(continued)*

Study	Sample size	Age	Type of sample	Diagnostic procedure[a]	Type of anxiety disorder studied/Prevalence (%) if obtained						
					ANX	SAD	AVD	SOC	OAD	GAD	SP
Warren et al. 2006	72	19 mo to 5 years	Mixed	Modified DSM-IV							
Wilens et al. 2002	200	2–6 yr	Pediatric psychiatry clinic	K-SADS:DSM-III-R		34		7	20		17
Wright et al. 2002	354	0–3 yr	Mental health clinic	DSM-IV	2–17						

Note. ANX=anxiety disorders generally; AVD=avoidant disorder; DC:0–3=Diagnostic Classification: Zero to Three; DICA=Diagnostic Interview for Children and Adolescents; DISC-R=Diagnostic Interview Schedule for Children-Revised; GAD=generalized anxiety disorder; K-SADS=Schedule for Affective Disorders and Schizophrenia for School-Age Children; OAD=overanxious disorder; PAPA=Preschool-Age Psychiatric Assessment; SAD=separation anxiety disorder, SOC=social phobia, SP=specific phobia; WIC=Women, Infants, and Children.

[a]Based on interview unless noted.

[b]Probability-based sample designed to be statistically representative of the population.

[c]Includes impairment.

[d]Implementation modifications made to criteria (see text).

[e]Subsample of 516 four- to six-year-olds.

[f]Diagnostic Classification: Zero to Three anxiety disorders diagnosis.

and impairment in family life as a result (Dunitz et al. 1996; Earls 1982; Hooks et al. 1988; Keenan et al. 1997; Lavigne et al. 1996; Lee 1987; Warren 2004). In reviewing the studies that describe children who seem to meet criteria for separation anxiety disorder, it is important to note that the duration criteria changed from 2 weeks in DSM-III-R (American Psychiatric Association 1987) to 4 weeks in DSM-IV (Rapoport and Ismond 1996). Only one study (Angold et al. submitted) has used the DSM-IV criteria with a probability-based sample; these authors found rates of separation anxiety disorder that were similar to those found for older children. For the younger children, the criteria were implemented in the following ways:

1. If a parent had changed plans in the past 3 months because of a child's distress or fear in anticipation of separation from a major attachment figure, this qualified as "recurrent excessive distress when separation from home or major attachment figures occurs or is anticipated";
2. No frequency criteria were required for "persistent reluctance or refusal to go to school or elsewhere because of fear of separation," but symptoms included trying to leave, refusing to go, and needing to be picked up early due to anxiety or worry; and
3. No frequency criteria were required for complaints of physical symptoms when separation occurred or was anticipated.

Because of concerns related to diagnosing young children, a group was formed to develop diagnostic criteria for disorders in young children called the Research Diagnostic Criteria—Preschool Age (Task Force on Research Diagnostic Criteria Infancy and Preschool 2003). Alternative criteria for separation anxiety disorder in young children were created but have not been tested. Therefore, it is not entirely clear at this time whether the criteria for the disorder require modification for young children

The diagnosis of social phobia in young children involves some of the same difficulties as were described for separation anxiety disorder. Because fear of strangers is generally considered to be developmentally appropriate until the end of the second year of life, clinicians have been reluctant to diagnose social phobia until after 2½ years of age (Rapoport and Ismond 1996). In addition, research suggests that children generally develop the capacity for being concerned about the evaluation of others at approximately 4 years of age (Asendorpf 1989). This would make the diagnosis of social phobia for infants and toddlers virtually impossible, because the diagnosis requires that an individual must fear that he or she will act in a way that will be humiliating or embarrassing. Previous versions of DSM had included a diagnosis called "avoidant disorder of childhood," which did not require such capabilities. This diagnosis was eliminated in DSM-IV because of an overlap with social phobia in older children (Francis et al. 1992; Rapoport and Ismond 1996). Few studies have investigated social phobia in young children. Some investigators (Keenan et al. 1997; Wilens et al. 2002) have described it in children older than 4 years of age. Angold et al. (submitted) studied younger children but did not require that the children fear humiliation or embarrassment. Warren et al. (2006) examined the Research Diagnostic Criteria—Preschool Age modifications, which eliminated determining whether the child feared humiliation or embarrassment and focused instead on observable behaviors by adding "excessive shrinking from contact with and persistent reluctance to approach unfamiliar people" to the A criterion. These modifications were supported by convergent validity with other reports of child anxiety and parental anxiety and discriminant validity with non-anxious behaviors (Warren et al. 2006). The research therefore suggests that such modifications to the social phobia criteria could be useful.

In DSM-IV-TR, the diagnosis of GAD requires excessive anxiety or worry about a number of events or activities, occurring more days than not for at least 6 months, with the person finding it difficult to control the worry or anxiety. For children, only one additional symptom related to the worry or anxiety is needed from a list that includes difficulty concentrating, restlessness, irritability, muscle tension, and sleep disturbance. GAD can be difficult to diagnose in young children because the hallmark of the disorders is worry, which must be reported by the child. Few studies have investigated GAD in young children. In a probability-based sample, Angold et al. (submitted) studied the DSM-IV criteria for GAD in young children. Their implementation required either worry about at least one topic that was intrusive into at least two activities and uncontrollable at least some of the time or that the child had experienced worry, situational anxious affect (fears), and/or free-floating anxious affect anxiety 90 times in the 3 months prior to the interview. To address the issue of young children's difficulties in reporting worries, Warren et al. (2006) proposed alternative criteria for young children that focused on fears instead of worries. However, the small pilot study did not support the modification (Warren et al. 2006). It would therefore appear that the diagnosis of GAD requires further study in terms of modifications needed for young children.

Young children can meet the criteria for specific phobia as outlined in DSM-IV-TR, although the requirement of a duration of 6 months signifies that this diagnosis would not be met by a child who experiences multiple specific fears that could be quite distressing and disabling but not of long-enough duration. Further research is needed regarding such a situation in young children as well as for the situation in which a child moves from one extreme and disabling fear to another over the course of development but does not meet the 6-month duration criteria for any one fear.

The issue of whether anxiety disorders should be parsed into multiple disorders has also been of concern not only for older children but also for younger children. For example, the Zero to Three/National Center for Clinical Infant Programs, which explicated criteria for diagnosing anxiety disorders in children younger than

3 years of age, proposed only one anxiety disorder (Zero to Three 1994). However, the newer version, released in the fall of 2005, included multiple disorders (Egger and Angold 2006), and recent studies have supported this. For example, Spence et al. (2001) studied anxiety symptoms in 755 preschoolers. Confirmatory factor analysis demonstrated a superior fit for a five-correlated factor model, reflecting separate areas of social phobia, separation anxiety, generalized anxiety, obsessive-compulsive disorder, and fears of physical injury along with high covariation between factors that could be explained by a general anxiety factor. Similarly, in a twin-study of preschool children, Eley et al. (2003) found evidence for five correlated factors: general distress, separation anxiety, fears, obsessive-compulsive behaviors, and shyness/inhibition. Genetic influences were found for all five factors, but the pattern of influences differed considerably among them. Thus, research is beginning to demonstrate that although there appears to be a common factor for anxiety disorders in young children generally, it is useful to study the disorders individually because they appear to show some differing aspects and etiologies.

In summary, research supports the diagnosis of different anxiety disorders in children younger than 5 years of age. Young children have generally seemed to meet the standard DSM-IV-TR criteria for specific phobia and separation anxiety disorder, although the criteria for the latter have not been fully studied. Modifications have been proposed for social phobia that have been supported by a small pilot study. Modifications also appear warranted for GAD but have not yet been identified. Much additional research is needed to more fully characterize and validate anxiety disorder diagnoses in young children.

Advances in Developmental Science

Developmental research concerning behaviors in response to new situations and strangers has been extremely helpful for understanding psychopathology. Behaviors in response to new situations and strangers have often been investigated in the context of studying temperament. The term *temperament* refers to relatively enduring behavioral and emotional reactions that appear early, differ among individuals, and have been thought to be associated with genetic constitution (Goldsmith et al. 1987). The type of temperament that has been most consistently studied in relation to anxiety disorders is *behavioral inhibition,* which refers to a child's tendency to exhibit quiet withdrawal in novel situations (Kagan 1994). When a behaviorally inhibited child is presented with an unfamiliar object, person, or situation, the child is quiet, retreats to the caregiver, and withdraws from the unfamiliar stimuli (Kagan 1994). Kagan and colleagues have measured behavioral inhibition by examining the latency of the child to talk to an unfamiliar examiner, tendency to retreat from novel objects and unfamiliar people, cessation of vocalization in new situations, and long periods of proximity to the caregiver, especially when not playing.

Several types of associations between behavioral inhibition and anxiety disorders have been described:

a. Young children of parents with anxiety disorders have been found to be more likely to show behavioral inhibition (Manassis et al. 1995; Rosenbaum et al. 1988, 2000), and because anxiety disorders tend to run in families (Biederman et al. 1991, 2001a; Hettema et al. 2001), behavioral inhibition could perhaps be an early manifestation of an anxiety disorder.
b. Children with behavioral inhibition have been found to subsequently develop anxiety disorders (Biederman et al. 1993; Schwartz et al. 1999).
c. Young children with behavioral inhibition have been found to have concurrent anxiety disorders (Biederman et al. 1990, 2001b; Hayward et al. 1998).

These associations could also support the possibility that behavioral inhibition is an early manifestation of an anxiety disorder.

In general, the clearest association between behavioral inhibition and anxiety disorders has been between behavioral inhibition and social phobia (Biederman et al. 2001b; Hayward et al. 1998; Schwartz et al. 1999). This makes sense because both refer to an individual's response to strangers and new social situations. Research concerning these associations has been extremely useful for understanding anxiety disorders, because young children with behavioral inhibition could be showing an early form of social phobia. Warren et al. (2006) utilized this research when modifying the social phobia criteria for young children.

The associations between behavioral inhibition and social phobia also have raised questions concerning how the two differ. In addition to the fact that they originated in different disciplines, several major distinctions are evident:

1. Social phobia occurs only in response to performance and social situations, whereas behavioral inhibition could occur in response to non-social stimuli.
2. As written in DSM-IV-TR, social phobia requires that an individual fear that he or she will act in a way that will be humiliating or embarrassing, whereas the definition of behavioral inhibition is based on observed behavior instead of on subjective feelings.
3. The diagnosis of social phobia requires that the anxiety persist for 6 months, whereas most measurements of behavioral inhibition occur only once.
4. According to the DSM-IV-TR criteria, social phobia symptoms must occur in peer settings, not just with adults, but behavioral inhibition is typically measured in relation to adults, although some researchers have included peers when studying preschoolers (Kagan 1994).
5. In meeting the distress or impairment criteria for social phobia, it would be expected that children with the disorder would be uncomfortable in a social situation for sustained periods, whereas behavioral inhibition only requires that

the child show difficulty initially in response to the stimuli or strangers—the difficulty need not persist.

6. The diagnosis of social phobia requires a high level of distress or impairment, but this is not part of the definition of behavioral inhibition. However, a child is often scored as having behavioral inhibition if he or she shows frequent distress in response to a standard protocol.

Research has not definitively established how children with behavioral inhibition differ from those with social phobia or even how typical fears differ from anxiety disorders. Some authors have defined *pathological anxiety* as fears or anxiety that are persistent, extreme, uncontrollable, irrational, and cause impairment in functioning (Ferrari 1986; Rosen and Schulkin 1998). Egger and Angold (2006) have described five qualities that could contribute to the characterization of clinically significant anxiety disorders: distressing, pervasive, uncontrollable, persistent, and impairing. Future research could thus focus on studying these criteria as applied to typical fears and anxious behaviors in order to more fully characterize anxiety disorders in young children.

Generating a Developmentally Informed Phenotype

Developmental psychopathology research has much to offer for generating a developmentally informed phenotype. Research on temperament has suggested two types of temperament related to anxiety in children: fearfulness and withdrawal (Rothbart et al. 2001). It has also identified potential biological markers associated with behavioral inhibition. Understanding how these different temperament types and biological markers are associated with psychopathology could provide further information concerning optimal diagnostic groupings.

Additional research is required to examine whether modifications to the DSM anxiety disorder criteria are needed and whether young children can meet the new proposed criteria. Utilizing the PAPA (Egger et al. 1999) appears to be promising because it examines specific symptoms in terms of intensity, frequency, onset, and duration. With this interview, researchers could establish different diagnostic symptom profiles by changing the specific symptoms used to make the diagnoses. Prevalence rates of the profiles could then be examined, and the profiles could be investigated in relation to validating criteria (such as family history) in order to determine the best diagnostic criteria for young children.

Longitudinal research is necessary to further establish the long-term significance and developmental trajectories of fearfulness and anxiety symptoms beginning in early childhood. Longitudinal studies examining outcomes at later ages for preschoolers meeting diagnostic criteria for anxiety disorders are also greatly needed.

The diagnosis of anxiety disorders in infants, toddlers, and preschoolers is challenging at this time but extremely important. Undiagnosed, these disorders create much suffering for children and their families (Hettema et al. 2001; Woodward and Fergusson 2001), and a delayed diagnosis may unnecessarily prolong this suffering. Many children have been found to not "grow out" of anxiety disorders and, in fact, may go on to develop additional psychopathology (Cole et al. 1998; Woodward and Fergusson 2001). Refinement of current diagnostic criteria for identifying anxiety disorders in young children is crucial for reducing current suffering and preventing additional psychopathology.

Commentary: Irene Chatoor, M.D. (Workgroup Co-Chair)

This review highlights the fact that anxiety disorders are prevalent and disabling conditions that occur in this young age group and explains the difficulty of diagnosing anxiety disorders in infants, toddlers, and preschool children. The extensive literature review points out that in spite of the many studies that have explored anxiety disorders in this young age group, the general lack of population-based samples and the lack of clear diagnostic criteria make it difficult to evaluate and compare these studies.

The diagnosis of anxiety disorders in this young age group is particularly challenging because it is difficult to differentiate anxiety disorders from typical developmental processes. In most situations it is not possible to have other informants in addition to the parents; infants, toddlers, and even preschoolers lack the verbal skills to express the worries and fear of embarrassment that are major diagnostic criteria for anxiety disorders in the older age group. In addition, it is very difficult to assess impairment in these young children, and the effect of the young child's anxiety disorder on the parents' functioning may have to be considered.

The review emphasizes the need for modifications to the diagnostic criteria in DSM-IV-TR, especially for social phobia and general anxiety disorder, in order to address the particular issues highlighted here. The review also explains the need for population-based studies that use multimodal assessment techniques, including biological measures and direct observation, to better understand the expression of anxiety disorders in this young age group.

References

American Psychiatric Association: Diagnostic and Statistical Manual of Mental Disorders, 3rd Edition Revised. Washington, DC, American Psychiatric Association, 1987

American Psychiatric Association: Diagnostic and Statistical Manual of Mental Disorders, 4th Edition. Washington, DC, American Psychiatric Association, 1994

American Psychiatric Association: Diagnostic and Statistical Manual of Mental Disorders, 4th Edition, Text Revision. Washington, DC, American Psychiatric Association, 2000

Angold A, Costello EJ: The Child and Adolescent Psychiatric Assessment (CAPA). J Am Acad Child Adolesc Psychiatry 39:39–48, 2000

Angold A, Egger H, Erkanli A, et al: Prevalence and comorbidity of psychiatric disorders in preschoolers attending a large pediatric service. Manuscript submitted for publication, 2005

Asendorpf J: Shyness as a final common pathway for two different kinds of inhibition. J Pers Soc Psychol 57:481–492, 1989

Beitchman JH, Wekerle C, Hood J: Diagnostic continuity from preschool to middle childhood. J Am Acad Child Adolesc Psychiatry 26:694–699, 1987

Biederman J, Rosenbaum JF, Hirshfeld DR, et al: Psychiatric correlates of behavioral inhibition in young children of parents with and without psychiatric disorders. Arch Gen Psychiatry 47:21–26, 1990

Biederman J, Rosenbaum JF, Bolduc EA, et al: A high risk study of young children of parents with panic disorder and agoraphobia with and without comorbid major depression. Psychiatry Res 37:333–348, 1991

Biederman J, Rosenbaum JF, Bolduc-Murphy EA, et al: A 3 year follow-up of children with and without behavioral inhibition. J Am Acad Child Adolesc Psychiatry 32:814–821, 1993

Biederman J, Faraone SV, Hirschfeld-Becker DR, et al: Patterns of psychopathology and dysfunction in high-risk children of parents with panic disorder and major depression. Am J Psychiatry 158:49–57, 2001a

Biederman J, Hirshfeld-Becker DR, Rosenbaum JF, et al: Further evidence of association between behavioral inhibition and social anxiety in children. Am J Psychiatry 158:1673–1679, 2001b

Briggs-Gowan MJ, Horwitz SM, Schwab-Stone ME, et al: Mental health in pediatric settings: distribution of disorders and factors related to service use. J Am Acad Child Adolesc Psychiatry 39:841–849, 2000

Cantwell DP, Baker L: The prevalence of anxiety in children with communication disorders. J Anx Disord 1:239–248, 1987

Cantwell DP, Baker L: Stability and natural history of DSM-III childhood diagnoses. J Am Acad Child Adolesc Psychiatry 28:691–700, 1989

Cole DA, Peeke LG, Martin JM, et al: A longitudinal look at the relation between depression and anxiety in children and adolescents. J Consult Clin Psychol 66:451–460, 1998

Cordeiro MJ, DaSilva PC, Goldschmidt T: Diagnostic classification: results from a clinical experience of three years with DC: 0–3. Infant Ment Health J 24:349–364, 2003

Dunitz M, Scheer PJ, Kvas E, et al: Psychiatric diagnoses in infancy: a comparison. Infant Ment Health J 17:12–23, 1996

Earls F: Application of DSM-III in an epidemiological study of preschool children. Am J Psychiatry 139:242–243, 1982

Egger HL, Angold A: Anxiety disorders, in Handbook of Preschool Mental Health: Development, Disorders, and Treatment. Edited by Luby J. New York, Guilford, 2006, pp 137–164

Egger HL, Ascher BH, Angold A: The Preschool Age Psychiatric Assessment. Durham, NC, Center for Developmental Epidemiology, Duke University Medical Center, 1999

Eley TC, Bolton D, O'Connor TG, et al: A twin study of anxiety-related behaviors in preschool children. J Child Psychol Psychiatry 44:945–960, 2003

Ferrari M: Fears and phobias in childhood: some clinical and developmental considerations. Child Psychiatry Hum Dev 17:75–87, 1986

Francis G, Last CG, Strauss CC: Avoidant disorder and social phobia in children and adolescents. J Am Acad Child Adolesc Psychiatry 31:1086–1089, 1992

Frankel KA, Boyum LA, Harmon RJ: Diagnoses and presenting symptoms in an infant psychiatry clinic: comparison of two diagnostic systems. J Am Acad Child Adolesc Psychiatry 43:578–587, 2004

Goldsmith HH, Buss AH, Plomin R, et al: Roundtable: what is temperament? Child Dev 58:505–529, 1987

Guédeney N, Guédeney A, Rabouam C, et al: The Zero-To-Three diagnostic classification: a contribution to the validation of this classification from a sample of 85 under-threes. Infant Ment Health J 24:313–336, 2003

Hayward C, Killen JD, Kraemer HC, et al: Linking self-reported childhood behavioral inhibition to adolescent social phobia. J Am Acad Child Adolesc Psychiatry 37:1308–1316, 1998

Hettema JM, Neale MC, Kendler KS: A review and meta-analysis of the genetic epidemiology of anxiety disorders. Am J Psychiatry 158:1568–1578, 2001

Hooks MY, Mayes LC, Volkmar FR: Psychiatric disorders among preschool children. J Am Acad Child Adolesc Psychiatry 27:623–627, 1988

Kagan J: Galen's Prophecy. New York, Basic Books, 1994

Keenan K, Shaw DS, Walsh B, et al: DSM-III disorders in preschool children from low-income families. J Am Acad Child Adolesc Psychiatry 36:620–627, 1997

Lavigne JV, Gibbons RD, Kristoffel KK, et al: Prevalence rates and correlates of psychiatric disorders among preschool children. J Am Acad Child Adolesc Psychiatry 35:204–214, 1996

Lee BJ: Multidisciplinary evaluation of preschool children and its demography in a military psychiatric clinic. J Am Acad Child Adolesc Psychiatry 26:313–316, 1987

Luby JL, Morgan K: Characteristics of an infant/preschool psychiatric clinic sample: implications for clinical assessment and nosology. Infant Ment Health J 18:209–220, 1997

Maldonado-Durán M, Helmig L, Moody C, et al: The Zero-To-Three diagnostic classification in an infant mental health clinic: its usefulness and challenges. Infant Ment Health J 24:378–397, 2003

Manassis K, Bradley S, Hood J, et al. Behavioural inhibition, attachment and anxiety in children of mothers with anxiety disorders. Can J Psychiatry 40:87–92, 1995

Minde K, Tidmarsh L: The changing practices of an infant psychiatry program: the McGill experience. Infant Ment Health J 18:135–144, 1997

Ost L-G, Treffers PDA: Onset, course, and outcome for anxiety disorders in children, in Anxiety Disorders in Children and Adolescents. Edited by Silverman WK, Treffers PDA. New York, Cambridge University Press, 2001, pp 293–312

Rapoport JL, Ismond DR (eds): DSM-IV Training Guide for Diagnosis of Childhood Disorders. New York, Brunner Mazel, 1996

Rosen J, Schulkin J: From normal fear to pathological anxiety. Psychol Rev 105:325–350, 1998

Rosenbaum JF, Biederman J, Gersten M, et al: Behavioral inhibition in children of parents with panic disorder and agoraphobia. Arch Gen Psychiatry 45:463–470, 1988

Rosenbaum JF, Biederman J, Hirshfeld-Becker DR, et al: A controlled study of behavioral inhibition in children of parents with panic disorder and depression. Am J Psychiatry 157:2002–2010, 2000

Rothbart MK, Ahadi SA, Hershey KL, et al: Investigations of temperament at three to seven years: the Children's Behavior Questionnaire. Child Dev 72:1394–1408, 2001

Schwartz CE, Snidman N, Kagan J: Adolescent social anxiety as an outcome of inhibited temperament in childhood. J Am Acad Child Adolesc Psychiatry 38:1008–1015, 1999

Spence SH, Rapee R, McDonald C, et al. The structure of anxiety symptoms among preschoolers. Behav Res Ther 39:1293–1316, 2001

Task Force on Research Diagnostic Criteria Infancy and Preschool: Research diagnostic criteria for infants and preschool children: the process and empirical support. J Am Acad Child Adolesc Psychiatry 42:1502–1512, 2003

Warren SL: Anxiety disorders, in Handbook of Infant, Toddler, and Preschool Mental Health Assessment. Edited by Del Carmen R, Carter A. New York, Oxford University Press, 2004, pp 355–375

Warren SL, Umylny P, Aron E, et al: Toddler anxiety disorders: a pilot study. J Am Acad Child Adolesc Psychiatry 45:859–866, 2006

Wilens TE, Biederman J, Brown S, et al: Patterns of psychopathology and dysfunction in clinically referred preschoolers. Dev Behav Pediatr 23:S31–S36, 2002

Woodward LJ, Fergusson DM: Life course outcomes of young people with anxiety disorders in adolescence. J Am Acad Child Adolesc Psychiatry 40:1086–1093, 2001

Wright H, Penny R, et al. DSM-IV diagnoses for infants and toddlers seen in an infant mental health clinic and community mental health center. Presented at the International Conference for Infant Studies, Toronto, Ontario, Canada, April 2002

Zero to Three: Diagnostic Classification: 0–3. Washington, DC, Zero to Three, 1994

18

CLASSIFYING SLEEP DISORDERS IN INFANTS AND TODDLERS

Thomas F. Anders, M.D.
Ronald Dahl, M.D.

Current State of the Science

Before we embark on a review of the classification of sleep disorders in infants, toddlers, and preschool children, it is worthwhile to consider the use of the designation "mental disorders" as a framework for what are often commonly perceived as behavioral problems. On the one hand, it can be misleading (and off-putting to pediatricians and family members) to regard these as categories of "mental disorder." On the other hand, there is growing evidence that even simple behavioral or medically based (e.g., sleep disturbances secondary to food allergy) sleep problems may have long-term consequences on behavioral and emotional health and the development of specific mental disorders. Thus, it is important to balance these contrasting views to maximize the usefulness of a system of categorization for pediatricians, epidemiologists, and a broader range of investigators conducting longitudinal studies that will ultimately help to inform these important developmental issues.

In the DSM-IV (American Psychiatric Association 1994) and its text update, DSM-IV-TR (American Psychiatric Association 2000), sleep disorders occurring in young children are not included in the special section "Disorders Usually First Diagnosed in Infancy, Childhood, or Adolescence." Rather, a diagnosis of sleep disorders in this age group requires that adult criteria for sleep disorders be applied.

For several of the sleep disorders, such as obstructive sleep apnea, narcolepsy, and the parasomnias, all of which have been well studied in children, these adult criteria are appropriate. However, for the most common disorders that affect infants, toddlers, and young children, namely the insomnias/dyssomnias—night waking and sleep onset disorders—the adult criteria are inadequate.

Addressing the "A" criterion, there are data to suggest that beginning in infancy, difficulties in night waking (maintaining sleep) develop at younger ages than difficulties in initiating sleep and that these two disorders, in addition to having different developmental trajectories, often do not co-occur in the same infant (Gaylor et al. 2005). Treatment strategies for each of the disorders differ as well.

Addressing the "B" criterion, clinically significant distress and impairment most often affect the parents, not the child. A young child rarely complains of distress related to sleep disruption. Impairment in functioning may be difficult to assess in the young child, especially in a preverbal infant and toddler. Daytime sleepiness/drowsiness is difficult to quantify. Other symptoms of possible sleep debt (e.g., hyperactivity, increased irritability, disturbed affect regulation, and/or attention) are also difficult to assess reliably in this age group. A distressed, sleep-deprived parent, however, may well exhibit increased fatigue, irritability, mood instability, and relational impairment within the family. Little data exist to address the B criterion in either the infant or family.

Moreover, there are differences between families with respect to the subjective experience and impact of the child's sleep patterns. For example, one family might be extremely distressed and actively seek professional assistance for their toddler who wakes up three times a night and requires parental help to return to sleep, whereas another family may express no concerns about dealing with their child, whose sleep characteristics are identical to the first. Does only the first infant have a disorder? Diverse cultural values and beliefs, unique parenting practices, and individual infant temperaments all affect the emergence and recognition of infant-toddler sleep disorders. Without more objective duration and intensity criteria and research-based impairment criteria (family and/or child), classification of sleep disorders in this age group remains problematic.

The American Academy of Sleep Medicine produced and published a coding manual (The International Classification of Sleep Disorders Diagnostic and Coding Manual [ICSD-DCM; American Sleep Disorders Association 1990]) in 1990 to be compatible with ICD-9 (World Health Organization 1977). The manual was revised in 1997 and 2001 (American Academy of Sleep Medicine 2001). A developmental section was provided by a work group focused on behavioral or environmental sleep disorders. In this section, a variety of descriptive subtypes were defined (e.g., environmental sleep disorder, adjustment sleep disorder). A second edition (ICSD-DCM2; American Academy of Sleep Medicine 2005) has recently been published that collapses the earlier subtypes of childhood dyssomnias into a single behavioral sleep disorder of children.

In ICSD-DCM, the subtypes were descriptive rather than quantitative and did not map well to DSM-IV. In ICSD-DCM2, the revised nosology maps are better but can be faulted, as can DSM-IV, for not being developmentally sensitive. There are also no specific subtypes that distinguish night waking disorders from sleep onset disorders, a major concern for parents.

Advances in Developmental Sciences

Review of the sleep literature in children indicates that some kind of sleep problem (insomnia/dyssomnia) affects from 10%–30% of families with young children (Adair et al. 1991; Lozoff et al. 1996; Moore and Ucko 1957; Ottaviano et al. 1996; Richman 1981; Thurnstrom 1999; Wolke et al. 1995, 1998). It has been reported that sleep problems tend to persist in up to 30% of children (Zuckerman et al. 1987). A few studies suggest that nighttime sleep disruption may affect daytime behavior, particularly with problems of irritability, hyperactivity, and attention (Dahl 1996; Lam et al. 2003; Lavigne et al. 1999; Marcotte et al. 1998). In general, children with neurodevelopmental disorders have a higher incidence of sleep disorders than children developing typically (Stores and Wiggs 2001). Yet given these many studies, we still do not have generally accepted, validated, objective criteria for the constructs of sleep "problems," "disruptions," or "disturbances" as they apply to the infant/toddler/preschool dyssomnias. Table 18–1 reviews some of the evidence regarding sleep problems in young children.

Few studies have attempted to define night waking and sleep onset disorders specifically at these ages, and these few have tended to have small sample sizes and relied primarily on clinic-referred rather than population based samples. Several researchers have attempted to quantify sleep problems in these age groups (Archbold et al. 2002; Owens et al. 2000; Richman 1981). For the most part, however, they have utilized structured questionnaires gathering data from parents instead of using more objective methods such as polysomnography, videosomnography, or actigraphy (Morrell 1999; Owens et al. 2000). Severity criteria (intensity and duration) vary from study to study, and studies of daytime impairment related to sleep debt have reported largely on attention-deficit/hyperactivity disorder outcomes concurrently (Marcotte et al. 1998) and at a later age.

Richman's (1981) quantitative criteria are the most widely used. She defined a "severe waking problem" in children 1–5 years of age when the problem persisted for at least 3 months and occurred at least five times a week. In addition, the child had to show one or more of the following: 1) waking three or more times a night, 2) waking for more than 20 minutes during the night, or 3) going into the parents' bed. Richman did not distinguish between a sleep-onset settling problem and a middle-of-the-night waking problem. She also did not propose age-related developmental refinements of these criteria and did not differentiate between reactive and proactive co-sleeping. For Richman, all co-sleeping constituted a problem.

TABLE 18–1. Research review of sleep disorders

Author	Subjects	Referred vs. nonclinic	Data instrument(s)	Nosology used	Impairment criteria	Daytime functioning
Richman 1981	*N*=777 returned questionnaires 1–2 years of age	Community	Parent questionnaire	Severe waking problem	Problem occurs ≥5x/week for 3 months, plus either: Waking ≥3x/night ≥20 minutes at a time in parents' bed	Behavior disorder
Zuckerman et al. 1987	*N*=308 8 months and 3 years of age	Community	Parent interview	Night waking, settling	≥3 night waking ≥1 hour to settle	10% night waking, 8% SO at 8 months, 29% had problems at 3 years (one or other) with 41% continuity; no daytime functioning assessed

TABLE 18–1. Research review of sleep disorders *(continued)*

Author	Subjects	Referred vs. nonclinic	Data instrument(s)	Nosology used	Impairment criteria	Daytime functioning
Gaylor et al. 2005	N=114–134 2–4 years of age	Nonclinic	Parent report by phone (RDC, SHQ, and Y/N)	Night waking protodysomnia SO protodysomnia	Quantitative	No relation between night and day
Archbold et al. 2002	N=1,038 399 preschoolers	Non-referred pediatric clinic while waiting appointment	PSQ	Insomnia (sleep onset and sleep maintenance), OSA, EDS, parasomnias	Cutoffs on PSQ	EDS (8.3%) associated most with snoring
Lam et al. 2003	3- to 4-year follow-up of 156 (114, 73%) infants who had been treated	Referred for sleep problems and treated between 8 and 10 months old	Maternal questionnaire about infant sleep, plus structured questionnaire	Persistent or recurrent "sleep problems" (night waking, nurse child to sleep)	7-point rating scale of severity, completed by mothers	CBCL and family function/ maternal depression scales; no infant, maternal, family factors predicted continuity of problem

TABLE 18–1. Research review of sleep disorders *(continued)*

Author	Subjects	Referred vs. nonclinic	Data instrument(s)	Nosology used	Impairment criteria	Daytime functioning
Thunstrom 1999	*N*=2,518 infants between 6 and 18 months, Sweden	Community sample	Parent report with structured questionnaire	Night waking (30%) and sleep onset (16%)	ICSD (6.2%)	None
Thunstrom 2002	Follow-up of 27 5-year-olds with severe sleep problems from previous study	Sleep problem sample	Clinical evaluation of ADHD	Past history of severe sleep onset problems and family dysfunction		7/27 had ADHD, no ADHD in matched control subjects
Lavigne et al. 1999	*N*=510 2–5 years of age	68 private pediatric practices	Parent report of amount of night and 24-hour sleep	Sleep duration and CBCL	DSM-III-R for behavior disorder	Less sleep associated with increase in behavior problems

Note. ADHD=attention-deficit/hyperactivity disorder; CBCL=Child Behavior Checklist; EDS=excessive daytime somnolence; ICSD=International Classification of Sleep Disorders; OSA=obstructive sleep apnea; PSQ=Pediatric Sleep Questionnaire; RDC=research diagnostic criteria; SHQ=Sleep Habits Questionnaire; SO=sleep onset; Y/N=sleep problem, yes/no.

Among the structured parent report instruments that are in popular use is the Children's Sleep Habit Questionnaire (Owens et al. 2000), which contains 46 items, answered by parents using a three-point Likert-like frequency/intensity scale, that then are reduced to eight subscales with cut points that define clinical sleep disorders. Sher et al. (1995) developed a 19-item questionnaire that describes a child's sleep over the past week. Two composite scores result: a night waking index that includes the number of interrupted nights, the average time spent awake, and the number of awakenings per night, and a sleep schedule index that includes the sleep onset time, the length of time to fall asleep (sleep latency), and the total sleep duration.

Pursuing a Developmentally Informed Genotype

So what do we know about sleep disorders in infants and toddlers? We actually know relatively little, and therefore, any proposed criteria for a nosology need to be viewed as research diagnostic criteria (RDC) at this time. The RDC should incorporate quantitative (duration and intensity) sleep disruption criteria for the infant/toddler/preschooler. They should be developmentally appropriate and should include associated infant and/or family impairment criteria. There are no generally acceptable infant/toddler/preschool dyssomnia criteria today that are suitable, per se, for inclusion into a formal DSM. The RDC should become the bases for further research. We propose intensity and duration criteria that are developmentally anchored (Tables 18–2 and 18–3) for both night waking and sleep onset dyssomnias. We have not identified impairment criteria for either the child or parent, but such criteria should be established and tested.

In studying sleep disruption in infants and young children, it will be important to bring a developmental neuroscience perspective to the research agenda. More specifically, there is growing evidence from both animal and human studies that sleep is a fundamental component of learning—it appears to be essential for the consolidation of both explicit and procedural learning, processes that are particularly important during early periods of maturation in relation to neural plasticity.

In general, adequate sleep appears to be important for optimal cognitive processing and affect regulation. Thus insufficient and/or disrupted sleep may have a negative impact on several neurobehavioral processes relevant to the development of behavioral and emotional problems. There is a compelling need for research to advance understanding of these developmental brain-behavior processes relevant to impaired function.

We also know that cultural attitudes and values affect the development of sleep-wake state organization, which may then affect brain development in significant ways. Therefore, these studies should incorporate a cross-cultural perspective.

TABLE 18–2. Night waking dyssomnia in toddlers and preschoolers

	Nighttime awakenings[a]	
Age	Frequency	Duration (total)
Perturbation (one episode per week for at least 1 month)		
12–24 months	≥3 awakenings/night	≥30 minutes
>24 months	≥2 awakenings/night	≥20 minutes
>36 months	≥2 awakenings/night	≥10 minutes
Disturbance (two to four episodes per week for at least 1 month)		
12–24 months	≥3 awakenings/night	≥30 minutes
>24 months	≥2 awakenings/night	≥20 minutes
>36 months	≥2 awakenings/night	≥10 minutes
Disorder (307.42.1) **(five to seven episodes per week for at least 1 month)**		
12–24 months	≥3 awakenings/night	≥30 minutes
>24 months	≥2 awakenings/night	≥20 minutes
>36 months	≥2 awakenings/night	≥10 minutes

Note. Awakenings occur after infant has been asleep for more than 10 minutes. In the Gaylor et al. 2005 paper, the criteria for night waking disorder were12–23 months of age: ≥2 awakenings/night, totaling ≥20 minutes; ≥ 24 months of age: ≥1 awakening/night, totaling ≥20 minutes.

[a]Awakenings require parental intervention.

Finally, it is often the parent–infant/child interactions and parent–child relationship factors (parent well being, effective parenting, and family stress) that affect the developmental outcomes of the child's sleep patterns, so that research needs to be directed at these transactional interactions. Similarly, it is often parent–child relationships that suffer as a consequence of sleep problems, particularly with respect to sleep deprivation, irritability, and negative affect in response to chronic night waking.

Research Agenda and Recommendations

A number of questions should be answered by a targeted research program. At what age should a sleep disorder in infants be diagnosed? If sleep disorders in infants are present in the first 3–6 months of life, what are cutoffs that differentiate them from normal "variability"? Can infants in the first year of life be too sleepy? Are hypersomnias (e.g., failure to maintain wakefulness and alertness, state regulation) present in this age group? Should parental impairment be sufficient grounds to classify a sleep disorder in infants and toddlers? Should daytime "sleepiness" or

TABLE 18–3. Sleep onset dyssomnia in toddlers and preschoolers

Age	Settling to sleep and reunions[a]
Perturbation (one episode per week for at least 1 month)	
12–24 months	1) >30 minutes to fall asleep
	2) Parent remains in room for sleep onset
	3) More than three reunions
>24 months	1) >20 minutes to fall asleep
	2) Parent remains in room for sleep onset
	3) More than two reunions
Disturbance (two to four episodes per week for at least 1 month)	
12–24 months	1) >30 minutes to fall asleep
	2) Parent remains in room for sleep onset
	3) More than three reunions
>24 months	1) >20 minutes to fall asleep
	2) Parent remains in room for sleep onset
	3) More than two reunions
Disorder[b] (307.42.2) (five to seven episodes per week for at least 1 month)	
12–24 months	1) >30 minutes to fall asleep
	2) Parent remains in room for sleep onset
	3) More than three reunions
>24 months	1) >20 minutes to fall asleep
	2) Parent remains in room for sleep onset
	3) More than two reunions

[a]Must meet any two of the three criteria; reunions reflect resistances going to bed (e.g., repeated bids, protests, struggles).
[b]Classify as 307.42.3 when sleep onset disorder and night waking disorder are coexistent.

behavioral disturbance be a requisite for making a diagnosis of sleep disorder in the child? When might an early childhood sleep disorder be considered a relationship sleep disorder rather than an infant sleep disorder?

We recommend three levels of study based on these questions: 1) developmental animal studies will be useful to look at brain and behavioral development; 2) clinical human studies can provide information about frequency, intensity, and cultural influences, including naturalistic longitudinal studies that illuminate the long-term consequences of early sleep problems; and 3) intervention research can provide information about outcomes/consequences. There should be a "multiaxial" approach to the research wherein structured instruments objectively assess the infant and infant's sleep (Axis 1); the parent, including family stress levels (Axis 4); and the infant–parent interaction (Axis 5).

Research needs to focus on the dyssomnias with the following objectives:

- Define infant/toddler/preschool sleep dyssomnias by using criteria based on quantitative, objective cut points (duration, frequency, intensity) that are developmentally appropriate.
- Include measures of daytime sleepiness and sleep-related behaviors (activity level, irritability, attention) as criteria of impairment for the child. Impairment criteria for the parent and/or the parent–child relationship need to be established.
- Determine the effect of culture, ethnicity, socioeconomic status, and gender by using large, population-based studies (perhaps multisite studies) of typically developing infants in the age range from 6 months to 5 years. Data about parental/family knowledge, attitudes, and values regarding infant sleep at these ages need to be collected and assessed in relation to how they affect emerging sleep-wake organization.
- Conduct multimethod data collection using both subjective parent reports (structured questionnaires and sleep diaries) and objective recording methods (video or actigraph). Data collection needs to occur over at least 5, but preferably 7, nights.
- Examine sleep context variables, including sleep location, family sleep times/problems, parenting stress, and so on.

In future editions of DSM, there are two options for classifying sleep disorders (and, in fact, for all early childhood disorders). If a separate section for "Disorders Usually First Diagnosed in Infancy, Childhood, or Adolescence" continues, then sleep disorders that affect this age group should be included in that section with developmentally appropriate criteria. If, on the other hand, developmentally appropriate criteria for the large majority of the psychiatric/behavioral disorders of this age group are adopted, then that separate section should be significantly curtailed and the developmentally appropriate criteria should be added as subsections to each of the adult disorders.

Commentary: Susan L. Warren, M.D.

This excellent review by Anders and Dahl notes that much additional research is needed concerning the classification of sleep disorders in young children. The authors raise several important points. First, difficulties in night waking (maintaining sleep) appear to be distinct from difficulties in initiating sleep. Such dissimilarities have been found not only with young children but also with the elderly (Klerman et al. 2004). Second, the authors note that it is very difficult to determine for sleep disorders in young children what constitutes clinically significant distress and impairment. One important area of investigation, suggested by the authors, would involve studying possible impairment in the children by utilizing developmental neuroscience approaches. Third, the authors propose compelling criteria for new disorders called "night waking dyssomnia" and "sleep onset dyssomnia." These criteria were developed by studying children's sleep patterns longitudinally (Gaylor et al. 2005). Investigating these criteria further—along with potential impairment and comorbid symptoms—utilizing longitudinal approaches in a large representative sample would seem to be beneficial to better characterize sleep disorders in young children.

References

Adair R, Bauchner H, Philipp B, et al: Night waking during infancy: role of parental presence at bedtime. Pediatrics 87:500–504, 1991

American Academy of Sleep Medicine: The International Classification of Sleep Disorders, Diagnostic and Coding Manual Revised. Westchester, IL, American Academy of Sleep Medicine, 2001

American Academy of Sleep Medicine: The International Classification of Sleep Disorders, Diagnostic and Coding Manual, 2nd Edition. Westchester, IL, American Academy of Sleep Medicine, 2005

American Psychiatric Association: Diagnostic and Statistical Manual of Mental Disorders, 4th Edition. Washington, DC, American Psychiatric Association, 1994

American Psychiatric Association: Diagnostic and Statistical Manual of Mental Disorders, 4th Edition, Text Revision. Washington, DC, American Psychiatric Association, 2000

American Sleep Disorders Association: The International Classification of Sleep Disorders, Diagnostic and Coding Manual. Kansas City, KS, Allen Press, 1990

Archbold KH, Pituch K, Panabi P, et al: Symptoms of sleep disturbances among children in two general pediatric clinics. J Pediatr 140:97–102, 2002

Dahl R: The impact of inadequate sleep on children's daytime cognitive function. Semin Pediatr Neurol 3:44–50, 1996

Gaylor EE, Burnham MM, Goodlin-Jones BL, et al: A longitudinal follow-up study of young children's sleep patterns using a developmental classification system. Behav Sleep Med 3:44–61, 2005

Klerman EB, Davis JB, Duffy JF, et al: Older people awaken more frequently but fall back asleep at the same rate as younger people. Sleep 27:793–798, 2004

Lam P, Hiscock H, Wake M: Outcomes of infant sleep problems: a longitudinal study of sleep, behavior and maternal well being. Pediatrics 111:e203–e207, 2003

Lavigne J, Arend R, Rosenbaum E, et al: Sleep and behavior problems among preschoolers. J Dev Behav Pediatr 20:164–169, 1999

Lozoff B, Askew G, Wolf A: Cosleeping and early childhood sleep problems: effects of ethnicity and socioeconomic status. J Dev Behav Pediatr 17:9–15, 1996

Marcotte A, Thacher P, Butters M, et al: Parental report of sleep problems in children with attentional and learning disorders. J Dev Behav Pediatr 19:178–186, 1998

Moore T, Ucko L: Night waking in early infancy, part 1. Arch Dis Child 32:333–342, 1957

Morrell J: The role of maternal cognitions in infant sleep problems as assessed by a new instrument, the maternal cognitions about infant sleep questionnaire. J Child Psychol Psychiatry 40:247–258, 1999

Ottaviano S, Giannotti F, Cortesi F, et al: Sleep characteristics in healthy children from birth to 6 years of age in the urban area of Rome. Sleep 19:1–3, 1996

Owens J, Spirito A, McGuinn M: The Children's Sleep Habits Questionnaire (CSHQ): psychometric properties of a survey instrument for school-aged children. Sleep 23:1043–1051, 2000

Richman N: A community survey of characteristics of one- to two-year-olds with sleep disruptions. J Am Acad Child Adolesc Psychiatry 20:281–291, 1981

Scher A, Tirosh E, Jaffe M, et al: Survey of sleep patterns of Israeli infants and young children. Int J Behav Dev 18:701–711, 1995

Stores G, Wiggs L (eds): Sleep Disturbance in Children and Adolescents with Disorders of Development: Its Significance and Management, No. 155. London, England, Mac Keith Press, 2001

Thunstrom M: Severe sleep problems among infants in a normal population in Sweden: prevalence, severity and correlates. Acta Pediatr 88:1318–1319, 1999

Thunstrom M: Severe sleep problems in infancy associated with subsequent development of attention-deficit/hyperactivity disorder at 5.5 years. Acta Paediatr 91:584–592, 2002

Wolke D, Meyer R, Ohrt B, et al: The incidence of sleeping problems in preterm and full-term infants discharged from neonatal special care units: an epidemiological longitudinal study. J Child Psychol Psychiatry 36:203–223, 1995

Wolke D, Sohne B, Riegel K, et al: An epidemiologic longitudinal study of sleeping problems and feeding experience of preterm and term children in southern Finland: comparison with a southern German population sample. J Pediatr 133:224–231, 1998

World Health Organization: International Classification of Diseases, 9th Revision. Geneva, Switzerland, World Health Organization, 1977

Zuckerman B, Stevenson J, Baily V: Sleep problems in early childhood: continuities, predictive factors and behavioral correlates. Pediatrics 80:664–671, 1987

19

CLASSIFYING FEEDING DISORDERS OF INFANCY AND EARLY CHILDHOOD

Irene Chatoor, M.D.
Massimo Ammaniti, M.D.

Current State of the Science

The term *feeding* is generally used to emphasize the dyadic nature of eating in infants and young children. It is estimated that 25%–50% of infants and young children have feeding problems (Carruth et al. 2004; Lindberg et al. 1994) and that severe feeding problems associated with poor weight gain occur in 1.4% of infants (Dahl and Sundelin 1986). Furthermore, longitudinal research has demonstrated that early food refusal and picky eating persist over time (Dahl et al. 1994; Jacobi et al. 2003). Some outcomes of early feeding problems are nontrivial, with "picky eating" in early childhood being related to symptoms of anorexia nervosa in adolescence; problem meals and pica in early childhood being significant risk factors for the development of bulimia nervosa in adolescence (Marchi and Cohen 1990); and early struggles with food and unpleasant meals as risk factors for the development of eating disorders during young adulthood (Kotler et al. 2001).

The research and preparation of this chapter has been supported by the National Institute of Mental Health grant awarded to Irene Chatoor (RO1-MH58219) and a grant from the National Center for Research Resources awarded to the Children's Clinical Research Center (RR132970).

TABLE 19–1. DSM-IV-TR diagnostic criteria for feeding disorder of infancy or early childhood

A. Feeding disturbance as manifested by persistent failure to eat adequately with significant failure to gain weight or significant loss of weight over at least 1 month.
B. The disturbance is not due to an associated gastrointestinal or other general medical condition (e.g., esophageal reflux).
C. The disturbance is not better accounted for by another mental disorder (e.g., Rumination Disorder) or by lack of available food.
D. The onset is before age 6 years.

Source. Reprinted from American Psychiatric Association: *Diagnostic and Statistical Manual of Mental Disorders,* 4th Edition, Text Revision. Washington, DC, American Psychiatric Association, 2000. Copyright 2000, American Psychiatric Association. Used with permission.

In spite of the high prevalence of feeding problems in early childhood and their extended course, it was not until 1994 that DSM-IV (American Psychiatric Association 1994) introduced "feeding disorder of infancy and early childhood" as a diagnostic category and for the first time provided a standard definition of feeding disorders. The DSM-IV-TR (American Psychiatric Association 2000) diagnostic criteria for this disorder are shown in Table 19–1.

Although this was a first step toward a definition of a feeding disorder, this definition does not address many important issues. First, it does not cover many types of feeding disorders, leading to confusion regarding what constitutes a feeding disorder. Second, perhaps as a result of the narrowness of the DSM-IV criteria, different diagnostic labels have been used to describe overlapping symptomatology, and the same label has been applied to describe different feeding problems (see Figure 19–1). Third, the relationship between failure to thrive and feeding disorders remains unclear. As a result, many reports of young children with feeding disorders describe only some clinical features of the disorders, but they fail to characterize distinctive features and how they are differentiated from more transient or subclinical feeding problems.

Advances in Understanding Feeding Disorders

To address the question of how to differentiate various severe feeding problems from one another and from transient or milder feeding difficulties, Chatoor et al. (2002) developed a classification system that describes the phenomenology and provides operational diagnostic criteria for six subtypes of feeding disorders in infants and young children. These criteria were modified by the American Academy of Child and Adolescent Psychiatry's Task Force for Research Diagnostic Criteria: Infants and Preschool (2003) and were further developed with the help of the current American Psychiatric Association work group. The diagnostic criteria include clinical symptoms and measures of impairment, which are primarily in the area of nutrition, for example, growth failure, specific dietary deficiencies, or inadequate food intake threatening the child's health and growth. Although the six subtypes of feeding disorders show some overlapping symptoms and some overlapping criteria for impairment, they reflect different symptom and impairment constellations that are believed to be related to different etiologies. The severity of the symptoms, and the impairment criteria, differentiate these feeding disorders from milder or transient feeding difficulties. Figure 19–1 lists these six feeding disorder subtypes and previously used names describing similar symptomatology.

The significance of differentiating the six feeding disorder subtypes lies in their different etiologies and treatment implications. For example, growth failure secondary to food refusal by the child (as seen in infantile anorexia) versus growth failure secondary to underfeeding by the mother (as seen in feeding disorder associated with lack of parent–infant reciprocity) require very different interventions. An effective therapeutic intervention for infantile anorexia that focuses on regulating mealtimes in order to help the child experience hunger (Chatoor et al. 1997b) is ineffective in overcoming the food refusal of children with a posttraumatic feeding disorder (Benoit et al. 2000). On the other hand, behavioral interventions that may be helpful to overcome a posttraumatic feeding disorder are counterproductive for infantile anorexia.

Generating Developmentally Informed Phenotypes

The first four feeding disorder subtypes listed in the following subsections tend to start during specific developmental periods and are arranged accordingly, whereas posttraumatic feeding disorder and feeding disorder associated with a concurrent medical condition can occur at various stages of the child's development.

FEEDING DISORDER OF STATE REGULATION

Proposed Diagnostic Criteria

A. The infant's feeding difficulties start in the first few months of life and should be present for at least 2 weeks.
B. The infant has difficulty reaching and maintaining a state of calm alertness for feeding; he or she is either too sleepy or too agitated to feed.
C. The infant fails to gain age appropriate weight or may show loss of weight.
D. The infant's feeding difficulties cannot be explained by a physical illness.

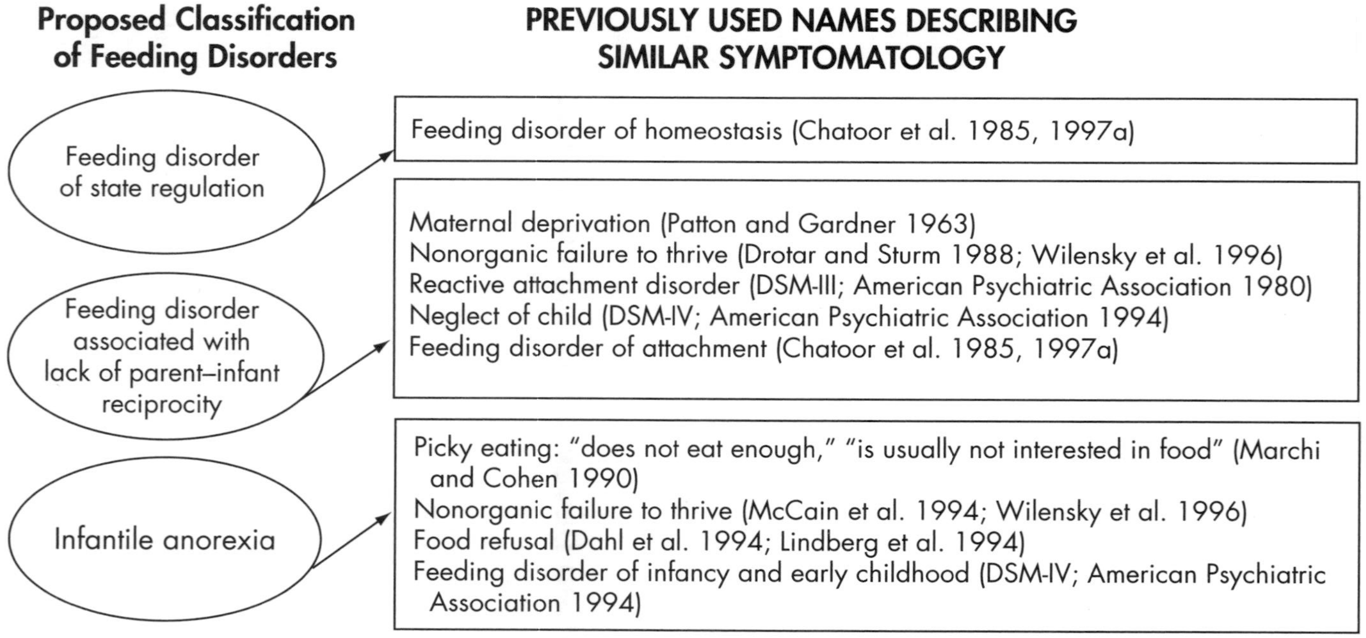
Proposed Classification of Feeding Disorders
PREVIOUSLY USED NAMES DESCRIBING SIMILAR SYMPTOMATOLOGY
Feeding disorder of state regulation
Feeding disorder of homeostasis (Chatoor et al. 1985, 1997a)
Feeding disorder associated with lack of parent–infant reciprocity
Maternal deprivation (Patton and Gardner 1963)
Nonorganic failure to thrive (Drotar and Sturm 1988; Wilensky et al. 1996)
Reactive attachment disorder (DSM-III; American Psychiatric Association 1980)
Neglect of child (DSM-IV; American Psychiatric Association 1994)
Feeding disorder of attachment (Chatoor et al. 1985, 1997a)
Infantile anorexia
Picky eating: "does not eat enough," "is usually not interested in food" (Marchi and Cohen 1990)
Nonorganic failure to thrive (McCain et al. 1994; Wilensky et al. 1996)
Food refusal (Dahl et al. 1994; Lindberg et al. 1994)
Feeding disorder of infancy and early childhood (DSM-IV; American Psychiatric Association 1994)

FIGURE 19–1. The Chatoor classification of feeding disorders and previously cited terminology.

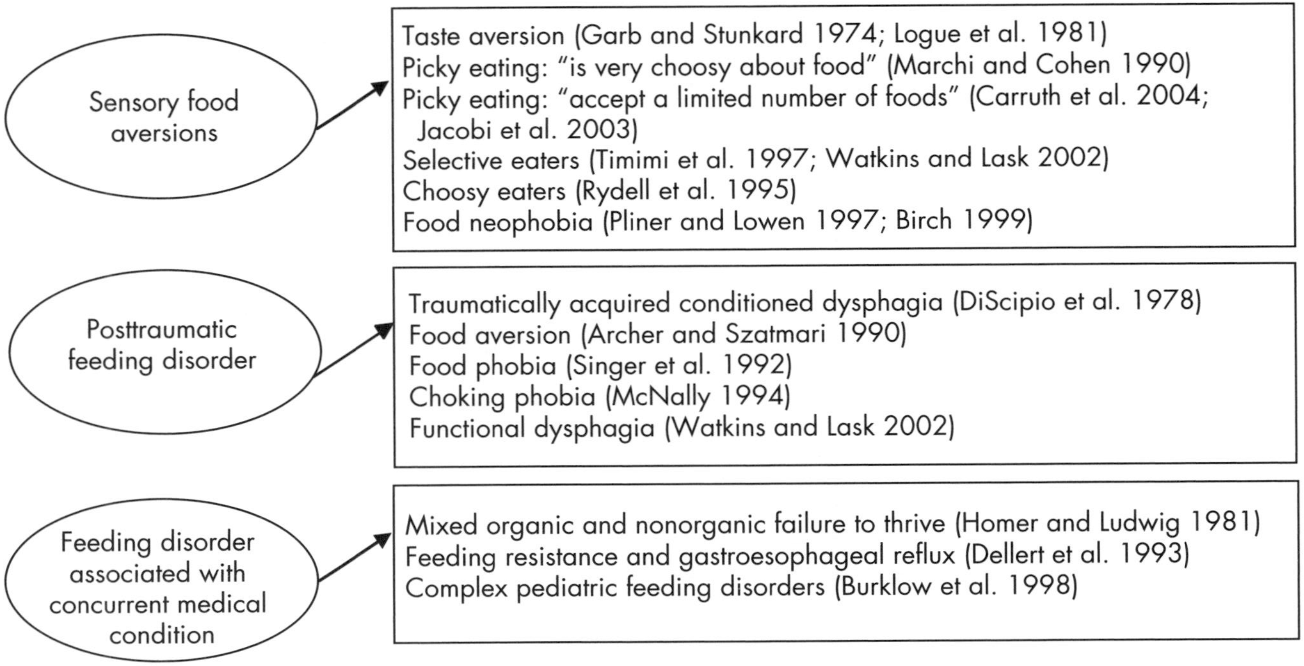

FIGURE 19–1. The Chatoor classification of feeding disorders and previously cited terminology *(continued)*.

Research Findings

Feeding disorder of state regulation was described in the past as "feeding disorder of homeostasis" because it usually begins in the postnatal period when infants need to transition from continuous feedings in utero through the umbilical cord to a new state of homeostasis characterized by the rhythms of sleep and wakefulness and feeding and elimination (Chatoor et al. 1985, 1997a). Observation of mother–infant interactions of a small group of infants revealed poor dyadic reciprocity to be associated with this feeding disorder (Chatoor et al. 1997a). However, more research is needed to better understand this disorder.

FEEDING DISORDER ASSOCIATED WITH LACK OF PARENT–INFANT RECIPROCITY

Proposed Diagnostic Criteria

A. This feeding disorder is usually observed in the first year of life, when the infant presents to the primary care physician or to the emergency department with some acute medical problem (commonly an infection), and the physician notices that the infant is malnourished.
B. The infant shows lack of developmentally appropriate signs of social responsivity (e.g., visual engagement, smiling, babbling) during feeding with primary caregiver.
C. The infant shows significant growth deficiency (acute and/or chronic malnutrition according to Waterlow et al. (1977); or the child's weight deviates across two major percentiles in a 2- to 6-month period).
D. The primary caregiver is often unaware of the feeding and growth problems of the infant.
E. The growth deficiency and lack of relatedness are not solely due to a physical illness or to a pervasive developmental disorder.

Research Findings

Feeding disorder associated with lack of parent–infant reciprocity was first described as "maternal deprivation" (Patton and Gardner 1963), suggesting that the infant does not thrive because of the emotional unavailability of the mother. Then DSM-III (American Psychiatric Association 1980) introduced the diagnosis of "reactive attachment disorder," which included weight loss or failure to gain appropriate amounts of weight. However, in DSM-III-R (American Psychiatric Association 1987), growth failure was no longer included in the diagnostic criteria of reactive attachment disorder, and this continued in DSM-IV and DSM-IV-TR. Although high rates of insecure attachment have been described in infants and young children with failure to thrive (Ward et al. 1993), it is clear that attachment disorders and failure to thrive are distinct and that the diagnostic term "non-organic failure to thrive" is overly vague and even misleading.

Previous publications referred to this disorder as "feeding disorder of attachment" (Chatoor et al. 1985, 1997a), but it was later changed to "feeding disorder of reciprocity" (Task Force on Research Diagnostic Criteria: Infancy and Preschool 2003) because the feeding disorder is primarily seen in young infants, and attachment is difficult to assess in infants younger than 1 year of age. Infants with this feeding disorder and their mothers were found to have less dyadic reciprocity during feeding than healthy eaters and their mothers. In addition, mothers of the infants with feeding disorder received higher maternal noncontingency ratings than mothers of healthy eaters (Chatoor et al. 1997a).

INFANTILE ANOREXIA

Proposed Diagnostic Criteria

A. Infantile anorexia is characterized by the infant's or toddler's refusal to eat adequate amounts of food for at least 1 month.
B. Onset of the food refusal often occurs during the transition to spoon and self-feeding, typically between 6 months and 3 years of age.
C. The infant or toddler rarely communicates hunger and lacks interest in food and eating but shows strong interest in play, exploration, and/or interaction with caregivers.
D. The infant or toddler shows significant growth deficiency (acute and/or chronic malnutrition according to Waterlow et al. (1977); or the child's weight deviates across two major percentiles in a 2- to 6-month period).
E. The food refusal does not follow a traumatic event to the oropharynx.
F. The food refusal is not due to an underlying medical illness.

Research Findings

Several studies have demonstrated that infantile anorexia can be diagnosed with high interrater reliability (Chatoor et al. 1998b, 2000, 2002). Mother–infant interactional patterns are characterized by less dyadic reciprocity, high dyadic conflict, struggle for control, and increased talk and distractions during feedings (Chatoor et al. 1988, 1998b, 2001; Lucarelli et al. 2003). Toddlers with infantile anorexia are rated by their parents as more negative, irregular, dependent, unstoppable, and difficult (Chatoor et al. 2000), and they exhibit more anxiety/depression, somatic complaints, and aggressive behaviors than healthy control children (Ammaniti et al. 2004a). More mothers of toddlers with infantile anorexia demonstrate insecure attachment patterns to their own parents (Chatoor et al. 2000) and dysfunctional eating attitudes, anxiety, depression, and hostility than do mothers of healthy control children (Ammaniti et al. 2004a). Additional studies have found that toddlers with infantile anorexia exhibited a higher rate of insecure attachment relationships than healthy eaters (Ammaniti et al. 2004b; Chatoor et al. 1998a), although the majority of anorexic toddlers (60%) showed secure attachment patterns. However, the significant correlation between the severity of malnutrition and the degree of attachment insecurity indicated that an insecure infant–mother relationship is associated with a more severe expression of infantile anorexia (Chatoor et al. 1998a). It is of interest that infantile anorexia appears to occur with the same frequency in boys and girls, in contrast to anorexia nervosa, which is seen predominantly in females.

On average, toddlers with infantile anorexia performed within the normal range of cognitive development. However, the Mental Developmental Index (MDI; Bayley 1969) scores of the healthy eaters were significantly higher than those of the infantile anorexia group. Within the infantile anorexia group, correlations between MDI scores and the toddlers' percent ideal body weight did not reach statistical significance, whereas across all groups, the toddlers' MDI scores showed a significant correlation with the quality of mother–child interactions and socioeconomic status of the family (Chatoor et al. 2004b).

In addition, results of a recent pilot study found increased physiological arousal and decreased ability to modulate physiological reactivity in toddlers with infantile anorexia compared with a control group of healthy eaters (Chatoor et al. 2004a). This study raised the question of whether the difficulty of recognizing hunger, which characterizes children with infantile anorexia, may be related to a different physiological arousal pattern—that is, that these children do not feel hunger because of their heightened physiological arousal. This study should be replicated with larger numbers of children to further explore this question.

In summary, these studies revealed specific child and parent vulnerabilities to be associated with infantile anorexia, and both child and parent characteristics were significantly correlated with the strained parent–child relationship during feeding. All of these studies were cross-sectional, and consequently they do not allow any firm conclusions about the causality of this feeding disorder. However, the developmental histories of these children reveal that from early infancy they display little interest in feeding and eat only small amounts, triggering parental anxiety and setting the stage for the ensuing parent–child struggles during feeding. Consequently, a transactional model for infantile anorexia was developed. According to this model, the infant or toddler with a poor hunger drive and refusal to eat elicits anxiety, especially in mothers who try to compensate for their infant's poor food intake by engaging in noncontingent behaviors. These behaviors may range from distracting the toddler with toys or television while feeding to forcing food into the toddler's mouth. These parental behaviors further interfere with the toddler's awareness of hunger and lead to increasingly conflictual interactions between mother and child, with both struggling for control. As a result of these struggles, the child does not learn to regulate eating internally, but eating becomes completely dependent on the interactions of the child with the environment.

This transactional model has served as a basis for an intervention to facilitate internal regulation of eating in toddlers with infantile anorexia. Parents are trained to help their toddlers recognize hunger and to learn to eat according to their internal signals of hunger and fullness. An initial pilot study (Chatoor et al. 1997b) was conducted, and a randomized, controlled treatment study is under way.

SENSORY FOOD AVERSIONS

Proposed Diagnostic Criteria

A. Sensory food aversion is characterized by the infant's or child's consistent refusal to eat specific foods with specific tastes, textures, smells, and/or appearances for at least 1 month.
B. The onset of the food refusal occurs during the introduction of a new type or taste of food (e.g., may drink one type of formula but refuse another; may eat carrots, but refuse green beans; may eat crunchy foods but refuse pureed food or baby food).
C. Eats well when offered preferred foods.
D. Does not show growth deficiency, but without supplementation, demonstrates specific dietary deficiencies (i.e., vitamins, iron, zinc, or protein); or displays oral motor and expressive speech delay; or starting during the preschool years, demonstrates anxiety around, and avoids, social situations that involve eating.
E. Refusal to eat specific foods is not related to food allergies or any other medical illness.

Research Findings

Several authors have described children's difficulty to eat certain foods but have used a variety of names (see Figure 19–1). These studies are usually based on parent reports and do not differentiate between milder or more severe forms of food selectivity. Consequently, some authors report very high numbers (25%–50%) of "picky eating" (Carruth et al. 2004; Marchi and Cohen 1990). A diagnostic study of feeding disorders (Chatoor et al. 2002) using the diagnostic criteria outlined here demonstrated excellent interrater reliability of the diagnosis of sensory food aversions.

Some studies have explored whether taste sensitivities are heritable, and various models of genetic transmission have been suggested, for example, a two locus model (Olson et al. 1989) and specific polymorphism of gene *Tas2r* on Chromosome 7q (Kim et al. 2003). Keller et al. (2002) reported on the relationship between genetic taste sensitivity to propylthiouracil and food selectivity in preschool children. Others (Birch 1999; Birch and Marlin 1982) have demonstrated that certain aspects of the eating environment can also have a strong influence on the development of food preferences and shape selective food refusal. It appears that both genetic predisposition and the eating environment affect toddler's food preferences, but much remains to be learned about both contributors and mechanisms.

POSTTRAUMATIC FEEDING DISORDER

Proposed Diagnostic Criteria

A. Posttraumatic feeding disorder is characterized by the acute onset of consistent food refusal.
B. The onset of the food refusal can occur at any age of the child from infancy onward.
C. The food refusal follows a traumatic event or repeated traumatic insults to the oropharynx or gastrointestinal tract (e.g., choking, severe vomiting, insertion of nasogastric or endotracheal tubes, suctioning) that trigger distress in the child.
D. Consistent refusal to eat manifests in one of the following ways, depending on the feeding experience of the child in association with the traumatic event:
    - Refuses to drink from the bottle, but may accept food offered by spoon (although consistently refuses to drink from the bottle when awake, may drink from the bottle when sleepy or asleep).
    - Refuses solid food, but may accept the bottle.
    - Refuses all oral feedings.
E. Reminders of the traumatic events cause distress, as manifested by one or more of the following:
    - May show anticipatory distress when positioned for feeding.
    - Shows intense resistance when approached with bottle or food.
    - Shows intense resistance to swallow food placed in his or her mouth.
F. Without supplementation (e.g., specific fortified formula preparations, intravenous fluids, nasogastric or gastrostomy tube feedings, or parenteral nutrition), the food refusal poses an acute and/or long-term threat to the child's health, nutrition, and growth and threatens the progression of age-appropriate feeding development of the child.

Research Findings

Using the diagnostic criteria listed here, a recent study demonstrated that posttraumatic feeding disorder can be diagnosed with high interrater reliability (Chatoor et al. 2002). Another study found that toddlers with the disorder showed intense mother–infant conflict during feeding and demonstrated the most intense resistance to swallowing food (Chatoor et al. 2001). One controlled, randomized treatment study demonstrated the effectiveness of a behavioral intervention in the treatment of this feeding disorder (Benoit et al. 2000).

FEEDING DISORDER ASSOCIATED WITH A CONCURRENT MEDICAL CONDITION

Proposed Diagnostic Criteria

A. This feeding disorder is also characterized by food refusal and inadequate food intake for at least 2 weeks.
B. The onset of the food refusal can occur at any age of the child and may wax and wane in intensity, depending on the underlying medical condition.
C. The infant or toddler readily initiates feeding, but over the course of the feeding shows distress and refuses to continue feeding.
D. The child has a concurrent medical condition that is believed to cause the distress (e.g., gastroesophageal reflux, cardiac or respiratory disease).
E. The child fails to gain age appropriate weight or may even lose weight.
F. Medical management improves but may not fully alleviate the feeding problems.

Research Findings

Since Homer and Ludwig (1981) described a third category of "failure to thrive" which was caused by a combination of various organic and non-organic problems, it has been accepted that organic conditions can be associated with psychological difficulties and lead to severe feeding problems. Co-occurrence of medical and severe feeding problems is now well established (Dellert et al. 1993; Lemons and Dodge 1998; Nelson et al. 1998). The implication is that medical and psychological factors can lead to complex feeding problems, requiring combined interventions.

One diagnostic study has demonstrated that feeding disorder associated with a concurrent medical condition can be diagnosed with high interrater reliability when the feeding history given by the mother and the observation of mother–infant interactions during feeding are combined (Chatoor et al. 2002).

Is There Comorbidity Between Various Feeding Disorder Subtypes?

In the diagnostic study by Chatoor et al. (2002), 20% of the infants and young children examined showed comorbidity of two or more feeding disorders. The most frequent comorbidity observed was between infantile anorexia and sensory food aversions (13%), although these feeding disorders occurred more frequently in the pure form (31% sensory food aversions and 21% infantile anorexia). This raises the question of whether these are two feeding disorders or the same feeding disorder with variable symptom expression. We argue that they are separate feeding disorders with different etiologies and different responses to treatment. Toddlers with infantile anorexia respond to the regulation of mealtimes with an increase of appetite and improved food intake (Chatoor et al. 1997b), whereas toddlers with sensory food aversions will eat less or nothing if offered aversive foods, regardless of hunger cues.

What Are the Next Steps for Validating These Six Feeding Disorder Diagnoses?

The validity of the six feeding disorder subtypes would be further increased if any one of the following five criteria is met:

1. *There is a reliably observed collection of typically co-occurring symptoms that are found less frequently in other disorders.* The diagnostic interrater reliabilities of the specific symptom constellations of four feeding disorder subtypes (infantile anorexia, sensory food aversions, posttraumatic feeding disorder, feeding disorder associated with a medical condition) have been established in one clinical center but must be replicated independently.
2. *There is an association with family history/genetic factors.* Clinical interviews indicate that two feeding disorder subtypes (infantile anorexia and sensory food aversions) frequently aggregate in other family members of the affected children. Family history and genetic studies should explore a genetic basis for each of these feeding disorders.
3. *The longitudinal course distinguishes the disorder from health and from other disorders.* The study of the longitudinal course of these six feeding disorder subtypes will be critical in understanding whether they are truly different feeding disorders with continuity of specific symptoms or whether symptoms change to a different condition, later merge, and are difficult to untangle. Ideally, prospective studies—starting from birth—would address these questions and would allow a better understanding of the child's and the parent's contribution to the unfolding of these feeding disorder subtypes. However, because severe feeding disorders are estimated to occur in only 1%–2% of the population (Dahl and Sundelin 1986), such studies would require very large sample sizes. On the other hand, follow-up studies of clinical populations, although they cannot answer questions of causality, will be able to address the question of the continuity of symptom constellations of the specific feeding disorder subtypes. Long-term follow-up studies should examine the relationship of early feeding disorders to eating disorders during childhood, adolescence, and adulthood and the development of associated psychopathology, for example, anxiety disorders and depression.
4. *The syndrome exhibits unique neurobiological correlates.* The pilot study by Chatoor et al. (2004a) showed that toddlers with infantile anorexia demonstrated

higher levels of physiological arousal and decreased ability to modulate physiological reactivity when compared with healthy eaters. Further studies should explore whether this arousal pattern is typical for infantile anorexia or can be seen in other feeding disorder subtypes as well. Another important question to be addressed is whether there is a special biological vulnerability that predisposes certain children to a posttraumatic feeding disorder, because not all children who experience traumatic events to the oropharynx (e.g., choking or intubation) develop the disorder.

5. *The syndrome shows a specific response to certain treatments.* A different response to treatment for two feeding disorder subtypes was demonstrated in two studies. A randomized, controlled study showed the effectiveness of a behavioral intervention and the ineffectiveness of regulating meals and appetite in the treatment of posttraumatic feeding disorders (Benoit et al. 2000). The second study, a pilot study, demonstrated that regulating meal times is an effective way to stimulate appetite and increase food intake in toddlers with infantile anorexia (Chatoor et al. 1997b). Chatoor and colleagues are further testing this treatment model for infantile anorexia in a larger randomized study with results still pending. Further studies are needed to develop effective treatments for the other feeding disorder subtypes, especially for sensory food aversions, which in clinical experience does not respond to the behavioral interventions used for posttraumatic feeding disorders or for infantile anorexia.

Commentary: Thomas F. Anders, M.D.

The classification of feeding disorders in infants and toddlers has been advanced significantly by the careful theoretical conceptualization and clinical investigation of these two authors. Previous classifications that included such labels as the organic and nonorganic failure to thrive syndromes provided little guidance to clinicians regarding etiology and/or treatment. These authors describe a developmentally sensitive nosology from which both etiological factors and treatment strategies can be inferred. The primary strength of the chapter lies in the long-standing clinical and research commitment to these disorders manifested by Dr. Chatoor. She has published extensively and has been most willing to modify criteria as indicated by data. Dr. Ammaniti brings confirmatory experience to bear on Dr. Chatoor's observations. Yet this primary strength is also a potential weakness. The data are derived principally from clinical patients referred to an expert feeding-disorders clinician. Larger-scale studies using multiple sites and investigators and involving community and clinical samples need to be undertaken to further establish the nosological distinctness of the Chatoor subtypes, to further refine the cut points that define disorder, and to better track the natural histories and responses to treatment.

All of the subtypes of feeding disorder may become more difficult to define as the weight loss and chronic malnutrition criteria that characterize them are ameliorated by pediatricians' facility with nasogastric and gastrostomy tubes. At the point of tube insertion, the infant's weight, growth, and nutrition are restored, but the underlying interactional problem persists and may be heightened because of the anxiety and "watchfulness" that results from the associated stress and preoccupation of managing the feeding tube. With the insertion of a feeding tube, the chronicity of the feeding disorder is increased because it becomes difficult, even with psychosocial and/or behavioral treatments, to get to a stable oral feeding routine with adequate appetite to support removing the tube.

Finally, although it is not within the purview of Dr. Chatoor's research, a comprehensive nosology of feeding disorders of infants, toddlers, and preschool children should include disorders that define overeating and overfeeding, especially given the alleged epidemic of obesity in the United States.

References

American Psychiatric Association: Diagnostic and Statistical Manual of Mental Disorders, 3rd Edition. Washington, DC, American Psychiatric Association, 1980

American Psychiatric Association: Diagnostic and Statistical Manual of Mental Disorders, 3rd Edition Revised. Washington, DC, American Psychiatric Association, 1987

American Psychiatric Association: Diagnostic and Statistical Manual of Mental Disorders, 4th Edition. Washington, DC, American Psychiatric Association, 1994

American Psychiatric Association: Diagnostic and Statistical Manual of Mental Disorders, 4th Edition, Text Revision. Washington, DC, American Psychiatric Association, 2000

Ammaniti M, Ambruzzi AM, Lucarelli L, et al: Malnutrition and dysfunctional mother–child feeding interactions: clinical assessment and research implications. J Am Coll Nutr 23:259–271, 2004a

Ammaniti M, Cimino S, Lucarelli L, et al: Infantile anorexia and the child caregiver relationship: an empirical study on attachment patterns. Funzione Gamma Journal 14:1–19, 2004b

Archer LA, Szatmari P: Assessment and treatment of food aversion in a four-year-old boy: a multidimensional approach. Can J Psychiatry 35:501–505, 1990

Bayley N: Bayley Scales of Infant Development. New York, The Psychological Corporation, 1969

Benoit D, Wang EE, Zlotkin SH: Discontinuation of enterostomy tube feeding by behavioral treatment in early childhood: a randomized control trial. J Pediatr 137:498–503, 2000

Birch LL: Development of food preferences. Annu Rev Nutr 19:41–62, 1999

Birch LL, Marlin DW: I don't like it; I never tried it: effects of exposure on two-year-old children's food preferences. Appetite 3:353–360, 1982

Burklow KA, Phelps AN, Schultz JR, et al: Classifying complex pediatric feeding disorders. J Pediatr Gastroenterol Nutr 27:143–147, 1998

Carruth BR, Ziegler PJ, Gordon A, et al: Prevalence of picky eaters among infants and toddlers and their caregivers' decisions about offering a new food. J Am Diet Assoc 104 (suppl):57–64, 2004

Chatoor I, Dickson L, Schaefer S, et al: A developmental classification of feeding disorders associated with failure-to-thrive: diagnosis and treatment, in New Directions in Failure to Thrive: Research and Clinical Practice. Edited by Drotar D. New York, Plenum, 1985, pp 235–258

Chatoor I, Egan J, Getson P, et al: Mother–infant interactions in infantile anorexia nervosa. J Am Acad Child and Adolesc Psychiatry 27:535–540, 1988

Chatoor I, Getson P, Menvielle E, et al: A feeding scale for research and clinical practice to assess mother–infant interactions in the first three years of life. Infant Ment Health J 18:76–91, 1997a

Chatoor I, Hirsch R, Persinger M: Facilitating internal regulation of eating: a treatment model for infantile anorexia. Infants Young Child 9:12–22, 1997b

Chatoor I, Ganiban J, Colin V, et al: Attachment and feeding problems: a reexamination of non-organic failure to thrive and attachment insecurity. J Am Acad Child Adolesc Psychiatry 37:1217–1224, 1998a

Chatoor I, Hirsch R, Ganiban J, et al: Diagnosing infantile anorexia: the observation of mother–infant interactions. J Am Acad Child Adolesc Psychiatry 37:959–967, 1998b

Chatoor I, Ganiban J, Hirsch R, et al: Maternal characteristics and toddler temperament in infantile anorexia. J Am Acad Child Adolesc Psychiatry 39:743–751, 2000

Chatoor I, Ganiban J, Harrison J, et al: Observation of feeding in the diagnosis of posttraumatic feeding disorder of infancy. J Am Acad Child Adolesc Psychiatry 40:595–602, 2001

Chatoor I, McWade L, Harrison J, et al: There is more than one feeding disorder: theoretical issues of diagnosis and classification. Presented at the 8th Congress of the World Association of Infant Mental Health, Amsterdam, The Netherlands, July 2002

Chatoor I, Ganiban J, Surles J, et al: Physiological regulation in infantile anorexia: a pilot study. J Am Acad Child Adolesc Psychiatry 43:1019–1025, 2004a

Chatoor I, Surles J, Ganiban J, et al: Failure to thrive and cognitive development in toddlers with infantile anorexia. Pediatrics 113:e440–e447, 2004b

Dahl M, Sundelin C: Early feeding problems in an affluent society, I: categories and clinical signs. Acta Paediatr 75:370–379, 1986

Dahl M, Rydell AM, Sundelin C: Children with early refusal to eat: follow-up during primary school. Acta Paediatr 83:54–58, 1994

Dellert SF, Hyams JS, Treem WR, et al: Feeding resistance and gastroesophageal reflux in infancy. J Pediatr Gastroenterol Nutr 17:66–71, 1993

Di Scipio WJ, Kaslon K, Ruben RJ: Traumatically acquired conditioned dysphagia in children. Ann Otol Rhinol Laryngol 87:509–514, 1978

Drotar D, Sturm L: Prediction of intellectual development in young children with early histories of nonorganic failure to thrive. J Pediatr Psychol 13:281–296, 1988

Garb JL, Stunkard AJ: Taste aversions in man. Am J Psychol 131:1204–1207, 1974

Homer C, Ludwig S: Categorization of etiology of failure to thrive. Am J Dis Child 135:848–851, 1981

Jacobi C, Agras WS, Bryson S, et al: Behavioral validation, precursors, and concomitants of picky eating in childhood. J Am Acad Child Adolesc Psychiatry 42:76–84, 2003

Keller KL, Steinmann L, Nurse RJ: Genetic taste sensitivity to 6-n-propylthiouracil influences food preference and reported intake in preschool children. Appetite 38:3–12, 2002

Kim U, Jorgenson E, Coon H, et al: Positional cloning of the human quantitative trait locus underlying taste sensitivity to phenylthiocarbamide. Science 299:1221–1225, 2003

Kotler LA, Cohen P, Davies M: Longitudinal relationships between childhood, adolescent, and adult eating disorders. J Am Acad Child Adolesc Psychiatry 40:1434–1440, 2001

Lemons PK, Dodge NN: Persistent failure-to-thrive: a case study. J Pediatr Health Care 12:27–32, 1998

Lindberg L, Bohlin G, Hagekull B: Early food refusal: infant and family characteristics. Infant Ment Health J 15:262–277, 1994

Logue AW, Ophir I, Strauss K: The acquisition of taste aversions in humans. Behav Res Ther 19:319–333, 1981

Lucarelli L, Ambruzzi AM, Cimino S, et al: Feeding disorders in infancy: an empirical study on mother–infant interactions. Minerva Pediatrica 55:243–259, 2003

Marchi M, Cohen P: Early childhood eating behaviors and adolescent eating disorders. J Am Acad Child Adolesc Psychiatry 29:112–117, 1990

McCann JB, Stein A, Fairburn CG, et al: Eating habits and attitudes of mothers of children with non-organic failure to thrive. Arch Dis Child 70:234–236, 1994

McNally RJ: Choking phobia: a review of the literature. Compr Psychiatry 35:83–89, 1994

Nelson SP, Chen EH, Syniar GM, et al: One-year follow-up of symptoms of gastroesophageal reflux during infancy. Pediatric Practice Research Group. Pediatrics 102:E67, 1998

Olson JM, Boehnke M, Neiswanger K, et al: Alternative genetic models for the inheritance of the phenylthiocarbamide (PTC) taste deficiency. Genet Epidemiol 6:423–434, 1989

Patton RG, Gardner LL: Growth Failure in Maternal Deprivation. Springfield, IL, Charles C Thomas, 1963

Pliner P, Lowen ER: Temperament and food neophobia in children and their mothers. Appetite 28:239–254, 1997

Rydell AM, Dahl M, Sundelin C: Characteristics of school children who are choosy eaters. J Genet Psychol 156:217–229, 1995

Singer LT, Ambuel B, Wade S, et al: Cognitive-behavioral treatment of health-impairing food phobias in children. J Am Acad Child Adolesc Psychiatry 31:847–852, 1992

Task Force on Research Diagnostic Criteria: Infancy and Preschool: Research diagnostic criteria for infants and preschool children: the process and empirical support. J Am Acad Child Adolesc Psychiatry 42:1504–1512, 2003

Timimi S, Douglas J, Tsiftsopoulou K: Selective eaters: a retrospective case note study. Child Care Health Dev 23:265–278, 1997

Ward MJ, Kessler DB, Altman SC: Infant–mother attachment in children with failure to thrive. Infant Ment Health J 14:208–220, 1993

Waterlow JC, Buzina R, Keller W, et al: The presentation and use of height and weight data for comparing the nutritional status of groups of children under the age of 10 years. Bull World Health Organ 55:489–498, 1977

Watkins B, Lask B: Eating disorders in school-aged children. Child Adolesc Psychiatr Clin North Am 11:185–199, 2002

Wilensky DS, Ginsberg G, Altman M, et al: A community based study of failure to thrive in Israel. Arch Dis Child 75:145–148, 1996

20

DISRUPTIVE BEHAVIOR DISORDERS AND ADHD IN PRESCHOOL CHILDREN

Characterizing Heterotypic Continuities for a Developmentally Informed Nosology for DSM-V

Lauren S. Wakschlag, Ph.D.
Bennett L. Leventhal, M.D.
Jean Thomas, M.D.
Daniel S. Pine, M.D.

The writing of this chapter was supported in part by support from the National Institute of Mental Health (grant support from MH068455 to Drs. Wakschlag and Leventhal; MH62437 to Dr. Wakschlag; and R23 RR018334 to Dr. Thomas) and by ongoing support to Drs. Leventhal and Wakschlag by the Walden and Jean Young Shaw Foundation, Irving B. Harris Foundation, Daniel X. and Mary Freedman Foundation, and the Children's Brain Research Foundation. Ideas put forth in this chapter have been significantly shaped by treasured collaborations and critical discussions with our colleagues, Drs. Adrian Angold, Edwin Cook, Margaret Briggs-Gowan, Alice Carter, Barbara Danis, Helen Egger, Deborah Gorman-Smith, Nathan Fox, Carri Hill, Kate Keenan, Ellen Leibenluft, Daniel Pine, Chaya Roth, and Patrick Tolan. We also gratefully acknowledge the thoughtful input from our student, Anil Chacko.

There is no longer doubt that disruptive behaviors emerge in early childhood and exhibit moderate stability (Briggs-Gowan et al. 2006; Shaw et al. 2003; Tremblay et al. 2004). Additionally, preschool children can exhibit behavioral patterns similar (but not necessarily identical) to those in older children with behavior disorders (Angold et al., manuscript submitted for publication; Keenan and Wakschlag 2000; Lahey et al. 1998; Speltz et al. 1999). These patterns of behavior often impair developmental functioning (Egger and Angold 2006; Wakschlag and Keenan 2001). Yet there remains significant controversy about *diagnosing* behavior disorders in young children, due to questions about the validity of identifying behaviors as symptoms during a developmental period marked by variability and instability (Campbell 2002). In this chapter, we critically review the validity of DSM-IV (American Psychiatric Association 1994) behavior disorders in preschoolers and generate a framework for a more developmentally informed nosology.

Increasingly, there is agreement that early childhood is a critical period for brain development and that early intervention is crucial for addressing cognitive and developmental delays and disorders (Institute of Medicine Committee on Integrating the Science of Early Childhood Development 2000). However, this agreement fades when it comes to mental disorders, because diagnosing psychopathology in young children is seen by many as overly deterministic (Silk et al. 2000). This is exemplified in the contradictory language of DSM-IV itself. On the one hand, DSM-IV cautions against diagnosing behavior disorders in young children due to behavioral variability common during this developmental period. On the other hand, DSM-IV 1) requires early onset to meet criteria for attention-deficit/hyperactivity disorder (ADHD) (younger than 7 years), 2) identifies "problematic temperament in the preschool years" as an "associated feature" of oppositional defiant disorder (ODD), and 3) notes that conduct disorder may have onset as early as age 5 (American Psychiatric Association 2000). Such inherent contradictions also reflect the fact that there are substantial methodological and conceptual challenges to distinguishing typical and atypical behavior in a developmental period with an onset heralded by the "terrible twos."

As the study of early childhood disruptive behavior has matured, it has spawned three generations of studies. Prior to clinically focused research, numerous developmental studies on preschool behavior problems were conducted (Campbell 2002). Disruptive behavior in these studies was generally assessed with dimensional measures, in terms of either specific, individual behaviors (e.g., "noncompliance," "aggression") or aggregated attentional, oppositional, and conduct problems under the rubric of "externalizing behaviors." These first-generation studies established that behavior problems in young children were stable and measurable. However, these studies lacked clinical sensitivity and specificity, making it difficult to examine trajectories over time in a clinically coherent manner.

Second-generation studies then applied DSM-IV concepts to the study of preschool behavior problems (Keenan and Wakschlag 2002). In contrast to externalizing constructs, DSM-IV behavior disorders distinguish ADHD—that is, problems modulating attention and activity—from the disruptive behavior disorders (DBDs; e.g., ODD and conduct disorder), which involve negativistic patterns of social interaction. At the broadest level, these second-generation studies demonstrated that DSM-IV DBD and ADHD nosology could be applied to preschool children. However, in the absence of validated measures of preschool psychopathology, these studies used diagnostic instruments designed for older children with only minor modifications. As a result, this approach was relatively uninformative for examining the fit between DSM symptom constellations and actual preschool phenomenology. Testing "goodness of fit" is a central theme of the third, and current, generation of studies, which include an emphasis on validation of developmentally sensitive clinical assessment methods.

When we attempt to bridge generations of research, it is difficult to find a common language. The distinction between attentional, oppositional, and conduct problems has been called into question in research on older children because of high rates of comorbidity. For heuristic purposes, however, we maintain this distinction. When collectively referring to all three disorders, we use the term "behavior disorders." We use the terms ADHD and DBDs (and further distinguish between ODD and conduct disorder where appropriate) when we are addressing disorder-specific issues.

In what follows, we present a synthesis of second- and third-generation studies. Our review of these studies—their contributions and their limitations—is designed to set the stage for our conceptualization of the next, and fourth, generation of studies for which the field is now poised. These fourth-generation studies must draw on fundamental DSM principles to generate a developmentally refined nosology with which to characterize behavior disorders in preschool children.

Current State of the Science

Over the past decade, significant progress has been made in establishing the validity of DSM-IV (American Psychiatric Association 1994) and DSM-IV-TR behavior disorders in preschool children. We organize our review around three central questions:

1. **Do DSM behavior disorder symptom constellations occur in young children, and are they clinically meaningful?** More than a dozen independent studies have demonstrated that DSM DBD and ADHD criteria identify preschool children with clinically significant behavior problems (Connor 2002; Keenan and Wakschlag 2002). There has been concern that applying clinical criteria to young children would result in overidentification, including the "'psychopathologizing' of childhood, and the inappropriate treatment of transient de-

velopmental problems" (McClellan and Speltz 2003, p. 128). In fact, this has not proven to be the case. For both DBDs and ADHD, symptoms are endorsed at significantly higher rates in clinically referred versus nonreferred children (Bryne et al. 2000; Keenan and Wakschlag 2004) and impaired versus nonimpaired children in community samples (Angold et al., manuscript submitted for publication; Kim-Cohen et al. 2005). For example, when developmentally sensitive probing about intensity, duration, and context is used, even the most seemingly normative ODD symptom for preschoolers, "often loses temper," is endorsed by only 4% of parents of nonreferred preschoolers compared with nearly 75% of parents of referred preschoolers (Keenan and Wakschlag 2004). As with clinic samples of older children, rates of diagnosis in referred preschool children are high but quite low in nonreferred comparison children (Keenan and Wakschlag 2004; Lahey et al. 2004). Similarly, in community samples, prevalence is comparable with that in older children: ADHD, 5.1%, ODD, 7.3%, and conduct disorder, 3.4%–6.6% (Angold et al., manuscript submitted for publication; Kim-Cohen et al. 2005). Finally, DBD and ADHD symptoms are impairing, including pervasive problems across school, home, and clinic settings (Angold et al., manuscript submitted for publication; Lahey et al. 2004; Wakschlag and Keenan 2001).

2. **Do DSM symptom constellations "behave" in a manner similar to behavior disorders in older children? That is, do they have similar risk profiles, demonstrate comparable stability, and respond to validated treatments?** Studies of construct, concurrent, predictive, and treatment validity of preschool behavior disorders have demonstrated patterns comparable to those of older children. DBD and ADHD diagnoses are significantly associated with scores on developmentally validated measures of behavior problems (Kim-Cohen et al. 2005; Wakschlag and Keenan 2001). High rates of comorbidity are also common (Angold et al., manuscript submitted for publication; Thomas and Guskin 2001). For example, nearly half of preschool children presenting with behavior problems also have clinically significant emotional problems (Thomas and Guskin 2001). Behavior-disordered preschool children also exhibit social-cognitive deficits and problems in inhibitory control (Coy et al. 2001; Sonuga-Barke et al. 2002). Preschool DBDs have also been associated with established parenting and parent–child relationship correlates (Thomas and Guskin 2001; Wakschlag and Keenan 2001; Webster-Stratton and Hammond 1999). Only a handful of studies have examined predictive validity (virtually all of them with older preschool children). Emerging evidence suggests that stability of preschool behavior disorders is similar to that in older children (Kim-Cohen et al. 2005; Lahey et al. 2004; Speltz et al. 1999), although instability of ADHD subtypes in preschool children has been reported (Lahey et al. 2005). In terms of treatment validity, there is increasing evidence that preschool ADHD is responsive to stimulant medication, with large-scale randomized trials currently under way

(Connor 2002; Kratochvil et al. 2004). A number of parent training programs have been validated for treatment of preschool DBDs (Webster-Stratton 1997).

3. **Have we achieved broad-based consensus about clinical criteria for preschool behavior disorders?** At first glance, one might conclude that the "work is done." This conclusion is premature. Existing studies have unequivocally demonstrated that behaviors recognizable as DSM-IV behavior disorder symptoms are evident and clinically meaningful in preschool children. These studies have done a superb job of setting the stage for the specification of valid clinical criteria for preschool behavior disorders. However, they are also limited in several fundamental ways. First, most samples have been small and nonrepresentative. Second, by necessity, early studies have used nonstandardized methods to assess behavior disorder symptoms. Third, systematic testing of clinical criteria has been lacking.

   Are these concerns "just details" or do they actually impede achievement of consensus? We contend the latter, because valid clinical criteria for preschool behavior disorders cannot be established until distinct features of this developmental period are incorporated into the nosology.

DURATION CRITERIA

Duration criteria distinguish normative behavior from "repetitive and persistent patterns" of behavior that have reached clinical significance (American Psychiatric Association 2000). One could argue that duration criteria for preschool behavior disorders should be *longer* because "problem behaviors" normally wax and wane rapidly within this developmental period. Conversely, one could make the case that duration criteria should be *shorter* because requiring that behavioral patterns be present for as much as 20%–30% of a preschool child's life span seems overly stringent. These alternatives must be systematically tested.

SYMPTOM DEFINITION

As noted in DSM-IV, establishing that a behavior is "maladaptive and inconsistent with developmental level" is requisite to determining clinical significance. Thus, establishing clinical significance within a developmental period rests on the central organizing principle that psychopathological conditions manifest "heterotypic continuity" (Cicchetti and Richters 1997). That is, the latent patterns of behavior that define specific types of psychopathology are coherent over time, although their phenomenology differs across developmental periods. Thus, accurate characterization within a developmental period requires translation of latent constructs into their developmentally specific manifestations. Yet, paradoxically, DSM-IV provides a single criteria set across the life span for most disorders. The "problem" of preschool behavior disorders highlights how the absence of developmentally specific criteria *fundamentally impedes* valid determination of clinical significance in young children.

In DSM-IV, behavior disorder symptoms are defined in terms of manifestations in older children; this is inadequate for characterizing preschool symptoms because these are

- *Developmentally impossible*—a number of conduct disorder symptoms are behaviors of which preschoolers are developmentally incapable (e.g., forcible sexual activity, truancy). In response, some studies have dropped these items without replacing them with appropriate early childhood manifestations, thereby creating a limited symptom pool.
- *Developmentally improbable*—a number of conduct disorder symptoms of which preschoolers are physically capable (e.g., stealing without confrontation) emphasize extreme behaviors, with a particular focus on their illegal nature. If these behaviors are present in preschoolers at all, they only occur in extreme cases and are unlikely to adequately capture defining features of DBDs in young children (e.g., sneakiness). Similarly, many ADHD inattentive symptoms are defined in terms of interference with academically oriented tasks. Because preschoolers are only just mastering the requisite skills (e.g., independent completion of sequential tasks), and because academic performance is not central to this period, such symptoms are not likely to identify developmentally inconsistent capacities for sustained attention in young children. This may lead to misspecification. For example, several recent studies of preschool ADHD have reported that the "inattentive subtype" is rare and that ADHD subtypes in preschool children exhibit relatively low stability (Egger and Angold 2006; Egger et al., manuscript submitted for publication; Lahey et al. 2005). Although this may be true, it is equally likely that inattention is stably present but overlooked in young children because the heterotypic continuity for these behaviors has not been well articulated across developmental periods.
- *Developmentally imprecise*—many behavior disorder symptoms (e.g., noncompliance and aggression) are also normative manifestations of young children's struggles to master the central developmental tasks of the preschool period, such as individuation and the acquisition of self-control (Wakschlag and Danis 2004). As a result, in contrast to older children, the presence of these behaviors does not necessarily connote clinical significance during this age period. In fact, their *absence* in preschoolers may be more concerning than their presence.

Thus, to distinguish symptoms from normative manifestations in young children, behaviors must be specified precisely for this developmental period. This has several key implications. First, behavior disorder symptoms reflect deficits in attentional and behavioral regulation, skills that are just being mastered during the preschool period (Kochanska et al. 2001). As a result, some symptoms may not be discriminative in preschool children due to normative variation in the acquisition of regulatory skills. For example, emerging efforts to examine this issue for ADHD suggest that the symptom "often interrupts or intrudes" is not clinically discriminative because it is endorsed for nearly 50% of typically developing preschoolers (Byrne et al. 2000; Egger and Angold 2006; Egger et al., manuscript submitted for publication). Second, a number of behaviors that are reflected as a single symptom in DSM-IV may require disaggregation and a shift from a frequency-based definition to a conceptualization resting on qualitative features. For example, the ODD symptom "often loses temper" is not likely to capture the clinically distinct features of problems in anger modulation in young children because temper tantrums are normative during this age period and normative frequency varies for younger and older preschoolers (Egger and Angold 2004; Egger et al., manuscript in preparation). The problems of developmental impossibility and improbability may lead to *underidentification,* whereas the problem of developmental imprecision may contribute to *overidentification.*

DIAGNOSTIC THRESHOLD AND DISTINCTIONS BETWEEN DISORDERS AND SUBTYPES

A number of behaviors in the DSM-IV nosology occur normatively in preschool children, but it is the accrual of a *constellation* of such behaviors that determines when preschool children have crossed the threshold to clinical disorder. Thus, it is conceivable that higher symptom thresholds are necessary to ensure valid discrimination. Sex differences and age differences within the preschool period must also be examined in determining valid diagnostic thresholds. Furthermore, it is not at all clear that DSM-IV categorical distinctions between ODD and conduct disorder are meaningful in preschool children. To a large extent, this distinction reflects variations in the seriousness of behaviors. Conduct disorder is defined in terms of older children's increasing capacity to commit illegal acts and harm others. Along these lines, ODD is conceptualized as a developmental precursor to conduct disorder in DSM, thus, by definition the two cannot co-occur. This conceptualization is illogical during a developmental period when disruptive behaviors are first manifest and disorders are in their earliest form. As an example, in DSM-IV, a primary distinction between ODD and conduct disorder is the presence of aggressive behavior. However, aggression is a very common feature in young children with behavioral symptoms, and there is no evidence that aggression is nosologically distinct from oppositional behaviors in this age period. Finally, the DBD spectrum of symptoms reflects problems in multiple domains of behavior, broadly construed as angry negativity, resistance to authority, violent aggression, and callousness. Yet unlike other DSM disorders, the *pattern* of behavior across these domains is not incorporated into diagnostic threshold criteria or reflected in subtypes. Given these concerns, systematic examination of diagnostic threshold and patterns is essential for clinically meaningful characterization in young children.

These and related challenges make it abundantly clear that specification of valid clinical criteria for preschoolers requires the application of the same rigorous standards that have been used historically to construct DSM criteria. As articulated in DSM-IV, these standards rest on replicable and replicated studies that use standardized methods in large, representative samples.

Generating a Developmentally Informed Nosology

> Considering normal and abnormal together is the essence of developmental psychopathology.
>
> Title of paper by Sroufe (1990)

Given that developmental processes in early childhood are well-described; behavior disorders are identifiable in preschool children; and novel instruments specifically developed for the clinical assessment of disruptive behavior in young children now exist, we are well situated to generate a developmentally informed nosology for preschool behavior disorders.

Generating such a nosology requires a paradigm shift from a "top-down" to a "bottom-up" approach. To illustrate, a top-down approach starts with existing constructs and *confirms their generalizability* to a new context. Using this approach, we would ask: is the DSM-IV ODD symptom "actively defies" (validated for older children) clinically discriminative for preschoolers? In contrast, a bottom-up approach *generates contextually specific questions* and then tests their validity. Taking this approach, we might ask: what are the central features of clinically significant oppositionality in young children that discriminate it from normative assertions of autonomy?

Implementing a bottom-up approach must begin with the generation of a conceptual model that is developmentally sensitive, clinically informed, and operationalized in an empirically testable manner. Drawing on the principle of heterotypic continuity, this requires an iterative process moving between latent constructs, knowledge of normative behavior in young children, and indicators that normative processes have gone awry. Table 20–1 provides an illustration of the result of this type of process for DBDs; here we propose the manifestation of the full range of DBD behaviors operationalized in terms of their expression in preschool children. For example, in operationalizing the latent construct "noncompliance," the first step was conceptualizing the features distinguishing symptoms from healthy assertions of independence in preschool children. Building on literature elucidating developmental processes of internalization and the implications of quality of compliance for adaptation (Kochanska and Aksan 1995), we theorized that qualitative

TABLE 20–1. Illustration of developmentally informed nosology for preschool disruptive behavior disorders

Temper loss	Noncompliance	Aggression	Lack of concern
Reflexive no Characteristically responds to a wide variety of social interactions in a negative manner (not only to limit-setting or directions). May include being contrary and argumentative, resistant to transitions, and controlling.	**Rude** Often speaks in disrespectful and sassy manner, including being brazen, mouthy, sarcastic, and/or cursing.	**Proactive aggression** Acts aggressively "out of the blue." Aggression is not an emotional reaction to immediate anger or frustration; aggression is used instrumentally to coerce or dominate. May include covert aggression, such as sneaky pinching.	**Incites** Deliberately attempts to provoke others to anger, including taunting or teasing to provoke conflict. Intentionally does things to irritate and annoy others.
Sullen Characteristically angry and/or surly. Frequently pouts and/or whines.	**Stubbornly defies** Often says "no" or outright refuses to do what is asked; defiance persists in the face of adult prompts.	**Intense aggression** Engages in driven, persistent aggression to hurt others on purpose; may use objects or exhibit serious aggressive behavior such as cutting, choking, stabbing, or forceful hitting.	**Cruelty** Purposely causes pain or distress to others. May include spiteful comments, doing something to get even, and cruelty to animals.
Easily angered Angry response is easily elicited across multiple social interactions and activities (not just in response to provocation or frustration). Is touchy, and anger is often surprising and out of context.	**Persistently ignores** Actively ignores directions and requests, even when repeated.	**Adult aggression** Behaves aggressively toward adults.	**Indifferent** Unconcerned about others' needs or feelings, including taking pleasure in others' distress and/or being indifferent to pleasing others.

TABLE 20–1. Illustration of developmentally informed nosology for preschool disruptive behavior disorders *(continued)*

Temper loss	Noncompliance	Aggression	Lack of concern
Explosive temper Reacts intensely when angry or upset, escalates rapidly, including out-of-control behavior, destructive tantrums, and/or loud tirades.	**Disregards rules** Often brazenly breaks rules, tests limits, does whatever he or she pleases. May provocatively engage in misbehavior in adult presence.	**Reactive aggression** Frequently retaliates with aggression when angry; aggression is in response to perceived provocation or frustration with others.	**Sabotages** Purposely thwarts others' play, plans, and activities, including knocking over, spilling, and wrecking. Enjoys spoiling things for others.
Insistent anger Anger is often sustained and unyielding. Once set off, child may relentlessly engage others in angry/negative interactions (won't "let up").	**Sneaky** Deliberately hides mistakes and/or misbehavior, including lying to avoid responsibility and blaming others. Also may include sneaking items such as items from a store or others' belongings.	**Destructive** Intentionally breaks and damages things, including smashing, tearing, and/or destroying others' belongings and fire setting.	**Intimidates** Picks on, bullies, and/or intimidates other children, including verbal threats and forceful grabbing.

features define preschool behavior as symptomatic (Wakschlag et al. 2005, in press). Salient features of noncompliance in young children were then operationalized (e.g., rudeness, brazen misbehavior, intransigence, and sneakiness). Similarly, because symptoms of lack of concern and aggression in DSM-IV conduct disorder reflect mature forms of these behaviors (e.g., forcible sexual activity, using a weapon to harm), we conceptualized principal features for preschoolers as deviations from age-expected norms for empathy, modulation of aggression, and the early emergence of conscience (Kochanska and Aksan 1995; NICHHD Early Child Care Network 2004; Tremblay et al. 2004). Atypical manifestations were then operationalized as purposeful efforts to harm and insensitivity (e.g., sabotaging others' activities; intense, proactive aggression; and taking pleasure in others' distress).

Clearly, methods specifically developed and standardized for the clinical assessment of young children are essential tools for establishing the validity and incremental utility of such conceptual models. Fortunately, such methods are being developed, and their validation is currently under way. Evolving interview methodologies include the Preschool Age Psychiatric Assessment (PAPA; Egger and Angold 2004), a comprehensive diagnostic interview for preschool children, and the Kiddie-DBDs (K-DBDs; Keenan et al. 2007), a preschool modification of the behavior disorders module of the Schedule for Affective Disorders and Schizophrenia for School-Age Children (K-SADS; Orvaschel and Puig-Antich 1995). These interviews are designed to deconstruct DSM-IV behavior disorder symptoms into their component parts so that clinically discriminative features for young children can be identified. This work has already led to a new perspective on the constituent behaviors of DBDs in preschool children. For example, for the ODD symptom "often loses temper," the PAPA probes include questions about frequency, duration, triggers, and content of temper tantrums. Data from the PAPA indicate that, for preschool children, destructive tantrums (e.g., hitting, kicking, or biting others and/or breaking objects) are symptomatic, but nondestructive tantrums (e.g., crying, stamping, holding breath) are not (Egger et al., manuscript in preparation).

Although the multi-informant, multimethod approach is the gold standard for diagnostic validation, this has yet to be applied to the study of preschool behavior disorders. To complement information about discrete behaviors derived from parent interviews, diagnostic observation methods are an essential tool for refining and testing a developmentally informed nosology. For example, the Disruptive Behavior Diagnostic Observation Schedule (Wakschlag et al. 2005; in press) provides a standardized method of direct clinical observation that yields nuanced and contextualized information about child behavior during interactions with both parent and examiner. Multiple levels of contextual information (e.g., situational, developmental, and social) and qualitative aspects of behavior (e.g., its flexibility and regulation) are taken into account in defining the clinical significance of behavior. For example, assessment of noncompliant behavior is based on observations of whether the behavior is typically elicited in response to limits or is characteristic regardless of situational demands; results from poor language comprehension; is restricted to interactions with the parent or occurs pervasively; is responsive to adult support; and is intense and poorly modulated. By enhancing the clarity and specificity of behavioral description in this manner, diagnostic observation can substantially advance phenotypic characterization.

Conclusions

Over the past decade, a substantial body of empirical work has unequivocally demonstrated that behavior disorders are identifiable and clinically meaningful in preschool children. Clarity about this issue represents a substantial advance that rests on a rare level of integration across developmental and clinical science. With this clarity to guide us, it is also abundantly evident that much work lies ahead to establish a sensitive and specific nosology that will allow DSM-V to accurately characterize clinical phenomena for young children. The promise of such work lies not only in its clinical significance for preschoolers but also in its capacity to serve as a paradigm for honoring the DSM imperative to conceptualize symptoms within developmental and social contexts. Such efforts will result in a well-characterized phenotype that serves as the basis for translational investigation of basic processes underlying early emerging behavior disorders and ultimately will enhance our capacity to treat and prevent these disorders.

Commentary: Daniel S. Pine, M.D.

Research on early childhood manifestations of behavior disorders provides an ideal guide for addressing more general questions concerning future research directions in the classification of preschool psychopathology. Considerable work already exists in this area. Indeed, for this age period, perhaps only in the area of pervasive developmental disorders has more research addressed the pertinent questions. Moreover, whereas extreme forms of pervasive developmental disorders can be clearly differentiated from typical development, major questions remain in preschoolers concerning differences between even moderately extreme disruptive behavior and typical oppositional behavior, inattention, or aggression. This chapter embraces the promise of research in preschool psychopathology, holding the hope of guiding a more developmentally informed nosology while recognizing the need to wade "with caution" into a field with such inherent pitfalls.

The current chapter comprehensively and concisely elucidates both the opportunities and potential dangers of addressing questions in this area. Given the breadth of available information and complexity of questions, it is easy to miss the dramatic impact of two particularly salient points raised in the chapter that are worth repeating. First, in all areas of nosology, refinements in measurement represent a vital initial step toward building an increasingly valid classification scheme. Not only will this mean adapting currently available tools but it also will mean devising novel techniques that address the unique burdens associated with preschool assessment.

The opportunity for such novel approaches is exemplified by the work of Wakschlag, Leventhal, and their colleagues in developing a structured clinical observational assessment, the Disruptive Behavior Diagnostic Observation Schedule. Second, criticism with the current DSM system has grown steadily louder in recent years due to failures to embrace developmental concepts. To address these criticisms, investigators must collect considerable data in young children to demonstrate the validity of alternative, developmentally focused classification schemes. This will require a "fresh look" at symptoms manifest among preschoolers within the unique social context of this developmental period.

In considering the material within this chapter, one cannot help but emerge with a great sense of excitement and opportunity, regardless of one's perspective, be it focused on development, psychiatric classification, or clinical care. In confronting the issue of preschool classification, research on behavior disorders demonstrates both the great promise and considerable work we face in producing a more informed, developmentally sensitive nosology.

References

American Psychiatric Association: Diagnostic and Statistical Manual of Mental Disorders, 4th Edition. Washington, DC, American Psychiatric Association, 1994

American Psychiatric Association: Diagnostic and Statistical Manual of Mental Disorders, 4th Edition, Text Revision. Washington, DC, American Psychiatric Association, 2000

Angold A, Egger H, Erkanli A, et al: Prevalence and comorbidity of psychiatric disorders in preschoolers attending a large pediatric service. Manuscript submitted for publication

Briggs-Gowan M, Carter AS, Bosson-Heenan J, et al: Are infant–toddler social-emotional and behavioral problems transient? J Am Acad Child Adolesc Psychiatry 45:849–858, 2006

Byrne J, Bawden H, Beattie T, et al: Preschoolers classified as having ADHD: DSM-IV symptom endorsement pattern. J Child Neurol 15:533–538, 2000

Campbell S: Behavior Problems in Preschool Children: Clinical and Developmental Issues, 2nd Edition. New York, Guilford, 2002

Cicchetti D, Richters J: Examining conceptual and scientific underpinnings of research in developmental psychopathology. Dev Psychopathol 9:189–191, 1997

Connor D: Preschool attention-deficit/hyperactivity disorder: a review of prevalence, diagnosis, neurobiology and stimulant treatment. J Dev Behav Pediatr 23:S1–S9, 2002

Coy K, Speltz M, DeKlyen M, et al: Social-cognitive processes in preschool boys with and without oppositional defiant disorder. J Abnorm Child Psychol 29:107–120, 2001

Egger H, Angold A: The Preschool Age Psychiatric Assessment (PAPA): a structured parent interview for diagnosing psychiatric disorders in preschool children, in Handbook of Infant, Toddler and Preschool Mental Health Assessment. Edited by Del Carmen-Wiggins R, Carter A. New York, Oxford, 2004, pp 223–246

Egger H, Angold A: Common emotional and behavioral disorders in preschool children: presentation, nosology and epidemiology. J Child Psychol Psychiatry 47:313–337, 2006

Egger H, Erkanli A, Angold A: Temper tantrums and preschool mental health: when to worry. Manuscript in preparation

Egger H, Kondo D, Erkanli A, et al: The nosology of preschool attention-deficit/hyperactivity disorder. Manuscript submitted for publication

Institute of Medicine (IOM) Committee on Integrating the Science of Early Childhood Development: From Neurons to Neighborhoods: The Science of Early Childhood Development. Washington, DC, National Academy Press, 2000

Keenan K, Wakschlag L: More than the terrible twos: the nature and severity of behavior problems in clinic-referred preschool children. J Abnorm Child Psychol 28:33–46, 2000

Keenan K, Wakschlag L: Can a valid diagnosis of disruptive behavior disorder be made in preschool children? Am J Psychiatry 59:351–358, 2002

Keenan K, Wakschlag L: Are oppositional defiant and conduct disorder symptoms normative behaviors in preschoolers? A comparison of referred and nonreferred children. Am J Psychiatry 161:356–358, 2004

Keenan K, Wakschlag L, Danis B, et al: Further evidence of the reliability and validity of DSM-IV ODD and CD in preschool children. J Am Acad Child Adolesc Psychiatry 46:457–468, 2007

Kim-Cohen J, Arseneault L, Caspi A, et al: Validity of DSM-IV conduct disorder in 4½ – 5 year-old children: a longitudinal epidemiological study. Am J Psychiatry 162:108–117, 2005

Kochanska G, Aksan N: Mother–child mutual positive affect, the quality of child compliance to requests and prohibitions, and maternal control as correlates of early internalization. Child Dev 66:236–254, 1995

Kochanska G, Coy K, Murray K: The development of self-regulation in the first four years of life. Child Dev 72:1091–1111, 2001

Kratochvil C, Greenhill L, March J, et al: The role of stimulants in the treatment of preschool children with ADHD. CNS Drugs 18:957–966, 2004

Lahey BB, Loeber R, Quay HC, et al: Validity of DSM-IV subtypes of conduct disorder based on age of onset. J Am Acad Child Adolesc Psychiatry 37:435–442, 1998

Lahey B, Pelham W, Loney J, et al: Three year predictive validity of DSM-IV attention-deficit/hyperactivity disorder in children diagnosed at 4–6 years of age. Am J Psychiatry 161:2014–2020, 2004

Lahey B, Pelham W, Loney J, et al: Instability of the DSM-IV subtypes of ADHD from preschool through elementary school. Arch Gen Psychiatry 62:896–902, 2005

McClellan J, Speltz M: Psychiatric diagnosis in preschool children (letter). J Am Acad Child Adolesc Psychiatry 42:127–128, 2003

National Institute of Child Health and Human Development (NICHHD) Early Child Care Network: Trajectories of Physical Aggression From Toddlerhood to Middle Childhood, Vol 278. Boston, MA, Blackwell, 2004

Orvaschel H, Puig-Antich J: Schedule for Affective Disorders and Schizophrenia for School-Age Children–Epidemiologic 5th Version. Fort Lauderdale, FL, Nova University, 1995

Shaw D, Gilliom M, Ingoldsby E, et al: Trajectories leading to school-age conduct problems. Dev Psychol 39:189–200, 2003

Silk J, Nath S, Siegel L, et al: Conceptualizing mental disorders in children: where have we been and where are we going? Dev Psychopathol 12:713–735, 2000

Sonuga-Barke EJ, Dalen L, Daley D, et al: Are planning, working memory, and inhibition associated with individual differences in preschool ADHD symptoms? Dev Neuropsychol 21:255–272, 2002

Speltz M, McMellan J, DeKlyen M, et al: Preschool boys with oppositional defiant disorder: clinical presentation and diagnostic change. J Am Acad Child Adolesc Psychiatry 38:838–845, 1999

Sroufe LA: Considering normal and abnormal together: the essence of developmental psychopathology. Dev Psychopathol 2:335–348, 1990

Thomas J, Guskin K: Disruptive behavior in young children: what does it mean? J Am Acad Child Adolesc Psychiatry 40:44–51, 2001

Tremblay R, Nagin D, Seguin J, et al: Physical aggression during early childhood: trajectories and predictors. Pediatrics 114:43–50, 2004

Wakschlag L, Danis B: Assessment of disruptive behavior in young children: a clinical-developmental framework, in Handbook of Infant, Toddler and Preschool Mental Health Assessment. Edited by Del Carmen R, Wiggins A. New York, Oxford University Press, 2004, pp 421–440

Wakschlag L, Keenan K: Clinical significance and correlates of disruptive behavior symptoms in environmentally at-risk preschoolers. J Clin Child Psychol 30:262–275, 2001

Wakschlag L, Leventhal B, Briggs-Gowan M, et al: Defining the "disruptive" in preschool behavior: what diagnostic observation can teach us. Clin Child Fam Psychol Rev 8:183–201, 2005

Wakschlag L, Briggs-Gowan M, Carter A, et al: A developmental framework for distinguishing disruptive behavior from normative misbehavior in preschool children. J Child Psychol Psychiatry (in press)

Webster-Stratton C: Early Intervention for Families of Preschool Children With Conduct Problems. Baltimore, MD, Brookes, 1997

Webster-Stratton C, Hammond M: Marital conflict management skills, parenting style, and early onset conduct problems: processes and pathways. J Child Psychol Psychiatry 40:917–927, 1999

21

DIAGNOSIS OF AUTISM AND RELATED DISORDERS IN INFANTS AND VERY YOUNG CHILDREN

Setting a Research Agenda for DSM-V

Fred Volkmar, M.D.
Kasia Chawarska, Ph.D.
Alice Carter, Ph.D.
Catherine Lord, Ph.D.

Current State of the Science

Autism and related disorders (referred to either as the pervasive developmental disorders [PDDs] or as autism spectrum disorders) are a distinctive set of conditions characterized by disturbance in early developmental processes—particularly in social and communication skills—in the first years of life (Volkmar and Klin 2005). Of the various conditions included in the class in DSM-IV-TR (American Psychiatric Association 2000), autistic disorder has been, by far, the most intensively and extensively studied. As a result, much more is known about the early features and clinical presentation of autism than of related disorders, and accordingly, autism is largely the focus of this review. (For recent reviews of knowledge on conditions related to autism, see Volkmar et al. 2005.)

Although there is a consensus that autism almost always develops before age 3 years, it is somewhat paradoxical that knowledge regarding the development of infants and very young children with autism has been quite limited, largely because diagnosis did not occur until preschool. Thus, until recently, most information on early symptoms and features was obtained retrospectively, for example, through parental reports. However, since the mid-1990s increased awareness, an appreciation of the importance of early intervention, and advances in research have made it possible to study autism in the first 3 years of life (National Research Council 2001; Volkmar et al. 2005). Additionally, the awareness of the strong genetic basis of autism and increased sibling risk (Rutter 2005) also stimulated research in this age group. This is also an important topic because findings help to clarify central features before confounding effects of treatment, development, and comorbidity arise.

As defined in DSM-IV-TR, a diagnosis of autistic disorder is based on characteristic features distributed in social development, communication and play, and restricted interests and behaviors. The emphasis on this triad of difficulties (Lord 1995) and their early onset is consistent with a large body of work beginning with Kanner's (1943) original report and its various modifications. The current DSM-IV-TR approach was based on an extensive field trial in which almost 1,000 individuals were evaluated by more than 100 raters at various sites around the world; this sample included a considerable group of preschoolers (but not infants) (Volkmar et al. 1994). At the time of its preparation (in the early 1990s), the study of very young children with autism was just beginning, and the criteria finally proposed for inclusion were designed to be widely applicable across the range of syndrome expression (both in terms of age and developmental level); given the concern for general applicability, items with strong developmental relationships were specifically excluded from DSM-IV (American Psychiatric Association 1994) and DSM-IV-TR.

There is strong evidence that, overall, the DSM-IV/ICD-10 (World Health Organization 1994) approach has worked quite well (Volkmar and Klin 2005). As a result of better overall agreement on essential diagnostic features, interest in early diagnosis has increased dramatically, and knowledge about the earliest manifestations of autism has similarly grown. For example, studies on parental recognition of developmental abnormalities in autism suggest that in one-third (De Giacomo and Fombonne 1998) to one-half (Volkmar et al. 1985) of cases parents are concerned about the child's development before the child is 1 year of age; at least 80%–90% recognize their child's abnormalities by 24 months (De Giacomo and Fombonne 1998). However, these data are retrospective and may be confounded by passage of time (telescoping effects), limited parental knowledge of child development, and so on and thus likely represent the upper-bound limit of the actual age of symptom onset.

The diagnoses and individual diagnostic criteria for autism in DSM-IV-TR have generally reasonably good sensitivity and specificity relative to the entire (broad) range of autism when compared against a criterion of expert clinician ratings (Volkmar et al. 1994); the use of individual DSM-IV-TR diagnostic criteria also significantly improves the accuracy of diagnosis among less experienced clinicians (Klin et al. 2000). However, the robustness of these criteria is most strongly established in children ages 4 years and older, and issues do arise with the applicability of current criteria to infants and very young children. For example, as Lord (1995) noted, whereas some 2-year-olds referred for autism do meet categorical diagnostic criteria, others do not—often because of a failure to exhibit threshold levels of symptoms in of the "restricted interests" domain, because these symptoms often do not emerge until around age 3 years (see also Stone et al. 1994). Agreement is generally stronger for broader PDD/autism spectrum vs. non–autism spectrum than for autism vs. PDD not otherwise specified (Lord 1995; Stone et al. 1999). Certain criteria, such as failure to develop peer relationships, impaired conversational skills, and stereotyped language, are not usually specifically applicable to infants (Stone et al. 1999), particularly when language delay is part of the clinical presentation; this effectively reduces the number of criteria that can be rated. Thus further research on the utility of the DSM-IV-TR criteria in children under the age of 3 is needed; for example, a different algorithm for infants may be needed (Stone et al. 1999), or other criteria more specifically applicable to infants and young children might be included, such as attachments to unusual objects (Volkmar and Klin 2005).

Although there is general agreement on the onset of difficulties before age 3 (as currently is required in DSM-IV-TR), issues about the onset of the condition arise with regard to the phenomenon of developmental regression as well as to the implications of the onset criterion for the definition of other PDDs, notably childhood disintegrative disorder and Asperger's disorder. A series of studies (Volkmar and Klin 2005) have suggested that perhaps 20%–25% of children with autism are reported to have some degree of developmental regression, typically involving some degree of loss of language abilities (Lord et al. 2004). Unfortunately, the issue of regression in autism is a complex one. For example, one recent large, multisite study of several hundred children with illnesses on the autism spectrum reported that children with words also were reported by caregivers to have shown more gestures and social participation before the loss of skills and fewer such skills after the loss; the same patterns of developmental loss were not reported in the relatively small sample of children with problems not on the autism spectrum (Luyster et al. 2005). Thus, developmental regression may involve losses in multiple developmental domains. In a chart review study, Siperstein and Volkmar (2004) noted that whereas parents of children with autism were more likely to report possible developmental skills loss than children with other developmental disabilities, the issue of actual loss was complicated—for example, parents often reported previous developmental delays prior to regression or reported developmental stagnation rather than a regression. For purposes of research, however, it may be the less common pattern of dramatic, major, and significant loss of skills that may be most important, such as the pattern observed in the relatively rare condition of childhood disintegrative disorder (Volkmar et al. 1997). Another issue relative to the inclusion of onset before age 3 as an essential diagnostic feature arises with respect to Asperger's disorder, a condition in which some aspects of language ability are preserved (or precious) in the face of significant social disability. Asperger (1944) suggested that the condition was not usually recognized before age 3, likely reflecting preservation of some aspects of language. Problems do arise, however, because the current DSM-IV-TR approach gives autism precedence, and the issue of onset before or after age 3 can be a source of confusion and may complicate distinctions between the disorders (Hippler and Klicpera 2003; Klin et al. 2005b, 2005c; Miller and Ozonoff 1997).

Advances in Developmental Science

In the decade subsequent to the publication of DSM-IV in 1994, a substantial body of work has accumulated on autism as it exists in infants and young children (Carter et al. 2005; Chawarska and Volkmar 2005). Using several different methods (e.g., retrospective parent report or videotape review), studies have identified a set of developmentally sensitive diagnostic signs of autism. These include decreased visual attention to people, diminished response to own name, and so forth; such signs can readily be viewed as early manifestations of the social-communicative difficulties formalized in DSM-IV-TR criteria and capitalized on in the development of screening instruments for autism (Coonrod and Stone 2005). However, disturbances in the third area of behavioral disturbance required by DSM-IV-TR (restricted, repetitive interests and behaviors) have been more difficult to document in infants and very young children. Behaviors like aversion to touch or other unusual sensitivities have been reported less consistently in the first year of life, although typically between ages 2 and 3 years such behaviors intensify and assume the form more typically expected in DSM-IV-TR (Chawarska and Volkmar 2005). It is also the case that during the second year of life the typical infant exhibits profound gains developmentally in terms of language, increasingly sophisticated social interaction and play, and so forth, whereas the development of the infant with autism typically becomes more dramatically deviant. Thus, among 2-year-olds with autism difficulties with diminished eye contact, lack of interest in peers, joint attention, a limited range of facial expression, vocal and motor imitation, and play become more obviously deviant and delayed (Chawarska and Volkmar 2005). In the area of communication, one of the most striking differences relates to difficulties in use and understanding of conventional gestures as well as a lack of spontaneous pointing to show; in general, at this time the delays in both receptive and expressive language become more striking, and children with autism who have some language may begin to exhibit the unusual language features of the type emphasized in DSM-IV-TR, that is, echolalia. Although relatively less frequent, some stereotypic and repetitive behaviors often begin to emerge, including hand and finger mannerisms as well as unusual sensory seeking or avoidant behaviors (Baranek et al. 2005; Chawarska and Volkmar 2005). Between 24 and 36 months of age, the more classic symptoms of autism typically become more pronounced, whereas the converse is often true for children whose difficulties do not ultimately appear to be on the autism spectrum.

Many of the findings from developmental research have been incorporated into screening procedures (Coonrod and Stone 2005). A detailed discussion of such screeners is beyond the scope of this review, but it should be noted that strong developmental effects may be observed (i.e., screeners are sometimes designed for specific age groups, given differences in presenting symptoms at different ages; Coonrod and Stone 2005).

There are now reasonably good data, from various sources, on the features of autism in the first 3 years of life. At the same time it is important to note the various limitations inherent in these data. Parental retrospective reports and/or analysis of retrospective videos of the child have been the primary sources of data. Various factors limit information regarding the earliest syndrome expression and continue to be parent retrospective reports and video diaries. Factors complicating the interpretation of parent report/interview data include selective recall, denial, and effects of parental knowledge (or lack thereof) of normal children's development. For example, Stone et al. (1994) compared parental report and the observations of expert clinicians and found parents to be more accurate in reporting negative symptoms but much worse in reporting positive ones, for example, failures of the child to engage in social routines were more reliably reported by parents than were problems in engaging in joint attention behaviors or pretend play. Unfortunately, the latter are apparently the more important features of autism in the second year of life (Charman et al. 2001). An additional problem arises when parental report is used to track developmental change, because it appears that a complicated interaction of true developmental change (e.g., in frequency or intensity of behaviors) occurs in interaction with parental expectations and heightened observation (Lord 1995).

Analysis of videotaped materials has many obvious advantages. However, the videotapes collected vary significantly in terms of their setting, location, timing, and so forth. The lack of consistency is further compounded by the possibility of selective bias (i.e., in terms of when tapes are made). For example, videotaped studies of babies with autism in their first year of life have not documented the problems in arousal and self regulation, unusual fussiness or placidity, or lack of stranger anxiety widely reported by parents. It is possible that these behaviors are not really specific to infants with autism, although it is equally possible that selective bias in taping accounts for this apparent discrepancy.

Our difficulty to make comparisons across studies is compromised by several factors. Studies differ in the degree to which they focus on the specific behaviors and, when the focus is on the same behaviors, operational definitions may vary, making comparisons problematic. Studies also differ in the degree and manner in which comparison groups are utilized; in many cases such groups are absent. In other instances children with autism are compared with children with language disorders or those with a mixed pattern of developmental delay. Other studies have used consecutive cases referrals, for example, to clinics specializing in children with developmental disabilities or autism, and then compared children diagnosed with PDD with those without PDD.

Generating a Developmentally Informed Phenotype

The vast majority of research on the neurobiological basis of autism (i.e., apart from genetic factors) has focused on older children, adolescents, and adults, with comparatively little work done in infants and very young children (Minshew et al. 2000). However, some results have been obtained in infants and young children or are quite relevant to this population.

Beginning with Kanner's (1943) original report, it has been known that macrocephaly (typically defined as greater than 2 standard deviations above the mean) is relatively common in autism (Minshew et al. 2000). Macrocephaly usually begins to develop in the first or second year of life, although the data are limited (Lainhart et al. 1997; Minshew et al. 2000). In their retrospective study, Courchesne et al. (2003) suggested that onset of macrocephaly was most frequently between birth and 6–14 months. This increase in head circumference reflects an increased brain volume; head size plateaus in mid-childhood and then normalizes (Minshew et al. 2000). The significance of increased head circumference remains unclear and there are no clear relationships to either severity or gender, although a family history of macrocephaly is apparently relatively common (Miles et al. 2000; Stevenson et al. 1997). The significance of the observed macrocephaly is unclear, and it cannot be used as a screening tool at present. Microcephaly appears relatively less common and may be more frequently present in association with a genetic or some other medical condition (Minshew et al. 2000).

Minor physical anomalies have been of some interest in autism, because these often reflect disruption of embryonic development during early pregnancy (either by genetic or environmental factors or both). A series of studies have noted an increased rate in such anomalies in autism (Minshew et al. 2000; Rutter 2005). Again the significance of these observations is unclear. No physical anomaly has been identified as being specific to autism. An accurate assessment may be accomplished only by a specifically trained geneticist, and careful examination of family members is also needed. Furthermore, rates of minor physical anomalies are increased in a range of other disorders. In one recent study (Rodier et al. 1997), about 50% of children with autism were found to have one such anomaly and in another study only 20% appear to have more than one (Miles and Hillman 2000). It is clear that infants and young children for whom autism is considered as a diagnostic possibility should be examined for minor physical anomalies, although such features do not yet have clear-cut screening or diagnostic implications.

Probably the most replicated neurobiological finding in autism relates to the high rate of epilepsy and abnormal encephalographic readings in individuals with autism, although comparatively little work has been done in infants and very young children (Minshew et al. 2000). It does appear that one of the two modal times of onset of seizures is in infancy and early childhood (Deykin and MacMahon 1979; Volkmar and Nelson 1990), although again, straightforward implications for screening have not emerged.

Another line of work has focused on more specific neuropsychological processes, for example, on aspects of joint attention, attention to prosody, and gaze (see Chawarska et al. 2003; Klin et al. 2005a; Paul et al. 2005). Infants who appear to be at high risk for autism have deviant patterns of scanning social scenes (Klin et al. 2005). Studies of automatic attention cuing stimulated by changes in gaze direction in 2-year-olds suggest that in both children with autism and those with typical development, visual attention is cued by perceived eye movement but that those with autism may rely on different underlying strategies for gaze processing. Similar strategies have been used in studies of perception and face recognition in infants and older children (Carver et al. 2003; McPartland et al. 2004; Schultz et al. 2000) and suggest the potential, in the future, for the development of performance-based screeners relevant to infants.

The limitations and uses of the current DSM-IV-TR categorical approaches have been noted previously. To date, systematic data on other possible categorical approaches are sparse. As mentioned earlier, certain potential DSM-IV-TR criteria were noted to have a strong relationship with age or developmental level and were thus excluded from the final DSM-IV/ICD-10 criteria set (e.g., attachments to unusual objects). It is possible that additional data on other potential criteria could now be collected that focuses on the behaviors and features that have become of greater interest since the publication of DSM-IV. It is also possible that even with such approaches, no significant gains would be made over and above the current (DSM-IV-TR) approach; in many instances infants and young children do indeed meet the criteria, and the fast pace of developmental change in this age group might limit the utility of any categorical system. It is also possible that some other procedures, such as using weighted criteria (with weights adjusted for clinical significance/relevance at different ages), might also be a useful approach.

Other conceptualizations of the difficulties of very young children with symptoms associated with the autism spectrum continue to be proposed (National Center for Clinical Infant Programs 1994), although the recognition that there must be some relation to diagnostic systems for school-age children has lessened enthusiasm for completely different classification systems, and the empirical basis of such systems remains very limited. Apart from its great significance for research, the issue of early diagnosis is also important in terms of treatment implications. A number of well-researched treatment programs have included 2-year-old children with autism or broader autism spectrum diagnoses, but published information about interventions with even younger children are quite rare (Handleman and Harris 2000). Descriptions of developmentally oriented, communication-based approaches appropriate for 2-year-olds with autism have been made (Wetherby et al. 1997), and there have been several recent reports of intervention studies of relatively brief, parent-oriented treatment approaches for enhancing joint attention skills and social-communicative behavior (Aldred et al. 2004; Charman et al. 2003).

Several behavioral programs have included children as young as 2 years and have suggested that children who begin treatment younger may make more rapid progress. A consistent finding is that children with milder difficulties and higher IQ scores at the beginning of treatment tend to make greater improvements (and, in some cases, account for almost all of the significant improvements) than children with more limited skills and/or more severe autism spectrum disorders (Smith and Lovaas 1997; Smith et al. 1997). However, at least some of the markers for good response to treatment in older children (such as learning to imitate sounds upon command) may not be appropriate in children younger than 2 years of age. As indicated earlier, the stability of social deficits and communication delays in children younger than 2 is not yet clear (Stone et al. 1999). Furthermore, a number of aspects of treatment that have seemed crucial for preschool children, such as intensity and structure, may need to be interpreted in different ways for infants and toddlers. This is an important area for future research.

In summary, in the years since the appearance of DSM-IV, the considerable progress in studies on early symptoms and diagnosis of autism has been impressive and marks the beginning of intensive and interdisciplinary research programs targeting infants and toddlers with PDD. Longitudinal studies of very young children with autism (e.g., 12–24 months of age) as well as studies on high-risk populations of younger siblings of children with autism will help elucidate these diagnostic conundrums in the near future.

Commentary: Adrian Angold, M.B., MRCPsych, and Helen Link Egger, M.D.

As Volkmar and colleagues' review shows, the past decade has seen significant advances in our understanding of the early symptoms and diagnosis of autism spectrum disorders in young children as well as associated features such as head circumference, abnormal encephalographic patterns, and genetic risk. Although it highlights the need for further research on the utility of the DSM-IV-TR criteria with children younger than 3 years old, it also demonstrates that the DSM-IV-TR criteria have worked quite well as a means of advancing our understanding of the presentation and course of autism spectrum disorders in spite of the lack of developmentally specific criteria.

Efforts are under way to define developmentally informed phenotypes for autism and other autism spectrum disorders, including PDD not otherwise specified and Asperger's disorder. Key questions are whether different diagnostic algorithms are needed for very young children and/or whether new criteria applicable only to young children need to be included. Although there are some indications that some of the current criteria are not appropriate for very young children (particularly those with language delays) and that alternative criteria may be indicated for young children, the authors emphasize that further data from longitudinal studies of young children with or at high risk for autism and autism-related disorders are needed before a case can be made to include developmentally specific algorithms and/or criteria in a diagnostic system such as DSM-V. The multidisciplinary and multisite approaches that characterize current research programs targeting infants and toddlers with autism spectrum disorders, as well as the careful and cautious approach to proposing new developmentally sensitive diagnostic algorithms and criteria, should serve as an example and guide for programs of research focusing on other areas of psychopathology in young children.

References

Aldred C, Green J, Adams C: A new social communication intervention for children with autism: pilot randomized controlled treatment study suggesting effectiveness. J Child Psychol Psychiatry 45:1420–1430, 2004

American Psychiatric Association: Diagnostic and Statistical Manual of Mental Disorders, 4th Edition. Washington, DC, American Psychiatric Association, 1994

American Psychiatric Association: Diagnostic and Statistical Manual of Mental Disorders, 4th Edition, Text Revision. Washington, DC, American Psychiatric Association, 2000

Asperger H: Die autistichen Psychopathen im Kindersalter. Archive fur Psychiatrie und Nervenkrankheiten 117:76–136, 1944

Baranek GT, Parham L, Bodfish JW: Sensory and motor features in autism: assessment and intervention, in Handbook of Autism and Pervasive Developmental Disorders. Edited by Volkmar F, Klin A, Paul R, et al. Hoboken, NJ, Wiley, 2005, pp 88–125

Carter AS, Davis NO, Klin A, et al: Social development in autism, in Handbook of Autism and Pervasive Developmental Disorders. Edited by Volkmar FR, Klin A, Paul R, et al. Hoboken, NJ, Wiley, 2005, pp 312–334

Carver LJ, Dawson G, Panagiotides H, et al: Age-related differences in neural correlates of face recognition during the toddler and preschool years. Dev Psychobiol 42:148–159, 2003

Charman T, Baron-Cohen S, Swettenham J, et al: Testing joint attention, imitation, and play as infancy precursors to language and theory of mind. Cognitive Development 15:481–498, 2001

Charman T, Howlin P, Aldred C, et al: Research into early intervention for children with autism and related disorders: methodological and design issues. Report on a workshop funded by the Wellcome Trust, Institute of Child Health, London, UK, November 2001. Autism 7:217–225, 2003

Chawarska K, Volkmar F: Autism in infancy and early childhood, in Handbook of Autism and Pervasive Developmental Disorders. Edited by Volkmar F, Klin A, Paul R, et al. Hoboken, NJ, Wiley, 2005, pp 223–246

Chawarska K, Klin A, Volkmar F: Automatic attention cueing through eye movement in 2-year-old children with autism. Child Dev 74:1108–1122, 2003

Coonrod E, Stone W: Screening for autism in young children, in Handbook of Autism and Pervasive Developmental Disorders. Edited by Volkmar F, Klin A, Paul R, et al. Hoboken, NJ, Wiley, 2005, pp 707–729

Courchesne E, Carper R, Akshoomoff N: Evidence of brain overgrowth in the first year of life in autism. JAMA 290:337–344, 2003

De Giacomo A, Fombonne E: Parental recognition of developmental abnormalities in autism. Eur Child Adolesc Psychiatry 7:131–136, 1998

Deykin EY, MacMahon B: The incidence of seizures among children with autistic symptoms. Am J Psychiatry 136:1310–1312, 1979

Handleman JS, Harris SL: Preschool Education Programs for Children with Autism. Austin, TX, Pro-Ed, 2000

Hippler K, Klicpera C: A retrospective analysis of the clinical case records of "autistic psychopaths" diagnosed by Hans Asperger and his team at the University Children's Hospital, Vienna. Philos Trans R Soc Lond B Biol Sci 358:291–301, 2003

Kanner L: Autistic disturbances of affective contact. Nervous Child 2:217–250, 1943

Klin A, Lang J, Cicchetti DV, et al: Brief report: interrater reliability of clinical diagnosis and DSM-IV criteria for autistic disorder. Results of the DSM-IV autism field trial. J Autism Dev Disord 30:163–167, 2000

Klin A, Jones W, Schultz R, et al: The enactive mind, or from actions to cognition: lessons from autism, in Handbook of Autism and Pervasive Developmental Disorders. Edited by Volkmar F, Klin A, Paul R, et al. Hoboken, NJ, Wiley, 2005a, pp 682–703

Klin A, McPartland J, Volkmar F: Asperger syndrome, in Handbook of Autism and Pervasive Developmental Disorders. Edited by Volkmar F, Klin A, Paul R, et al. Hoboken, NJ, Wiley, 2005b, pp 88–125

Klin A, Pauls D, Schultz R, et al: Three diagnostic approaches to Asperger syndrome: implications for research. J Autism Dev Disord 35:221–234, 2005c

Lainhart JE, Piven J, Wzorek M, et al: Macrocephaly in children and adults with autism. J Am Acad Child Adolesc Psychiatry 36:282–290, 1997

Lord C: Follow-up of two-year-olds referred for possible autism. J Child Psychol Psychiatry 36:1365–1382, 1995

Lord C, Shulman C, DiLavore P: Regression and word loss in autistic spectrum disorders. J Child Psychol Psychiatry 45:936–955, 2004

Luyster R, Richler J, Risi S, et al: Early regression in social communication in autism spectrum disorders: a CPEA study. Dev Neuropsychol 27:311–336, 2005

McPartland J, Dawson G, Webb SJ, et al: Event-related brain potentials reveal anomalies in temporal processing of faces in autism spectrum disorder. J Child Psychol Psychiatry 45:1235–1245, 2004

Miles J, Hillman R: Value of a clinical morphology examination in autism. Am J Med Genet 91:245–253, 2000

Miles J, Hadden HL, Takahashi TN, et al: Head circumference is an independent clinical finding associated with autism. Am J Med Genet A 95:339–350, 2000

Miller J, Ozonoff S: Did Asperger's cases have Asperger disorder? A research note. J Child Psychol Psychiatry 38:247–251, 1997

Minshew N, Sweeney J, Bauman ML: Neurologic aspects of autism, in Handbook of Autism and Pervasive Developmental Disorders. Edited by Volkmar F, Klin A, Paul A, et al. Hoboken, NJ, Wiley, 2000, pp 453–472

National Center for Clinical Infant Programs: Diagnostic Classification of Mental Health and Developmental Disorders of Infancy and Early Childhood. Washington, DC, National Center for Clinical Infant Programs, 1994

National Research Council: Educating Young Children with Autism. Washington, DC, National Academy Press, 2001

Paul R, Augustyn A, Klin A, et al: Perception and production of prosody by speakers with autism spectrum disorders. J Autism Dev Disord 35:205–220, 2005

Rodier PM, Bryson SE, Welch JP: Minor malformations and physical measurements in autism: data from Nova Scotia. Teratology 55:319–325, 1997

Rutter M: Genetic influences and autism, in Handbook of Autism and Pervasive Developmental Disorders. Edited by Volkmar F, Klin A, Paul R, et al. Hoboken, NJ, Wiley, 2005, pp 425–452

Schultz RT, Gauthier I, Klin A, et al: Abnormal ventral temporal cortical activity during face discrimination among individuals with autism and Asperger syndrome. Arch Gen Psychiatry 57:331–340, 2000

Siperstein R, Volkmar F: Brief report: parental reporting of regression in children with pervasive developmental disorders. J Autism Dev Disord 34:731–734, 2004

Smith T, Lovaas O: The UCLA Young Autism Project: a reply to Gresham and MacMillan. Behav Disord 22:202–218, 1997

Smith T, Eikeseth S, Klevstrand M, et al: Intensive behavioral treatment for preschoolers with severe mental retardations and pervasive developmental disorder. Am J Ment Retard 102:238–249, 1997

Stevenson RE, Schroer RJ, Skinner C, et al: Autism and macrocephaly. Lancet 349:1744–1745, 1997

Stone WL, Hoffman HL, Lewis SE, et al: Early recognition of autism: parental reports vs clinical observation. Arch Pediatr Adolesc Med 148:174–179, 1994

Stone WL, Lee EB, Ashford L, et al: Can autism be diagnosed accurately in children under 3 years? J Child Psychol Psychiatry 40:219–226, 1999

Volkmar FR, Klin A: Issues in the classification of autism and related conditions, in Handbook of Autism and Pervasive Developmental Disorders, 2nd Edition. Edited by Volkmar FR, Klin A, Paul R, et al. Hoboken, NJ, Wiley, 2005, pp 5–41

Volkmar F, Nelson D: Seizure disorders in autism. J Am Acad Child Adolesc Psychiatry 29:127–129, 1990

Volkmar F, Stier D, Cohen D: Age of recognition of pervasive developmental disorder. Am J Psychiatry 142:1450–1452, 1985

Volkmar F, Klin A, Siegel B, et al: Field trial for autistic disorder in DSM-IV. Am J Psychiatry 151:1361–1367, 1994

Volkmar FR, Klin A, Marans W, et al: Childhood disintegrative disorder, in Handbook of Autism and Pervasive Developmental Disorders. Edited by Volkmar F, Klin A, Paul R, et al. Hoboken, NJ, Wiley, 1997, pp 60–93

Volkmar F, Chawarska K, Klin A: Autism in infancy and early childhood. Annu Rev Psychol 56:315–336, 2005

Wetherby A, Schuler A, Prizant B: Enhancing language and communication development: theoretical foundations, in Handbook of Autism and Pervasive Developmental Disorders. Edited by Cohen D, Volkmar F. New York, Wiley, 1997, pp 513–538

World Health Organization: Diagnostic Criteria for Research. Geneva, Switzerland, World Health Organization, 1994

PART III

THE ELDERLY

22

AGING-RELATED DIAGNOSTIC VARIATIONS

Need for Diagnostic Criteria Appropriate for Elderly Psychiatric Patients

Dilip V. Jeste, M.D.
Dan G. Blazer, M.D., M.P.H., Ph.D.
Michael B. First, M.D.

There have been relatively few studies estimating the incidence and prevalence of serious mental illnesses in elderly populations (Hybels and Blazer 2003). These studies in community samples document that many older adults who experience clinically significant psychopathology do not fit easily into our existing nomenclature (Diefenbach et al. 2002; Gallo et al. 1997). Furthermore, the published studies have had a number of methodological problems, including improper definitions and diagnostic criteria for older persons (Jeste et al. 1999). Nonetheless, these studies have led to a popular lore that the prevalence of most psychiatric disorders other than dementia is considerably lower among the elderly than among younger adults (Blazer 1994b). Existing diagnostic categories do not capture a significant portion of the burden of psychiatric symptoms. Studies of subjects in epidemiological sur-

This work was supported, in part, by grants from the National Institute of Mental Health (MH49671, MH43693, and MH59101) and by the Department of Veterans Affairs.

veys who experience subsyndromal symptoms of disorders such as major depression (often labeled minor depression), for example, have reported more disability days (Broadhead et al. 1990) and experiencing more functional disability than control subjects (Hybels et al. 2001).

It is also commonly believed that new onset of noncognitive psychiatric disorders in late life is rare. A likely consequence of these misconceptions is that clinically significant and potentially treatable mental illnesses may be overlooked, misdiagnosed, and mistreated in elderly patients who do not present with a cluster of symptoms typical for younger patients. There is a need to develop aging-appropriate diagnostic criteria for major psychiatric disorders. In this chapter, we discuss the potential causes of this diagnostic confusion leading to possible underdiagnosis, overdiagnosis, and misdiagnosis. Four specific classes of disorders—schizophrenia and related psychotic disorders, mood (specifically depressive) disorders, anxiety disorders, and substance use disorders—are given as examples. Finally, we suggest some future steps for reducing the potential for diagnostic confusion in the elderly.

Potential Causes of Diagnostic Confusion in the Elderly

TRUE AGE-RELATED DIFFERENCES

The symptoms of a disorder may actually vary by age. In such cases, application of the DSM-IV-TR (American Psychiatric Association 2000) criteria sets, which describe diagnostic presentations characteristic of the disorder occurring at a younger age, would result in under-, over-, or misdiagnosis when applied to the elderly. In the case of major depression and anxiety disorders, there is not much evidence in favor of major age-associated differences in pathognomonic features when comorbidity is taken into account (Charles et al. 2001). For these two disorders, the core symptoms do not appear to vary with age unless a disorder, such as vascular dementia, co-occurs with the depressive or anxious episode. Some subtypes of disorders, such as paranoid schizophrenia (Harris and Jeste 1988), vascular depression (Alexopoulos et al. 1997), and "depression without sadness" (Alexopoulos et al. 1997; Gallo et al. 1997), are more prevalent in late life.

PHYSICAL AND PSYCHIATRIC COMORBIDITY

Older adults experiencing psychiatric disorders such as major depression are more likely to experience comorbidity with general medical conditions (such as congestive heart failure; Sullivan et al. 1997) and other psychiatric disorders (such as dementia of the Alzheimer's type) (Lyketsos et al. 1997). Other comorbidities are probably no more frequent (such as the comorbidity of major depression and generalized anxiety disorder; Blazer 2000). Diagnosing depression in the medically ill is complicated by the overlap of many symptoms, and therefore, difficulty arises in disaggregating symptoms of the underlying medical illness, depressive symptoms that result from a response to the medical illness, and depressive symptoms independent of the medical illness. For example, sleep problems may be the direct result of an illness such as chronic obstructive pulmonary disease, a natural response to the burden of the illness, and/or be independent of the illness. Depression in chronically medically ill persons can result from an interpersonal problem or a recurrence of unipolar recurrent depression that preceded the medical illness.

UNDERREPORTING OF SYMPTOMS

Older persons may be less likely to report symptoms of a disorder, thus biasing both epidemiological and clinically based studies in the direction of underdiagnosis. Evidence suggests, for example, that the threshold for reporting symptoms of depression is higher in the elderly compared with those in middle age (Tweed et al. 1992). Older adults in one community study were less likely to report dysphoric symptoms than were younger adults (Gallo et al. 1999).

VARIATION THROUGH TIME OF ONSET

Symptoms of major depression may vary by time of onset—that is, late-onset depression (first onset in late life) may be associated with different symptoms than early onset depression that recurs in late life (Salloway et al. 1996). Nevertheless, the symptoms of depression typically "breed true" when comorbid disorders do not intervene. Few studies, especially of community based samples, have followed the patterns of presentation of depression over time. New statistical models, such as latent class analysis, will permit investigators to determine if the trajectories of symptom presentation through time vary in meaningful ways. Another confounding factor is the cohort effect. Unfortunately, different methods of assessing depressive symptoms from one generation of epidemiological studies to another undermine our ability to determine changing frequencies of clinically significant depression and changing patterns of symptom presentation.

SUBTHRESHOLD PRESENTATIONS

Older people, like people across the life cycle, may experience clinically significant symptoms of psychiatric disorders that fall below the diagnostic thresholds set by the DSM-IV-TR criteria sets that define the disorders (Kessler et al. 2003). Yet the clinical significance of these symptoms may be different for the elderly than for younger persons, suggesting that the diagnostic thresholds in DSM-IV-TR may be resulting in diagnostic errors. For example, "minor generalized anxiety disorder" may have a different significance and outcome in the elderly than in younger adults (Diefenbach et al. 2002).

Disorders Associated With Diagnostic Confusion

MOOD DISORDERS (SPECIFICALLY DEPRESSIVE DISORDERS)

Clinicians and clinical investigators do not agree about what constitutes clinically significant depression regardless of age, nor is there universal agreement about how depression should be divided into homogeneous subtypes (Blazer 2003). The subtypes most cogent to late-life depression are reviewed here. There is considerable overlap across these subtypes, because the differentiations often reflect particular orientations toward dissecting the syndrome—that is, different ways of "slicing the pie." When the factor structure for the range of depressive symptoms is examined across the life cycle, however, there are no major differences between whites and African Americans (Blazer et al. 1998a), between males and females (Berkman et al. 1986; Blazer et al. 1998a), or between older and younger adults (Berkman et al. 1986; Ross and Mirowsky 1984).

Among the older adults diagnosed with major depression, the symptoms of moderate to severe depression presented to the clinician are similar across older adults and persons in midlife if there are no comorbid conditions (Blazer et al. 1987). Yet there may be subtle differences in symptom subtypes by age. For example, melancholia (symptoms of noninteractiveness and psychomotor retardation or agitation) appears to have a later age of onset for the first episode than nonmelancholic depression in clinical samples, with psychomotor disturbances being more distinct in older persons (Parker 2000; Parker et al. 2001).

Minor depression (also known as subsyndromal or subthreshold depression) is diagnosed, according to an appendix of DSM-IV-TR, when depressed mood or loss of interest is present along with one to three additional symptoms (Blazer 2003). Other operational definitions of these less severe variants of depression include a score of 16 or more on the Center for Epidemiologic Studies Depression Scale (CES-D; Radloff 1977) but not meeting criteria for major depression (Beekman et al. 1995); a primarily biogenic depression not meeting criteria for major depression yet responding to antidepressant medication (Snaith 1987); or a score of 11–15 on the CES-D (Hybels et al. 2001) and therefore not meeting the CES-D criteria for clinically significant depression. Minor depression, as variously defined, has been associated with impairment similar to that of major depression, including impaired physical functioning, disability days, poorer self-rated health, use of psychotropic medications, perceived low social support, female gender, and being unmarried (Beekman et al. 1995; Hybels et al. 2001). Studies indicate that subsyndromal depression may be followed or preceded by major depression (Judd and Akiskal 2002). The construct of subsyndromal disorders has been useful to stimulate further study of subjects who do not meet standard criteria. It is, however, important to stress that the terms *subsyndromal, subthreshold,* and *minor depression* do not have clear boundaries, and their definitions are operational and vary from one study to another. Clearly this is an area that warrants more research in elderly persons.

Other investigators have suggested a syndrome of *depression without sadness,* thought to be more common in older adults (Blazer 2003; Gallo et al. 1997, 1999), or a depletion syndrome manifested by withdrawal, apathy, and lack of vigor (Adams 2001; Newman 1989; Newman et al. 1991). *Dysthymic disorder* is a long-lasting chronic disturbance of mood, less severe than major depression, that lasts for 2 years or longer (American Psychiatric Association 2000). It rarely begins in late life but may persist from midlife into late life (Blazer 1994a; Devenand et al. 1994). These diagnostic categories are actually truncated from all the different potential subtypes of depression that have been suggested for geriatric depression, both past and present. Modern psychiatry has been criticized for its tendency to split syndromes into so many different subtypes without adequate empirical (especially biological) data to justify such splitting (Horowitz 2002). One investigator has suggested that the only meaningful split of the depressive spectrum is a split between the more physical symptoms of depression (such as anhedonia, agitation, and perhaps some of the symptoms of executive dysfunction) and the more psychological symptoms (e.g., feelings of worthlessness) (Parker and Hadzi-Pavlovic 1996).

Depression in late life is frequently *comorbid* with other physical and psychiatric conditions, especially in the oldest old (i.e., generally 85 years of age or older; Blazer 2000, 2003). For example, depression is common in older patients recovering from myocardial infarction and other heart conditions (Blazer 2000; Sullivan et al. 1997), in diabetes (Blazer et al. 2002), following hip fracture (Magaziner et al. 1997), and after stroke (Robinson and Price 1982). In community-dwelling Mexican American elders, depression was associated with diabetes, arthritis, urinary incontinence, bowel incontinence, kidney disease, and ulcers (a profile different from whites, who exhibit comorbidities such as hip fracture and stroke) (Black et al. 1998). Major depression is generally thought to be present in about 20% of Alzheimer's disease patients (Krishnan et al. 1997; Patterson et al. 1990; Reifler et al. 1982). In some studies, however, the rates are much lower (1%–5%), probably due to different approaches to case ascertainment (Weiner et al. 1994). Depressive symptoms may be common even in elders with mild dementia of the Alzheimer's type (Rubin et al. 2001).

Some differences have been reported between *early onset* (first episode before the age of 60) and *late-onset* (first episode after the age of 60) depression. Personality dysfunction, a family history of psychiatric illness, and dysfunctional past marital relationships were significantly more common in early onset depression (Brodarty et al. 2001). Yet when compared in terms of severity, phenomenology, history of a previous episode, and neuropsychological performance, there were no differences between early onset and late-onset depression in the elderly (Brodarty et al. 2001).

Interest in differentiating early vs. late-onset depression in late life has arisen in large part because some have speculated that contributors to etiology may vary by age at onset. For example, *vascular depression* (depression proposed to be due to vascular lesions in the brain) may be much more common with late-onset depression, and the clinical presentation may differ, even if only in subtle ways (Alexopoulos et al. 1997; Krishnan et al. 1997; Salloway et al. 1996). Severely depressed older adults exhibit impairment in set shifting, verbal fluency, psychomotor speed, recognition memory, and planning (executive cognitive function; Beats et al. 1996). The clinical presentation of elderly patients with this "depression-executive dysfunction syndrome" is characterized by psychomotor retardation and reduced interest in activities but a less pronounced vegetative syndrome than is seen in the depressed persons without executive dysfunction. The dysfunction consists of impaired verbal fluency, impaired visual naming, and poor performance on tasks of initiation and perseveration (Alexopoulos et al. 1996; Lockwood et al. 2002). Vascular depression, which may lead to executive dysfunction (but may not be the only cause), is associated with an absence of psychotic features, less likelihood of a family history, more anhedonia, and greater functional disability when compared with nonvascular depression (Alexopoulos et al. 1997; Hickie et al. 2001; Krishnan et al. 1997; Salloway et al. 1996)

Psychotic depression, in contrast to nonpsychotic depression, occurs in 20%–45% of hospitalized elderly depressed patients (Meyers 1992) and 3.6% of persons in the community with depression (Kivela et al. 1988). Psychotic depression is similar to schizophrenia and different from nonpsychotic depression in terms of neurocognitive deficits (Jeste et al. 1996). Recently, a group of investigators proposed a *depression of (due to) Alzheimer's disease.* In persons who meet the DSM-IV-TR criteria for dementia of the Alzheimer's type, at least three of a series of symptoms—including depressed mood, anhedonia, social isolation, poor appetite, poor sleep, psychomotor changes, irritability, fatigue or loss of energy, feelings of worthlessness, and suicidal thoughts—must be present for the diagnosis to be made (Olin et al. 2002). These criteria were developed (similar to those for psychosis of Alzheimer's disease as noted later) to describe a psychopathological (mood) state that is not captured by current diagnostic criteria, and they need to be validated by future research.

SCHIZOPHRENIA AND RELATED PSYCHOTIC DISORDERS

Schizophrenia

Although schizophrenia typically has its onset during late adolescence or early adulthood, a sizeable minority of patients manifest symptoms for the first time in middle or old age (Howard et al. 2000). Inconsistencies in nosology and a tendency among clinicians and researchers to attribute late-onset psychoses to "organic" factors have led to a likely underdiagnosis of schizophrenia in these cases. A central question here is how to be certain about the validity of the diagnosis of schizophrenia in a patient with late-onset, nonorganic, nonaffective chronic psychotic disorder. There are no clinical or laboratory tests that can reliably establish or rule out schizophrenia in any person, regardless of the age of onset of the symptoms. However, studies have shown that patients whose presentations meet strict clinical criteria for late-onset schizophrenia are similar to those with early onset schizophrenia in clinical symptomatology, family history, cognitive deficits, nonspecific brain imaging abnormalities, course of illness, and treatment response and do not manifest mood disorders, and they are at no elevated risk for dementia when followed over a number of years (Harris and Jeste 1988; Howard et al. 1993, 1994, 2000; Jeste et al. 1995, 1997; Palmer et al. 2001; Pearlson et al. 1993; Rabins et al. 1984; Sachdev et al. 1997). At the same time, there are some important and consistent differences between early- and late-onset schizophrenia that suggest that the latter should be identified as a distinct subtype of schizophrenia (Jeste et al. 1997; Pearlson et al. 1993). Such differences include a markedly higher prevalence of late-onset schizophrenia in women, its association with paranoid symptoms, less severe cognitive impairment, and a need for lower doses of antipsychotics.

A second issue to consider in determining the best classification scheme is what age at onset should be called "late." A review of the literature showed that 13% of all cases of schizophrenia had onset in the fifth decade (ages 41–50), 7% in the sixth decade, and only 3% after the age of 60 (Pearlson et al. 1993). In contrast, most studies of *late paraphrenia* (a term used for nonaffective psychoses characterized by paranoid delusions and auditory hallucinations that symptomatically resemble schizophrenia) conducted in Europe have been with patients in whom onset was after age 65. Differences in age at onset between studies of late-onset schizophrenia and studies of late paraphrenia may help explain some of the diagnostic confusions that have persisted.

A few years ago, an international late-onset schizophrenia group met to review published data on chronic, late-onset, nonaffective, nonorganic psychoses and to develop a consensus statement regarding diagnostic labeling (Howard et al. 2000). The group concluded that, in terms of epidemiology, symptom profiles, and identified pathophysiologies, there was face validity and clinical utility for two separate categories: late-onset (mostly, middle-age-onset) schizophrenia (illness onset after 40 years of age) and very-late-onset schizophrenia-like psychosis (onset after 60 years).

Similarities between late-onset groups and early onset schizophrenia cover areas such as type of symptoms (Jeste et al. 1997; Pearlson et al. 1989), family history, brain imaging findings (Jeste et al. 1998; Pearlson et al. 1993), and the nature of cognitive deficits. These strong similarities support a diagnosis of schizophrenia in the late-onset (mostly middle-age-onset) group. On the other hand, a distinction between those with middle-age-onset and geriatric-onset psychoses in terms of epidemiological, etiological, and symptom differences suggests that very-late-onset schizophrenia-like psychosis is a different category. It differs from both early and late-onset schizophrenia in being associated with sensory impairment, social isolation, and visual hallucinations but not with formal thought disorder, affective blunting, or familial aggregation of schizophrenia.

Although they agreed about the nomenclature, the members of the International Late-Onset Schizophrenia Group were not unanimous in their support of the particular age cutoffs given in the consensus statement (Howard et al. 2000). It was stressed that although the age cutoffs have clinical utility, they are inevitably arbitrarily defined, need to be viewed with caution, and warrant further research.

Regardless of the specific age cutoffs to be used, a subtyping of schizophrenia based on age of onset of illness may be more useful in terms of premorbid indicators, neurobiological underpinnings, prognostic considerations, and management issues than the current DSM classification based on symptom differences such as paranoid, catatonic, or disorganized types.

Other Psychotic Disorders in Late Life

Late-onset schizoaffective disorder. On the basis of recent research, late-onset schizoaffective disorder appears to share a majority of critical clinical and demographic features with late-onset schizophrenia (Evans et al. 1999). Thus, late-onset schizoaffective disorder appears to be a subtype of late-onset schizophrenia in which mood symptoms are also present. Late-onset delusional disorder, by contrast, can be distinguished from late-onset schizophrenia by a preoccupation with non-bizarre delusions in the context of preserved affective and personality functioning in other domains (Evans et al. 1996). In addition, treatment of these individuals may be more challenging than that of patients with schizophrenia due to their typical lack of insight about their delusionality. Cognitive function, however, is somewhat more preserved in older patients with delusional disorder than in those with schizophrenia. Unfortunately, there is a lack of research comparing early and late-onset delusional disorder.

Psychosis of Alzheimer's disease. Specific diagnostic criteria have been proposed for psychosis of Alzheimer's disease, based on the concept that this is a distinct disorder different from schizophrenia and other primary or secondary psychoses (Jeste and Finkel 2000). These criteria have been modeled after those for schizophrenia. They include

1. Characteristic symptoms: presence of visual or auditory hallucinations or delusions
2. Primary diagnosis: dementia of the Alzheimer's type
3. Chronology: onset of dementia precedes or coincides with that of psychosis
4. Duration and severity: symptoms have been present, at least intermittently, for 1 month or longer and are severe enough to cause some disruption in functioning
5. Exclusion of schizophrenia, delusional disorder, psychotic mood disorder, another general medical condition, or substance- or medication-induced psychosis
6. Delirium: psychosis does not occur exclusively during the course of a delirium

ANXIETY DISORDERS

Epidemiological studies suggest that the prevalence of anxiety disorders among the elderly is lower than that among younger adults and that anxiety disorders rarely have onset in late life (Blazer et al. 1991; Flint 1994; Regier et al. 1988). Unfortunately, these conclusions are based on diagnostic criteria that may not be optimal for elderly persons (Palmer et al. 1997). A number of differences have been reported between anxiety disorders in younger versus older adults (Lindesay 1991; Palmer et al. 1997; Parmlee et al. 1993; Rogers et al. 1994; Sheikh 1992). For example, older phobic patients are more likely to have fear of situations or inanimate stimuli such as heights or lightning, whereas younger patients may be more likely to have a fear of animals. Physical and psychosocial changes associated with aging may make it difficult to distinguish between phobias and nonpathological avoidance behaviors in elderly patients. Thus, a new-onset agoraphobic disorder would be less obvious (and therefore, underdiagnosed) in elderly individuals who are less mobile and tend to leave their houses less frequently. Similarly, social phobias may be attributed to diminished physical abilities, including visual problems, that make elderly persons afraid to go out at night or into cities where they could be victims of crime. There is a need for epidemiological studies of elderly persons using well-defined, age-appropriate diagnostic criteria that distinguish between anxiety disorders and behaviors that are secondary to reality-based factors.

Several reports suggest that older adults may be more likely than younger patients to manifest a mixture of anxiety and depression (Palmer et al. 1997; Parmlee et al. 1993). One possibility is that physical and psychosocial changes associated with aging may influence the very nature of syndrome clusters. The comorbidity could be a result of a co-occurrence of two common conditions or could reflect one being an epiphenomenon or a complication of the other. Attempts to separate anxiety and depression in mixed-age populations using cluster analytic techniques have met with mixed success. A syndrome of "mixed anxiety-depressive disorder" may have both heuristic and clinical utility for older patients. Proposed criteria for such a disorder are listed within DSM-IV-TR Appendix B (pp. 780–781).

SUBSTANCE USE DISORDERS

Studies using currently available diagnostic criteria for substance dependence and abuse are likely to underestimate the prevalence of mental illnesses in the elderly because these criteria were developed and validated on young and middle-aged samples and thus may have only limited utility among elderly populations (Patterson and Jeste 1999).

There are specific examples of inappropriateness of DSM-IV-TR criteria for substance use disorders in the elderly (Ellor and Kurz 1982; King et al. 1994; Miller et al. 1991). For instance, DSM-IV-TR criteria for substance dependence include increased tolerance to the effects of the substance leading to increased levels of consumption over time. Yet changes in pharmacokinetics and pharmacodynamics lower drug tolerance in the elderly, making it more difficult for the "tolerance" criterion for substance dependence to apply to this population. Similarly, a DSM-IV-TR criterion for substance abuse is the substance-related failure to fulfill major role obligations as manifested by absences or poor work performance; suspensions or expulsions from school; and neglect of children. Each of these occurrences fails to consider psychosocial changes seen with aging. A large proportion of the elderly do not have a major role obligation to fulfill—that is, they usually do not have full-time paid employment, do not go to school, and do not raise children; hence, these criteria would not apply to an elderly person who may be abusing substances. This makes it harder for the elderly to meet criteria for substance abuse.

Suggestions for an Age-Related Research Agenda

Further research is needed to clarify the classification of a number of late-life psychiatric disorders. Thus, longitudinal follow-up studies are necessary to determine how the course, neurobiology, psychosocial aspects, and management of psychiatric disorders in the elderly compare with those in younger patients.

EPIDEMIOLOGY

Epidemiological studies should use standardized criteria that are age specific or at least age modified. When comparisons are made by age at onset, first-onset episodes should be clearly defined based on clinical and historical assessment. Because cases of late-onset disorders may be somewhat uncommon, multicenter studies would be necessary. Long-term follow-up investigations can provide valuable information and test the hypothesis that patients tend to have a similar course regardless of age at onset (Howard et al. 2000).

Both risk factors and protective factors should be sought. Studies of the correlates of the subsyndromal disorders are warranted to determine whether they are associated with functional difficulties (Broadhead et al. 1990) or whether they respond to treatment (Williams et al. 2000).

SYMPTOMATOLOGY

Appropriate statistical analysis is necessary for determining relationship of specific symptoms to variables such as age at onset of illness. For example, because late-onset schizophrenia has a higher proportion of women than early onset illness, and because gender interacts with symptom variables such as emotional expressiveness and social activity, it is important to control for gender when comparing the prevalence of symptoms by age at onset.

Ample use should be made of secondary data analysis of clinical and community-based samples using new cluster procedures. For example, it would be useful to determine if clusters differ by age for symptoms among persons with diagnoses of the disorders under study, such as Grade of Membership analysis (Blazer et al. 1998b).

PATHOPHYSIOLOGY

Specific cognitive models should be tested in patients with onset in childhood, young adulthood, middle age, and old age to establish whether identified cognitive abnormalities are truly similar across the age-at-onset span (Howard et al. 2000). Sophisticated neurocognitive tests that allow for fine distinctions of performance should be used in combination with functional brain imaging to test hypotheses of differential neurocircuitry involvement. In very-late-onset cases, the possible role of sensory impairment should be further examined.

ETIOLOGY

Functional brain imaging studies involving adequate numbers of subjects should be conducted with patients across the age-at-onset span. The role of neurohormonal changes at menopause should be explored, as should genetic, viral, and degeneration-related factors. Large existing data sets should be explored with reference to late- and very-late-onset groups. Both developmental and degenerative processes that affect specific brain circuitry should be studied.

TREATMENT

Appropriately designed clinical trials of pharmacological and psychological treatments are required. Single-photon emission computed tomography and positron emission tomography receptor occupancy studies that compare early and late-onset cases would be valuable for understanding drug action and treatment response across age groups. Multisite investigations of combined pharmacological and psychosocial/behavioral management approaches—with meaningful outcome measures such as quality of life and everyday functioning—are warranted. Modern moderator and mediator analyses are warranted for examining how risk factors may work together to influence an outcome, especially as moderators and mediators (Kraemer et al. 2001, 2002). A *moderator* is a baseline or pre-randomization characteristic (e.g., age of onset of illness) that can be shown to have an interactive effect with the treatment on the outcome; moderators specify in whom a medication may produce specific therapeutic or adverse effects. A *mediator* is a change that occurs during (and is related to) treatment that has an effect on outcome (e.g., treatment-induced improvement in cognition that enhances everyday functioning); mediators would help identify possible mechanisms through which the specific effects of a treatment are produced.

Conclusions

Although it is generally thought and taught that most psychiatric disorders other than dementia are less common in the elderly than among younger adults, there are several reasons to question the data on which such assertions are based. Further research is needed to determine the degree to which DSM-IV-TR criteria for specific psychiatric disorders need modification or reclustering of symptoms to better describe the typical patterns of clinically significant syndromes in the elderly. Most of the gaps in the current knowledge outlined here can be filled via systematic research and better attention to the potential presence of these disorders in elderly patients.

References

Adams K: Depressive symptoms, depletion, or developmental change? Withdrawal, apathy, or lack of vigor in the Geriatric Depression Scale. Gerontologist 41:768–777, 2001

Alexopoulos GS, Vrontou C, Kakuma T, et al: Disability in geriatric depression. Am J Psychiatry 153:877–885, 1996

Alexopoulos GS, Meyers BS, Young RC, et al: "Vascular depression" hypothesis. Arch Gen Psychiatry 54:915–922, 1997

American Psychiatric Association: Diagnostic and Statistical Manual of Mental Disorders, 4th Edition, Text Revision. Washington, DC, American Psychiatric Association, 2000

Beats B, Sahakian B, Levy R: Cognitive performance in tests sensitive to frontal lobe dysfunction in the elderly depressed. Psychol Med 26:591–603, 1996

Beekman AT, Deeg DJ, van Tilburg T: Major and minor depression in later life: a study of prevalence and risk factors. J Affect Disord 36:65–75, 1995

Berkman LF, Berkman CS, Kasl S: Depressive symptoms in relation to physical health and functioning in the elderly. Am J Epidemiol 124:372–388, 1986

Black S, Goodwin J, Markides K: The association between chronic diseases and depressive symptomology in older Mexican Americans. J Gerontol Med Sci 53:M118–M194, 1998

Blazer D: Dysthymia in community and clinical samples of older adults. Am J Psychiatry 151:1567–1569, 1994a

Blazer D: Is depression more frequent in late life? An honest look at the evidence. Am J Geriatr Psychiatry 2:193–199, 1994b

Blazer D: Psychiatry and the oldest old. Am J Psychiatry 157:1915–1924, 2000

Blazer D: Depression in late life: review and commentary. Med Sci 58A:249–265, 2003

Blazer D, Bachar J, Hughes D: Major depression with melancholia: a comparison of middle-aged and elderly adults. J Am Geriatr Soc 35:927–932, 1987

Blazer D, George LK, Hughes D: The epidemiology of anxiety disorders: an age comparison, in Anxiety in the Elderly: Treatment and Research. Edited by Salzman C, Lebowitz BD. New York, Springer, 1991, pp 17–30

Blazer D, Landerman L, Hays J, et al: Symptoms of depression among community-dwelling elderly African-American and White older adults. Psychol Med 28:1311–1320, 1998a

Blazer D, Swartz M, Woodbury M, et al: Depressive symptoms and depressive diagnoses in a community population: use of a new procedure for analysis of psychiatric classification. Arch Gen Psychiatry 45:1078–1084, 1998b

Blazer D, Moody-Ayers S, Craft-Morgan J, et al: Depression in diabetes and obesity: racial/ethnic/gender issues in older adults. J Psychosom Res 52:1–4, 2002

Broadhead WE, Blazer DG, George LK, et al: Depression, disability days, and days lost from work: a prospective epidemiologic survey. JAMA 264:2524–2528, 1990

Brodarty H, Luscombe G, Parker G, et al: Early and late onset depression in old age: different aetologies, same phenomenology. J Affect Disord 66:225–236, 2001

Charles S, Reynolds C, Gatz M: Age-related differences and changes in positive and negative affect over 23 years. J Pers Soc Psychol 80:136–151, 2001

Devenand D, Noble M, Singer T, et al: Is dysthymia a different disorder in the elderly? Am J Psychiatry 151:1592–1599, 1994

Diefenbach G, Hopko D, Feigon S, et al: "Minor GAD": characteristics of subsyndromal GAD in older adults. Behav Res Ther 41:481–487, 2002

Ellor JR, Kurz DJ: Misuse and abuse of prescription and nonprescription drugs by the elderly. Nurs Clin North Am 17:319–330, 1982

Evans JD, Paulsen JS, Harris MJ: A clinical and neuropsychological comparison of delusional disorder and schizophrenia. J Neuropsychiatry Clin Neurosci 8:281–286, 1996

Evans JD, Heaton RK, Paulsen JS, et al: Schizoaffective disorder: a form of schizophrenia or affective disorder? J Clin Psychiatry 60:874–882, 1999

Flint AJ: Epidemiology and comorbidity of anxiety disorders in the elderly. Am J Psychiatry 151:640–649, 1994

Gallo J, Rabins PV, Lyketsos CG, et al: Depression without sadness: functional outcomes of nondysphoric depression in later life. J Am Geriatr Soc 45:570–578, 1997

Gallo J, Rabins P, Anthony J: Sadness in older persons: 13-year follow-up of a community sample in Baltimore, Maryland. Psychol Med 29:341–350, 1999

Harris MJ, Jeste DV: Late-onset schizophrenia: an overview. Schizophr Bull 14:39–55, 1988

Hickie I, Scott E, Naismith S, et al: Late-onset depression: genetic, vascular and clinical contributions. Psychol Med 31:1403–1412, 2001

Horowitz A: Creating Mental Illness. Chicago, IL, University of Chicago Press, 2002

Howard R, Castle D, Wessely S, et al: A comparative study of 470 cases of early and late-onset schizophrenia. Br J Psychiatry 163:352–357, 1993

Howard R, Almeida O, Levy R: Phenomenology, demography and diagnosis in late paraphrenia. Psychol Med 24:397–410, 1994

Howard R, Rabins PV, Seeman MV, et al: Late-onset schizophrenia and very-late-onset schizophrenia-like psychosis: an international consensus. Am J Psychiatry 157:172–178, 2000

Hybels C, Blazer D: Epidemiology and geriatric psychiatry, in Psychiatric Epidemiology. Edited by Tsuang M, Tohen M. New York, John Wiley and Sons, 2003, pp 603–628

Hybels C, Blazer D, Pieper C: Toward a threshold for subthreshold depression: an analysis of correlates of depression by severity of symptoms using data from an elderly community survey. Gerontologist 41:357–365, 2001

Jeste DV, Finkel SI: Psychosis of Alzheimer's disease and related dementias: diagnostic criteria for a distinct syndrome. Am J Geriatr Psychiatry 8:29–34, 2000

Jeste DV, Harris MJ, Krull A, et al: Clinical and neuropsychological characteristics of patients with late-onset schizophrenia. Am J Psychiatry 152:722–730, 1995

Jeste DV, Heaton SC, Paulsen JS, et al: Clinical and neuropsychological comparison of psychotic depression with nonpsychotic depression and schizophrenia. Am J Psychiatry 153:490–496, 1996

Jeste DV, Symonds LL, Harris MJ, et al: Non-dementia non-praecox dementia praecox? Late-onset schizophrenia. Am J Geriatr Psychiatry 5:302–317, 1997

Jeste DV, McAdams LA, Palmer BW, et al: Relationship of neuropsychological and MRI measures with age of onset of schizophrenia. Acta Psychiatr Scand 98:156–164, 1998

Jeste DV, Alexopoulos GS, Bartels SJ, et al: Consensus statement on the upcoming crisis in geriatric mental health: research agenda for the next two decades. Arch Gen Psychiatry 56:848–853, 1999

Judd LL, Akiskal HS: The clinical and public health relevance of current research on subthreshold depressive symptoms to elderly patients. Am J Geriatr Psychiatry 10:233–238, 2002

Kessler R, Merikangas K, Berglund P, et al: Mild disorders should not be eliminated from DSM-V. Arch Gen Psychiatry 60:1117–1122, 2003

King CJ, VanHasselt VB, Segal DL, et al: Diagnosis and assessment of substance abuse in older adults: current strategies and issues. Addict Behav 19:41–55, 1994

Kivela S, Pahkala K, Laippala P: Prevalence of depression in an elderly Finnish population. Acta Psychiatr Scand 78:401–413, 1988

Kraemer H, Stice E, Kazdin A, et al: How do risk factors work together? Mediators, moderators, and independent, overlapping, and proxy risk factors. Am J Psychiatry 158:848–856, 2001

Kraemer HC, Wilson T, Fairburn CG, et al: Mediators and moderators of treatment effects in randomized clinical trials. Arch Gen Psychiatry 59:877–883, 2002

Krishnan K, Hays J, Blazer D: MRI-defined vascular depression. Am J Psychiatry 154:497–501, 1997

Lindesay J: Phobic disorders in the elderly. Br J Psychiatry 159:531–541, 1991

Lockwood KA, Alexopoulos GS, Van Gorp WG: Executive dysfunction in geriatric depression. Am J Psychiatry 159:1119–1126, 2002

Lyketsos C, Baker L, Warren A, et al: Major and minor depression in Alzheimer's disease: prevalence and impact. J Neuropsychiatry Clin Neurosci 9:556–561, 1997

Magaziner J, Simonsick E, Kashner M: Predictors of functional recovery in the year following hospital discharge for hip fracture. J Gerontol Med Sci 45:M107-M110, 1997

Meyers BS: Geriatric delusional depression. Clin Geriatr Med 8:299–308, 1992

Miller N, Belkin B, Gold M: Alcohol and drug dependence among the elderly: epidemiology, diagnosis, and treatment. Compr Psychiatry 32:153–165, 1991

Newman J: Aging and depression. Psychol Aging 4:150–165, 1989

Newman J, Engel R, Jensen J: Age differences in depressive symptom experiences. J Gerontol 46:224–235, 1991

Olin JT, Katz IR, Meyers BS, et al: Provisional diagnostic criteria for depression of Alzheimer disease: rationale and background. Am J Geriatr Psychiatry 10:129–141, 2002

Palmer BW, Jeste DV, Sheikh JI: Anxiety disorders in the elderly: DSM-IV and other barriers to diagnosis and treatment. J Affect Disord 46:183–190, 1997

Palmer BW, McClure F, Jeste DV: Schizophrenia in late-life: findings challenge traditional concepts. Harv Rev Psychiatry 9:51–58, 2001

Parker G: Classifying depression: should paradigms lost be regained? Am J Psychiatry 157:1195–1203, 2000

Parker G, Hadzi-Pavlovic D: Melancholia: A Disorder of Movement and Mood. New York, Cambridge University Press, 1996

Parker G, Roy K, Hadzi-Pavlovic D, et al: The differential impact of age on the phenomenology of melancholia. Psychol Med 31:1231–1236, 2001

Parmlee P, Katz I, Lawton MP: Anxiety and its association with depression among institutionalized elderly. J Geriatr Psychiatry 1:46–58, 1993

Patterson M, Schnell A, Martin R, et al: Assessment of behavioral and affective symptoms in Alzheimer's disease. J Geriatr Psychiatry Neurol 3:21–30, 1990

Patterson TL, Jeste DV: The potential impact of the baby-boom generation on substance abuse among elderly persons. Psychiatr Serv 50:1184–1188, 1999

Pearlson GD, Kreger L, Rabins RV, et al: A chart review study of late-onset and early onset schizophrenia. Am J Psychiatry 146:1568–1574, 1989

Pearlson GD, Tune LE, Wong DF, et al: Quantitative D_2 dopamine receptor PET and structural MRI changes in late onset schizophrenia. Schizophr Bull 19:783–795, 1993

Rabins PV, Pauker S, Thomas J: Can schizophrenia begin after age 44? Compr Psychiatry 25:290–293, 1984

Radloff LS: The CES-D Scale: A self-report depression scale for research in the general population. Applied Psychological Measurement 1:385–401, 1977

Regier DA, Boyd JH, Burke JDJ, et al: One-month prevalence of mental disorders in the United States: based on five Epidemiologic Catchment Area sites. Arch Gen Psychiatry 45:977–986, 1988

Reifler B, Larson E, Hanley R: Coexistence of cognitive impairment and depression in geriatric outpatients. Am J Psychiatry 139:623–626, 1982

Robinson R, Price T: Post-stroke depressive disorders: a follow-up study of 103 patients. Stroke 13:635–641, 1982

Rogers MP, White K, Warshaw MG, et al: Prevalence of medical illness in patients with anxiety disorders. Int J Psychiatry Med 24:83–96, 1994

Ross C, Mirowsky J: Components of depressed mood in married men and women: The Center for Epidemiologic Studies Depression Scale. Am J Epidemiol 122:997–1004, 1984

Rubin E, Veiel L, Kinscherf D, et al: Clinically significant depressive symptoms and very mild to mild dementia of the Alzheimer type. J Geriatr Psychiatry 16:694–701, 2001

Sachdev P, Brodaty H, Rose N, et al: Regional cerebral blood flow in late-onset schizophrenia: a SPECT study using 99mTc-HMPAO. Schizophr Res 27:105–117, 1997

Salloway S, Malloy P, Kohn R, et al: MRI and neuropsychological differences in early and late-life onset geriatric depression. Neurology 46:1567–1574, 1996

Sheikh JI: Anxiety disorders and their treatment. Clin Geriatr Med 8:411–426, 1992

Snaith R: The concepts of mild depression. Br J Psychiatry 150:387–393, 1987

Sullivan M, LaCroix A, Baum C: Functional status in coronary artery disease: a one year prospective study of the role of anxiety and depression. Am J Med 103:348–356, 1997

Tweed D, Blazer D, Ciarlo J: Psychiatric epidemiology in elderly populations, in The Epidemiologic Study of the Elderly. Edited by Wallace RB, Woolson RF. New York, Oxford University Press, 1992, pp 213–233

Weiner MF, Edland SD, Luszczynska H: Prevalence and incidence of major depression in Alzheimer's disease. Am J Psychiatry 151:1006–1009, 1994

Williams JW, Barrett J, Oxman T, et al: Treatment of dysthymia and minor depression in primary care: a randomized controlled trial in older adults. JAMA 284:1519–1526, 2000

23

LATE-LIFE DEPRESSION

A Model for Medical Classification

George S. Alexopoulos, M.D.
Susan K. Schultz, M.D.
Barry D. Lebowitz, Ph.D.

The principal function of medical diagnosis is to guide treatment. Effective treatment strategies depend on the physicians' ability to identify a clinical picture with distinct underlying biological and nonbiological contributors, which can be targeted with the available interventions. Despite the advantages of the medical diagnostic system, psychiatric nosology consists of phenomenologically defined syndromes that are either biologically heterogeneous or have unknown biological contributors. We argue that geriatric psychiatric syndromes, and geriatric depression in particular, can serve as the starting point for a medical classification in psychiatry because these syndromes occur in the context of medical and neurological comorbidity and are accompanied by clinical, neuropsychological, and neuroimaging findings pointing to specific brain abnormalities. In this chapter, we review relevant literature and propose a model and a research agenda that may lead to a medical classification.

This paper was supported by NIMH grants P30 MH 68638 and RO1 MH65653 and the Sanchez Foundation.

The DSM-III Revolution

Historically, DSM-III (American Psychiatric Association 1980) was created to provide an operational framework for the classification of clinical observations during an era in which diagnoses had previously been made on the basis of clinicians' individual views and even feelings. Indeed, DSM-III and its successors revolutionized the field by creating a common language for clinicians to use in characterizing their patients. An equally profound change occurred in psychiatric research, where systematic assessment of psychopathology became standard practice. Like all landmark ideas, DSM-III soon began to be used for purposes beyond its original raison d'étre; it became a nosology without a medical basis. One of the reasons for this development has been the absence of definitive knowledge of biological contributors to most of the major DSM syndromes.

A diagnostic system that relies exclusively on phenomenology has significant limitations. Phenomenology strives for syndromic homogeneity. However, syndromic homogeneity is neither feasible nor desirable. First, use of DSM-II (American Psychiatric Association 1968) or DSM-IV (American Psychiatric Association 1994) criteria results in nonhomogeneous syndromes because different symptom permutations may qualify for the same diagnosis. Second, psychiatric disorders need not have homogeneous clinical presentations any more than medical illnesses do. Authoritative textbooks of medicine, such as *Harrison's Principles of Internal Medicine,* permit a variety of accompanying features in describing the clinical picture of medical illnesses—for example, pneumonia may be accompanied by dyspnea, fever, and so on. The typical presentation of a syndrome rarely occurs in all patients with the same medical illness—for example, myocardial infarction without precordial pain is common among older adults. Some diseases are, in fact, characterized by their clinical heterogeneity. Syphilis has so many diverse clinical presentations that it was once referred to as "the great imitator." The diverse clinical presentations of mycoplasma pneumonia led to the early term *atypical pneumonia.* Insistence on uniform clinical presentation can be counterproductive, because it may classify as "non-syndromes" conditions with common pathogenetic contributors. Nonetheless, improved understanding of specific contributors to the pathogenesis of a larger syndrome may provide information on specific symptoms. For example, subjects with frontostriatal dysfunction and depression may exhibit executive function deficits, whereas individuals with early-onset depression with significant genetic contribution may exhibit other clinical features.

Readiness for a Medical Classification

The etiology of psychiatric disorders remains unknown. However, advancements in understanding biological correlates of psychiatric disorders and the context in which they occur place us in a better position to propose a research agenda that would eventually lead to a medical classification of psychiatric disorders.

Medical classification requires that some of the clinical manifestations of a disorder are mediated by biological mechanisms rather than mandating a unitary biological explanation for all aspects of the disorder. Therefore, medical classification allows nonbiological factors to contribute to the development of a disorder. For example, severe acute respiratory syndrome (SARS) is a viral respiratory infection with diverse clinical presentation, a higher incidence during the cold months of the year, and a higher mortality among elders and medically compromised patients. Therefore, even in an infectious disorder like SARS, environmental facilitation and noninfectious medical burden (nonspecific to the SARS virus) play a role in the development and course of the disease.

Geriatric psychiatric syndromes, and depression in particular, occur in patients with medical and neurological disorders and offer an opportunity for research leading to a model medical classification. Like disorders complying with the demands of medical classification, biological research on psychiatric syndromes needs to take into consideration the biological and nonbiological context in which geriatric psychiatric disorders occur.

Although medical/neurological comorbidity offers a research window to the brain, it is unreasonable to expect a direct lesion–syndrome relationship. There are at least five reasons for the absence of such a one-to-one relationship. First, the most likely brain abnormalities associated with behavioral disorders affect high-level neural systems. These systems are redundant and interactive. Unlike peripheral nerve lesions and, to a lesser extent, lesions of the internal capsule and some brain stem areas, lesions of high-level cortical and subcortical structures do not result in identical behavioral abnormalities. Neural system redundancy and plasticity may explain the heterogeneity in symptom expression because other centers assume some of the function of the lesioned circuitry. In addition, the complex interactions among neural systems (lateral prefrontal cortex, anterior thalamus, anterior cingulate, subgenual cingulate, orbitofrontal cortex, hippocampus, and medial frontal cortex) may explain why different brain lesions or pathological processes can lead to similar syndromes. Moreover, there is evidence that differences in limbic-cortical activation are associated with differential response to antidepressant treatments; more limited limbic-cortical and cortical-cortical connections differentiate responders to cognitive-behavioral therapy from responders to pharmacotherapy (Seminowicz et al. 2004). A second reason for a lack of a direct central nervous system (CNS) lesion–syndrome relationship is the contribution of non-CNS medical burden that either directly or through the resultant disability facilitates the development of psychopathology. Third, the premorbid competencies that each person possesses at the time of the CNS insult may influence the character and course of psychopathology. These competencies can be behavioral (e.g., skills relevant to problem solving and dealing with stress) or cognitive (e.g., ability of a person to assess risks and benefits of specific situations and decisions and act accordingly). A fourth reason is that environmental adversity may lead to adaptation problems and enhance abnormal behavioral patterns. Environmental adversity needs to be viewed in the context of the individual's physical, behavioral, and cognitive skills, because a mild environmental change may overwhelm a person with underdeveloped skills. Finally, genetic makeup is an important contributor in early onset depression but also increases the risk of depression in patients with late-onset depression occurring after a brain insult. For example, personal or family history of a depressive disorder has been shown to increase the incidence of poststroke depression as much, if not more, than the site of the vascular lesion (Morris et al. 1992).

Accordingly, research aiming to generate the grounds for a medical classification of psychiatric disorders needs to focus on CNS abnormalities that confer a morbid vulnerability to psychopathology development rather than leading to a distinct behavioral syndrome (Figure 23–1). The affected neural systems may determine to some extent the clinical presentation and course of the ensuing behavioral disorder. However, medical burden, cognitive and behavioral competence, and their relationship to the individual's environment and genetic makeup may also influence the neurobiology as well as the clinical presentation and outcomes of the behavioral disorder. Additional studies may focus on the mechanisms mediating the expression of syndromic states in predisposed individuals.

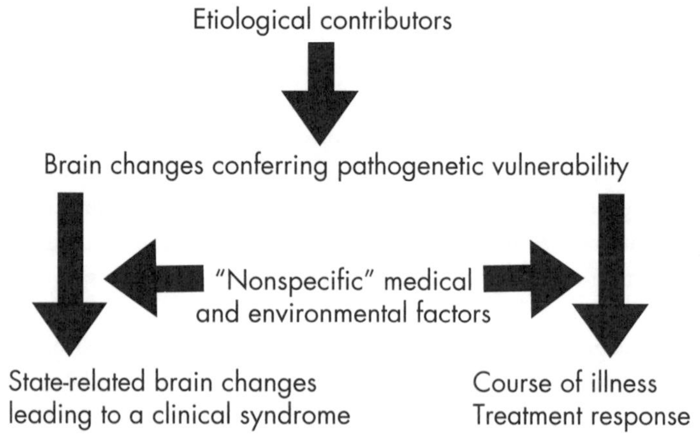

FIGURE 23–1. A model for late-life psychiatric disorders.

Geriatric Depression

Geriatric depression may serve as a model entity for the work needed toward a medical classification of psychiatric disorders. First, geriatric depression resembles medical diseases. Along with changes in mood, ideation, and behavior, geriatric depression is associated with peripheral body changes. These include the vegetative syndrome as well as hypercortisolemia, increased abdominal fat, decreased bone density, and increased risk for type II diabetes and hypertension (Brown et al. 2004). Depression of older adults often is accompanied by cognitive impairments resulting from abnormally functioning neural systems; dysfunction of frontostriatal pathways, the amygdala, and the hippocampus have been implicated. In addition to CNS pathology, geriatric patients have multiple medical illnesses requiring treatment with agents crossing the blood–brain barrier; experience disability; and often are presented with difficulties in negotiating their environment. Each of these factors may contribute to the heterogeneity of the clinical presentation and the course of geriatric depression.

Although geriatric depressed patients vary in their clinical presentation and course, most of them have aging-related CNS changes. Thus an appropriate first step for research relevant to medical classification is the search for CNS pathology predisposing to depressive symptoms and influencing their course (Figure 23–1). This work needs to be followed by studies examining the relationships of CNS pathology to the context in which geriatric depression occurs (e.g., non-neurological medical burden, disability, poor matching of the depressed person to his or her habitat, psychiatric history).

Abnormalities in more than one brain region may predispose to depression. There are least two reasons for this assumption. First, abnormalities in one region may influence other functionally connected regions. Second, elderly patients may have abnormalities in more than one brain region, with complex interactions leading to vulnerability to depression. In the following sections we discuss three examples of brain structure abnormalities for which available findings suggest that they increase vulnerability to depression. However, it should be emphasized that these may not be the only brain structures whose compromise predisposes to depression.

FRONTOSTRIATAL DYSFUNCTION

Two sets of clinical findings suggest a relationship between frontostriatal dysfunction and geriatric depression. First, executive dysfunction, a disturbance resulting from compromised integrity of frontal structures and their subcortical connections, is common in geriatric depression (Lockwood et al. 2002; Nebes et al. 2001) and persists after improvement of mood-related symptoms (Murphy and Alexopoulos 2004; Nebes et al. 2003). Second, disorders compromising frontostriatal pathways are often complicated by depression. Subcortical dementing disorders, including vascular dementia, Parkinson's disease, and Huntington's disease, are more likely to result in depression than cortical dementias (Sobin and Sackeim 1997). Moreover, development of depression is more likely to occur in Alzheimer's patients with subcortical atrophy (Starkstein et al. 1995).

Along with clinical observations, structural neuroimaging studies have documented that neurologically unimpaired depressed patients have low volumes of structures of frontostriatal networks, including the subgenual anterior cingulate (Drevets et al. 1997), caudate head (Krishnan et al. 1992), and putamen (Husain et al. 1991). Moreover, low volumes of the anterior cingulate, orbitofrontal cortex, and rectus gyrus have been reported in geriatric depression (Ballmaier et al. 2004), and hyperintensities in subcortical structures and their frontal connections are prevalent in geriatric depression (Coffey et al. 1990; Krishnan et al. 1997; Steffens et al. 1999). Subcortical hyperintensities have been associated with executive dysfunction (Aizenstein et al. 2002; Boone et al. 1992), the clinical expression of frontostriatal dysfunction. Reduction in glia of the subgenual anterior cingulate gyrus (Rajkowska et al. 1999), as well as abnormalities in neurons of the dorsolateral prefrontal cortex, have been observed in unipolar depressed patients (Ongur et al. 1998b).

Cognitive neuroscience studies suggest that dysfunction in certain parts of frontostriatal circuitry—that is, the prefrontal cortices and the anterior cingulate—is relevant to the development of depressive symptoms. A model of the prefrontal cortex function proposes that this brain structure maintains the representation of an individual's goals and sends signals to other brain areas to facilitate the expression of task-appropriate response (Davidson et al. 2002). Such signals facilitate the expression of the most adaptive response to a stimulus at the expense of an immediately rewarding response. Theoretically, abnormalities in prefrontal circuitry responsible for positive affect-guided anticipation may predispose to some types of depression and result in failure to anticipate positive incentives. The left medial orbitofrontal cortex is activated in response to reward and the right orbitofrontal cortex in response to punishment (O'Doherty et al. 2001); both these functions are relevant to depression. The anterior cingulate gyrus has connections to brain structures relevant to the expression of depressive symptoms and is responsible for functions that are often impaired in depression. Accordingly, the affective cingulate subdivision is connected to the orbitofrontal cortex, the amygdala, the lateral hypothalamus, the anterior insula, the periaqueductal grey, and some autonomic stem centers (Bush et al. 2000; Ongur et al. 1998a). The affective cingulate assesses conflicts between current function and information with motivational consequences and integrates affective and cognitive information. The cognitive cingulate subdivision has connections with the dorsolateral prefrontal cortex, the posterior cingulate, the parietal cortex, and the supplementary motor cortex. Its principal function is to monitor competing responses and modulate attention and executive functions in collaboration with the dorsolateral cortex (Bush et al. 2000; Whalen et al. 1998).

Frontostriatal dysfunction may influence the clinical presentation of geriatric depression. Among elderly depressed patients, those with executive dysfunction have more pronounced psychomotor retardation and reduced interest in activities than depressed patients without executive dysfunction (Alexopoulos et al. 1997a, 2002; Krishnan et al. 1997), a clinical presentation resembling medial frontal lobe syndromes. Nonetheless, depressed patients with executive dysfunction have sad mood, hopelessness, helplessness, and worthlessness of similar severity to that of depressed patients without executive dysfunction (Alexopoulos et al. 2002) and meet the criteria for major depression.

Clinical and laboratory studies suggest that frontostriatal abnormalities influence the course of depression. Executive dysfunction, a clinical expression of frontostriatal abnormalities, predicts slow, poor (Alexopoulos et al. 2004; Dunkin et al. 2000; Kalayam and Alexopoulos 1999; Potter et al. 2004; Simpson et al. 1998), and unstable response (Alexopoulos et al. 1999) to antidepressants, although some disagreement exists (Butters et al. 2004). White matter abnormalities have been associated with both executive dysfunction (Aizenstein et al. 2002; Boone et al. 1992) and poor outcomes of geriatric depression (Alexopoulos 2002; Hickie et al. 1995, 1997; O'Brien et al. 1998; Simpson et al. 1998; Steffens et al. 2001). Hypometabolism of the rostral anterior cingulate was reported in treatment-resistant depression, whereas cingulate hypermetabolism was associated with favorable response (Mayberg 2001). Anterior cingulate activity is a predictor of the extent of treatment response in depressed young adults (Pizzagalli et al. 2001). Finally, increased left frontal error negative wave amplitude following a response inhibition task (mediated by the anterior cingulate) predicts limited or slow change in depressive symptoms in elders receiving citalopram treatment (Kalayam and Alexopoulos 2003).

AMYGDALAR DYSFUNCTION

Patients experiencing their first depressive episode have larger amygdalar volumes than patients with recurrent depression and healthy control subjects (Frodl et al. 2003). In contrast, decline in amygdalar volume has been documented in recurrent depression (Sheline et al. 1998). Along these lines, a hypermetabolic state of the amygdala has been associated with greater depressive symptoms and negative emotions (Drevets 1999, 2003). It has been hypothesized that increased activation of the amygdala is a result of inadequate inhibition of this structure by prefrontal centers (Drevets 1999). Thus the combination of increased amygdalar metabolism with failure of cortical modulation of the emotional input may confer vulnerability to depression.

The association of amygdala to depression is further supported by its role in the processing of stimuli. A series of studies suggests that the amygdala is integral to the modulation of mood states because it mediates the perception of emotion and particularly the processing of aversive stimuli (Davidson 2001). The amygdala integrates negative emotions and signals to centers responsible for coping behavior and autonomic activity (LeDoux 1993).

The pathways associated with emotional perception are affected by aging-related changes. Changes associated with a loss or attenuation of emotional perception may contribute to a depressed or apathetic clinical presentation. Brain diseases, such as stroke and subcortical disorders such as Parkinson's disease, may damage the connections between regions of the amygdala, the medial dorsal thalamic nucleus, and the orbital and medial prefrontal cortex and predispose to depression (Drevets 1999). Finally, hypercortisolemia occurring during chronic medical illnesses is associated with increased activity of the amygdala, and conversely, amygdalar activation stimulates cortisol release, representing yet another mechanism by which comorbid illnesses may increase the risk of a depressive syndrome (Erickson et al. 2003).

HIPPOCAMPAL DYSFUNCTION

Growing evidence suggests that hippocampal abnormalities confer vulnerability to depression (Bremner et al. 2000; Sheline 2003). Hippocampal volume was found to be reduced in individuals in their first episode of depression, raising the possibility that hippocampal abnormalities represent a premorbid risk factor (Frodl et al. 2002). However, some disagreement exists (Campbell et al. 2004; Hastings et al. 2004). Studies have documented that reduced hippocampal size is correlated with the total length of time spent in a depressed state (Brown et al. 2004; Sheline 2000). Moreover, a rapid decline in hippocampal volume has been documented over several years after the first depressive episode, even when treatment was offered (MacQueen et al. 2003).

Abnormalities of the hippocampus are relevant to the aging population, because this structure is particularly vulnerable to aging and aging-related changes. Genetics determine only 40% of the variance in the size of hippocampus, whereas the rest of the variance is determined by environmental factors (Sullivan et al. 2001). Advanced age is associated with hippocampal atrophy. Moreover, the CA1 hippocampal region and the subiculum are vulnerable to ischemia (MacQueen et al. 2003) and to the effect of hypercortisolemia resulting from stress and chronic medical illness (Miller and O'Callaghan 2003).

MECHANISMS OF THE DEPRESSIVE SYNDROME

The findings dicussed in the previous section suggest that frontostriatal, amygdalar, and hippocampal dysfunction occur in some patients with geriatric depression. However, depressed elders with clinical or laboratory evidence of dysfunction in these systems have neither a homogeneous clinical presentation nor a homogeneous course of illness. For this reason, frontostriatal, amygdalar, and hippocampal dysfunction are best conceptualized as a morbid vulnerability that predisposes to depression and increases its propensity for chronicity and relapse. This conceptualization allows for other factors to contribute to the development of the syndrome and influence its course, including overall medical burden, disability interfering with adaptation, psychosocial adversity, prior psychiatric history, and so on.

Predisposition to depression need not be identical to the mechanisms of symptom expression during depressive states. Accordingly, frontostriatal, amygdalar, and hippocampal dysfunction need not be the exact final mechanisms that directly mediate symptom expression during depressive episodes. Functional neuroimaging studies converge to the conclusion that, during depressive states, dorsal neocortical structures are hypometabolic and ventral limbic structures are hypermetabolic (Alexopoulos 2002; Drevets 2000). Similar changes occur in experimentally induced sadness (Mayberg 2001). So the expression of depressive symptoms may be mediated by a common pathway, but the predisposing factor—in this case frontostriatal, amygdalar, or hippocampal dysfunction—may be unique to a subgroup of depressed patients. In contrast, nondepressed individuals who develop sadness at will may have a quick normalization of the sadness-associated brain metabolic changes because they have no predisposing factors to sustain symptoms of depression.

ETIOLOGY OF GERIATRIC DEPRESSION

Frontostriatal, amygdalar, and hippocampal dysfunction can be caused by various processes. Degenerative and vascular as well as immune and inflammatory processes may lead to dysfunction of subcortical structures and thus be the etiological factors underlying vulnerability to depression. Depression often occurs in degenerative disorders of subcortical structures with a long preclinical phase (Sobin and Sackeim 1997). Similarly, depression is common in patients with vascular risk factors and disorders resulting in subcortical lesions (Alexopoulos et al. 1997b; Krishnan et al. 1997). Finally, levels of proinflammatory cytokines, including interferon-gamma, interleukin-6, and tumor necrosis factor–alpha, and C-reactive protein are elevated during depressed states (Schiepers et al. 2005; Thomas et al. 2005). Interferon administration often leads to development of depressive symptoms or syndromes as well as cognitive and electrophysiological changes (Amodio et al. 2005).

This paradigm follows the traditional medical conceptualization of disease, that is, etiologic contributors → brain changes conferring pathogenetic vulnerability → interaction with nonspecific medical and environmental factors → state-related brain changes → clinical syndrome. Moreover, vulnerability-inducing brain changes may influence the course of illness (Figure 23–1).

TREATMENT IMPLICATIONS

Identifying neural systems whose abnormalities contribute to depression may guide pharmacological research in selecting candidate antidepressants for specific subgroups of depressed elders. For example, depressed elders with evidence of frontostriatal impairment may be candidates for dopamine-enhancing agents, whereas use of such agents in a broader group of depressives may dilute the therapeutic signal and lead to the erroneous conclusion that dopaminergic agents have no antidepressant properties for any patients (Alexopoulos 2001). Similarly, research may examine whether adjunct pharmacotherapy with agents enhancing the metabolism of frontostriatal structures, such as modafinil (Scammell et al. 2000), can improve the outcomes of depressed patients with evidence of anterior cingulate dysfunction. Although these approaches are sensible, their efficacy must be clinically tested. The reason is that direct lesion-to-syndrome relationships are unlikely in late-life depression. Moreover, even "selectively acting drugs" have broader effects and change the function of systems other than those on which they exert their immediate action (Millan 2004). Finally, treatment and prevention studies need to investigate the efficacy of behavioral approaches, such as problem solving therapy, that remedy behavioral deficits originating from executive dysfunction (Alexopoulos et al. 2003).

Understanding the role of amygdalar pathology as a predisposing condition to depression has treatment implications relevant to a medical model classification approach. Preliminary evidence suggests that a persistently hypermetabolic state of the amygdala is associated with increased relapse risk or inadequate response to antidepressant treatment (Drevets 1999). Further research in this area may document that amygdalar hyperactivity demonstrated through neuroimaging studies or its associated hypercortisolemia predict unstable antidepressant response and dictate a cautious course of clinical action.

As in the case of frontostriatal systems and the amygdala, studies of the role of hippocampus in predisposing to depression can guide the development of focused therapies. For example, a treatment study utilizing cognitive-behavioral therapy for adults with major depression demonstrated that treatment response was associated with increases in metabolism in the hippocampus and dorsal cingulate (Goldapple et al. 2004). Understanding these regional changes may also influence the selection of treatment, because new data suggest that cellular plasticity may be enhanced by antidepressant treatment in a way that intercedes in hippocampal loss by inducing regional neurogenesis (Kempermann and Kronenberg 2003). Specifically, serotonergic antidepressants have been shown to increase neurogenesis in the dentate gyrus of the rat hippocampus (Malberg et al. 2000).

Implications for Geriatric Psychiatric Syndromes Other Than Depression

In the previous sections, we discussed brain abnormalities predisposing to depression. However, discrete brain abnormalities may predispose to a variety of behavioral syndromes, including psychosis, disinhibition, and delirium. For example, the presence of Lewy bodies in limbic and neocortical regions in patients with Lewy body dementia is thought to account for the neuropsychiatric symptoms of this disorder, such as visual hallucinations, whereas the more subcortical distribution of Lewy bodies observed in Parkinson's disease accounts for the predominance of motor symptoms (Barber et al. 2001). Along the same lines, progressive supranuclear palsy (PSP) and Parkinson's disease have different patterns of regional brain degeneration and present rather distinct behavioral pathology (Aarsland et al. 2001). PSP leads to degeneration of many subcortical regions (e.g., putamen, globus pallidus, caudate, subthalamus) as well as orbitofrontal and medial frontal regions. In contrast, Parkinson's disease primarily leads to degeneration of mesocortical dopaminergic and other monoaminergic regions. Consistent with these regional differences, patients with PSP are more likely to develop disinhibition and apathy syndromes, whereas patients with Parkinson's disease are more likely to present hallucinations, delusions, and depression. Differences in behavioral pathology between PSP and Parkinson's disease persist even after dopaminergic medications are accounted for (Aarsland et al. 2001). Finally, discrete brain abnormalities may predispose to side effects, as in the case of Parkinson's disease, in which degeneration of the mesocortical dopaminergic system may increase vulnerability to L-dopa and lead to delirium.

Toward a Research Agenda

Psychiatric syndromes consist of complex and heterogeneous behaviors unlikely to follow a simple lesion–syndrome relationship. We posit that aging-related changes in specific brain structures interacting with personal vulnerability (either genetic, neurodevelopmental, or early trauma) or any other individual biological or cultural vulnerabilities (e.g., gender or ethnicity) and environmental factors create a propensity for development of certain psychiatric syndromes. The predisposing factors may be distinct from the actual mechanisms operating during the expression of a syndromic state, much like hypertension is distinct from stroke but represents a predisposing vulnerability.

We argue that research seeking to identify both morbid vulnerabilities to psychiatric syndromes and the mediating mechanisms of symptomatology has the potential to lead to a medical classification of psychiatric disorders. In turn, a medical classification can guide the effort to improve treatment and prevention of psychiatric disorders by focusing therapeutic efforts to the underlying predisposing abnormalities as well as to the syndrome-mediating mechanisms.

The proposed model parallels the etiopathogenesis of syndromes such as myocardial infarction, in which obesity, hypertension, cholesterol, and emotional stress are all multimodal risk factors compromising vascular integrity and predisposing to infarction. Similarly, CNS aging or vascular disease, as well as behavioral disability, physical deconditioning, and psychosocial adversity, may compromise frontostriatal, amygdalar, or hippocampal integrity and confer vulnerability to depression. A similar model has been articulated by McEwen (2003), who described the cumulative effects of these risk factors as "allostatic load" resulting from the individual's inability to accommodate to extrinsic stressors.

The research agenda suggested here, in addition to focusing on mechanisms, can guide treatment research targeting persons with specific vulnerabilities. For example, an intervention may involve medication geared toward discrete neural systems predisposing to psychiatric syndromes, treatments preventing further damage to these neural systems (e.g., treatment of hypertension, hyperlipidemia, hypercortisolemia as well as health-promoting behaviors, including stress-reduction, exercise, and perhaps antioxidants), and behavioral approaches aimed at improving coping with adversity and remedying disability. Thus we propose the following:

1. Studies aimed at understanding the role of specific brain structure abnormalities in predisposing to late-life behavioral pathology. Such studies need to focus on interactions among aging-related changes in brain structures, personal vulnerability (either genetic, neurodevelopmental, or early trauma), other individual biological or cultural vulnerabilities (e.g., gender or ethnicity), and environmental factors.
2. Studies aimed at understanding aging-related processes leading to brain structure damage predisposing to psychiatric disorders.
3. Studies aimed at understanding the mechanisms mediating psychiatric symptom expression in elderly patients.
4. Treatment and prevention studies targeting the predominant neurotransmitter-system abnormalities of pathways conferring vulnerability to psychiatric disorders. Such studies should focus on patients with evidence of specific neural network impairment rather than the whole elderly population with similar symptoms.
5. Studies of psychosocial interventions targeting the behavioral deficits produced by abnormalities in neural networks that predispose to late-life behavioral pathology.

References

Aarsland D, Litvan I, Larsen JP: Neuropsychiatric symptoms of patients with progressive supranuclear palsy and Parkinson's disease. J Neuropsychiatry Clin Neurosci 13:42–49, 2001

Aizenstein HJ, Nebes RD, Meltzer CC, et al: The relation of white matter hyperintensities to implicit learning in healthy older adults. Int J Geriatr Psychiatry 17:664–669, 2002

Alexopoulos G: "The depression-executive dysfunction syndrome of late life": a specific target for D3 agonists? Am J Geriatr Psychiatry 9:22–29, 2001

Alexopoulos G: Frontostriatal and limbic dysfunction in late-life depression. Am J Geriatr Psychiatry 10:687–695, 2002

Alexopoulos G, Meyers BY, Kakuma T, et al: Clinically defined vascular depression. Am J Psychiatry 154:562, 1997a

Alexopoulos G, Meyers BS, Young RC, et al: The "vascular depression" hypothesis. Arch Gen Psychiatry 54:915–922, 1997b

Alexopoulos G, Bruce ML, Hull J, et al: Clinical determinants of suicidal ideation and behavior in geriatric depression. Arch Gen Psychiatry 56:1048–1053, 1999

Alexopoulos G, Kiosses DN, Klimstra S, et al: Clinical presentation of the "depression-executive dysfunction syndrome" of late life. Am J Geriatr Psychiatry 10:98–106, 2002

Alexopoulos G, Raue P, Arean P: Problem-solving therapy versus supportive therapy in geriatric major. Am J Geriatr Psychiatry 11:46, 2003

Alexopoulos G, Kiosses DN, Murphy C: Executive dysfunction, heart disease burden, and remission of geriatric depression. Neuropsychopharmacology 29:2278–2284, 2004

American Psychiatric Association: Diagnostic and Statistical Manual of Mental Disorders, 2nd Edition. Washington, DC, American Psychiatric Association, 1968

American Psychiatric Association: Diagnostic and Statistical Manual of Mental Disorders, 3rd Edition. Washington, DC, American Psychiatric Association, 1980

American Psychiatric Association: Diagnostic and Statistical Manual of Mental Disorders, 4th Edition. Washington, DC, American Psychiatric Association, 1994

Amodio P, Toni EN, Cavaletto L, et al: Mood, cognition and EEG changes during interferon alpha (alpha-INF) treatment for chronic hepatitis C. J Affect Disord 84:93–98, 2005

Ballmaier M, Toga AW, Blanton RE, et al: Anterior cingulate, gyrus rectus, and orbitofrontal abnormalities in elderly depressed patients: an MRI-based parcellation of the prefrontal cortex. Am J Psychiatry 161:99–108, 2004

Barber R, Panikkar A, McKeith IG: Dementia with Lewy bodies: diagnosis and management. Int J Geriatr Psychiatry 16:S12–S18, 2001

Boone KB, Miller BL, Lesser IM, et al: Neuropsychological correlates of white-matter lesions in healthy elderly subjects: a threshold effect. Arch Neurol 49:549–554, 1992

Bremner J, Narayan M, Anderson E, et al: Hippocampal volume reduction in major depression. Am J Psychiatry 157:115–118, 2000

Brown ES, Varghese FP, McEwen BS: Association of depression with medical illness: does cortisol play a role? Biol Psychiatry 55:1–9, 2004

Bush G, Luu P, Posner MI: Cognitive and emotional influences in anterior cingulate cortex. Trends Cogn Sci 4:215–222, 2000

Butters M, Whyte E, Nebes R, et al: The nature and determinants of neuropsychological functioning in late-life. Arch Gen Psychiatry 61:587–595, 2004

Campbell S, Marriott M, Nahmias C, et al: Lower hippocampal volume in patients suffering from depression: a meta-analysis. Am J Psychiatry 161:598–607, 2004

Coffey CE, Figiel GS, Djang WT, et al: Subcortical hyperintensity on magnetic resonance imaging: a comparison of normal and depressed elderly subjects. Am J Psychiatry 147:187–189, 1990

Davidson RJ: Toward a biology of personality and emotion. Ann NY Acad Sci 935:191–207, 2001

Davidson RJ, Pizzagalli D, Nitschke JB: Depression: perspectives from affective neuroscience. Annu Rev Psychol 53:545–574, 2002

Drevets WC: Prefrontal cortical-amygdalar metabolism in major depression. Ann NY Acad Sci 877:614–637, 1999

Drevets WC: Neuroimaging studies of mood disorders. Biol Psychiatry 48:813–819, 2000

Drevets WC: Neuroimaging abnormalities in the amygdala in mood disorders. Ann NY Acad Sci 985:420–444, 2003

Drevets WC, Price JL, Simpson JR Jr, et al: Subgenual prefrontal cortex abnormalities in mood disorders. Nature 386:824–827, 1997

Dunkin JJ, Leuchter AF, Cook IA, et al: Executive dysfunction predicts nonresponse to fluoxetine in major depression. J Affect Disord 60:13–23, 2000

Erickson K, Drevets W, Schulkin J: Glucocorticoid regulation of diverse cognitive functions in normal and pathological emotional states. Neurosci Biobehav Rev 27:233–246, 2003

Frodl T, Meisenzahl E, Zetzsche T, et al: Hippocampal changes in patients with a first episode of major depression. Am J Psychiatry 159:1112–1118, 2002

Frodl T, Meisenzahl EM, Zetzsche T, et al: Larger amygdala volumes in first depressive episode as compared to recurrent major depression and healthy control subjects. Biol Psychiatry 53:338–344, 2003

Goldapple K, Segal Z, Garson C, et al: Modulation of cortical-limbic pathways in major depression: treatment-specific effects of cognitive behavior therapy. Arch Gen Psychiatry 61:34–41, 2004

Hastings R, Parsey R, Oquendo M, et al: Volumetric analysis of the prefrontal cortex, amygdala, and hippocampus in major depression. Neuropsychopharmacology 29:952–959, 2004

Hickie I, Scott E, Mitchell P, et al: Subcortical hyperintensities on magnetic resonance imaging: clinical correlates and prognostic significance in patients with severe depression. Biol Psychiatry 37:151–160, 1995

Hickie I, Scott E, Wilhelm K, Brodaty H: Subcortical hyperintensities on magnetic resonance imaging in patients with severe depression: a longitudinal evaluation. Biol Psychiatry 42:367–374, 1997

Husain MM, McDonald WM, Doraiswamy PM, et al: A magnetic resonance imaging study of putamen nuclei in major depression. Psychiatry Res 40:95–99, 1991

Kalayam B, Alexopoulos GS: Prefrontal dysfunction and treatment response in geriatric depression. Arch Gen Psychiatry 56:713–738, 1999

Kalayam B, Alexopoulos GS: A preliminary study of left frontal region error negativity and symptom improvement in geriatric depression. Am J Psychiatry 160:2054–2056, 2003

Kempermann G, Kronenberg G: Depressed new neurons—adult hippocampal neurogenesis and a cellular plasticity hypothesis of major depression. Biol Psychiatry 54:499–503, 2003

Krishnan KR, McDonald WM, Escalona PR, et al: Magnetic resonance imaging of the caudate nuclei in depression: preliminary observations. Arch Gen Psychiatry 49:553–557, 1992

Krishnan KR, Hays JC, Blazer DG: MRI-defined vascular depression. Am J Psychiatry 154:497–501, 1997

LeDoux J: Emotional memory: in search of systems and synapses. Ann NY Acad Sci 702:149–157, 1993

Lockwood KA, Alexopoulos GS, van Gorp WG: Executive dysfunction in geriatric depression. Am J Psychiatry 159:1119–1126, 2002

MacQueen GM, Macdonald K, Amano S, et al: Course of illness, hippocampal function and hippocampal volume in major depression. Proc Natl Acad Sci USA 100:1387–1392, 2003

Malberg J, Eisch A, Nestler E, et al: Chronic antidepressant treatment increases neurogenesis in the adult rat hippocampus. J Neurosci 20:9104–9110, 2000

Mayberg H: Depression and frontal-subcortical circuits: focus on prefrontal-limbic interactions, in Frontal-Subcortical Circuits in Psychiatric and Neurological Disorders. Edited by Lichter DC, Cummings JL. New York, Guilford, 2001, pp 177–206

McEwen B: Mood disorders and allostatic load. Biol Psychiatry 54:200–207, 2003

Millan MJ: The role of monoamines in the actions of established and novel antidepressant agents: a critical review. Eur J Pharmacol 500:371–384, 2004

Miller DB, O'Callaghan JP: Effects of aging and stress on hippocampal structure and function. Metabolism 52:17–21, 2003

Morris PL, Robinson RG, Raphael B, et al: The relationship between risk factors for affective disorder and poststroke depression in hospitalised stroke patients. Aust N Z J Psychiatry 26:208–217, 1992

Murphy CF, Alexopoulos GS: Longitudinal association of initiation/perseveration and severity of geriatric depression. Am J Geriatr Psychiatry 12:50–56, 2004

Nebes RD, Butters MA, Houck PR, et al: Dual-task performance in depressed geriatric patients. Psychiatry Res 102:139–151, 2001

Nebes RD, Pollock BG, Houck PR, et al: Persistence of cognitive impairment in geriatric patients following antidepressant treatment: a randomized, double-blind clinical trial with nortriptyline and paroxetine. J Psychiatr Res 37:99–108, 2003

O'Brien J, Ames D, Chiu E, et al: Severe deep white matter lesions and outcome in elderly patients with major depressive disorder: follow up study. BMJ 317:982–984, 1998

O'Doherty J, Kringelbach ML, Rolls ET, et al: Abstract reward and punishment representations in the human orbitofrontal cortex. Nat Neurosci 4:95–102, 2001

Ongur D, An X, Price JL: Prefrontal cortical projections to the hypothalamus in macaque monkeys. J Comp Neurol 401:480–505, 1998a

Ongur D, Drevets WC, Price JL: Glial reduction in the subgenual prefrontal cortex in mood disorders. Proc Natl Acad Sci USA 95:13290–13295, 1998b

Pizzagalli D, Pascual-Marqui RD, et al: Anterior cingulate activity as a predictor of degree of treatment response in major depression: evidence from brain electrical tomography analysis. Am J Psychiatry 158:405–415, 2001

Potter GG, Kittinger JD, Wagner HR, et al: Prefrontal neuropsychological predictors of treatment remission in late-life depression. Neuropsychopharmacology 29:2266–2271, 2004

Rajkowska G, Miguel-Hidalgo JJ, Wei J, et al: Morphometric evidence for neuronal and glial prefrontal cell pathology in major depression. Biol Psychiatry 45:1085–1098, 1999

Scammell TE, Estabrooke IV, McCarthy MT, et al: Hypothalamic arousal regions are activated during modafinil-induced wakefulness. J Neurosci 20:8620–8628, 2000

Schiepers OJ, Wichers MC, Maes M: Cytokines and major depression. Prog Neuropsychopharmacol Biol Psychiatry 29:201–217, 2005

Seminowicz DA, Mayberg HS, McIntosh AR, et al: Limbic-frontal circuitry in major depression: a path modeling meta-analysis. Neuroimage 22:409–418, 2004

Sheline Y: 3D MRI studies of neuroanatomic changes in unipolar depression: the role of stress and medical comorbidity. Biol Psychiatry 48:791–800, 2000

Sheline Y: Neuroimaging studies of mood disorder effects on the brain. Biol Psychiatry 54:338–352, 2003

Sheline Y, Gado M, Price J: Amygdala core nuclei volumes are decreased in recurrent major depression. Neuroreport 9:2023–2028, 1998

Simpson S, Baldwin RC, Jackson A, et al: Is subcortical disease associated with a poor response to antidepressants? Neurological, neuropsychological and neuroradiological findings in late-life depression. Psychol Med 28:1015–1026, 1998

Sobin C, Sackeim HA: Psychomotor symptoms of depression. Am J Psychiatry 154:4–17, 1997

Starkstein SE, Migliorelli R, Teson A, et al: Prevalence and clinical correlates of pathological affective display in Alzheimer's disease. J Neurol Neurosurg Psychiatry 59:55–60, 1995

Steffens DC, Helms MJ, Krishnan KR, et al: Cerebrovascular disease and depression symptoms in the cardiovascular health study. Stroke 30:2159–2166, 1999

Steffens DC, Conway CR, Dombeck CB, et al: Severity of subcortical gray matter hyperintensity predicts ECT response in geriatric depression. J ECT 17:45–49, 2001

Sullivan EV, Pfefferbaum A, Swan GE, et al: Hereditability of hippocampal size in elderly twin men: equivalent influence from genes and environment. Hippocampus 11:754–762, 2001

Thomas AJ, Davis S, Morris C, et al: Increase in interleukin-1beta in late-life depression. Am J Psychiatry 162:175–177, 2005

Whalen PJ, Bush G, McNally RJ, et al: The emotional counting Stroop paradigm: a functional magnetic resonance imaging probe of the anterior cingulate affective division. Biol Psychiatry 44:1219–1228, 1998

24

CHALLENGES OF DIAGNOSING PSYCHIATRIC DISORDERS IN MEDICALLY ILL PATIENTS

Ira Katz, M.D., Ph.D.
Linda Ganzini, M.D., M.P.H.

Old age is marked by an increase in medical disorders outside the central nervous system, particularly of the heart, lungs, kidneys, and musculoskeletal system, as well as cancer. As people age, the diagnosis of some mental disorders and the relationship between mental disorders and medical illnesses becomes increasingly complex. DSM-IV-TR (American Psychiatric Association 2000) defines a *mental disorder* as a behavioral or psychological syndrome or pattern that occurs in an individual that is associated with distress, disability, or an increased risk of suffering, death, or an important loss of freedom. In examining the relationship between advanced medical illness and mental disorders in the elderly we consider the following questions:

1. Are there limits of parsimony, wherein one particular medical illness is hypothesized to cause a specific mental disorder?
2. Have all of the distressing and disabling syndromes that could be considered mental disorders been identified?
3. Are there contexts in which some psychological syndromes that might be considered pathological in a young, healthy person would not be in a medically ill elderly person?

4. Are the current models of disability, suffering, loss of freedom, and increased risk of death adequate for determining thresholds of diagnosis among elderly medically ill patients, especially for those in the final period of life?
5. Are there some geriatric syndromes such as frailty and sickness behaviors that, although primarily of a medical nature, have such strong overlap with mental disorders that they deserve more consideration for DSM-V?
6. How can our understanding of the role of mental disorders in worsening the course of physical illness be strengthened?
7. How might research agendas be modified to answer these questions?

The Limits of Parsimony

Both medical disorders and treatments for them can cause a variety of mental syndromes, including depression, anxiety, psychosis, dementia, and delirium. DSM-IV-TR allows diagnosis of mood, psychotic, and anxiety disorders all secondary to a general medical condition if, in the clinician's assessment, the symptoms are etiologically related to the disorder through physiological mechanisms. This is a rare case in which DSM-IV-TR allows an etiological diagnosis. Commonly seen examples of these diagnoses include anxiety secondary to hyperthyroidism or stimulants; mood disorder secondary to hypothyroidism or corticosteroids; and psychosis secondary to levodopa or other dopamine antagonist medications. These categories are useful in leading to appropriate discovery and treatment of the underlying medical disorder, which may theoretically help avoid other unnecessary psychopharmacological and psychotherapeutic interventions.

Yet this parsimonious notion wherein one particular medical disease results in one specific mental disorder through an identifiable pathophysiological mechanism may be neither valid nor reliable in old age. For example, the incidence of major depressive disorder is substantial following a myocardial infarction or a cerebrovascular accident, and development of depression predicts poor outcomes, including death. Researchers are currently attempting to clarify the pathophysiological association between stroke location and the development of depression and to discover biochemical abnormalities that may mediate the high rate of depression (Berkman et al. 2003; Jorge et al. 2003; Lesperance et al. 2004; Narushima et al. 2003; Robinson et al. 1999). As reviewed in other chapters in this volume, these studies support that distinguishing between diseases of the central nervous system and those of peripheral systems may be difficult and that many disorders of other systems can give rise to psychiatric symptoms through structural or metabolic effects on the brain. Yet even when physiological mechanisms are present, they do not, in general, act in isolation. A myocardial infarction or cerebrovascular accident may bring about existential concerns, threaten relationships, and cause disability, resulting in a change of residence and decreased ability to pursue pleasurable activities. Whether depression results from specific illness, ill health in general, or even a patient's perception of the meaning of the disease is unclear. Furthermore, mental disorders in old age often occur within the context of multiple medical illnesses and medications, functional decline, bereavement, and loss of meaning and control, all of which may contribute to psychiatric difficulties. Studies that examine the reliability and frequency of mental disorders secondary to medical conditions and their usefulness in leading to appropriate therapies are needed. Even more significant may be studies evaluating the extent to which these conditions respond to "standard" therapies.

Similarly, depression and related symptoms are listed as side effects of a significant number of medications that are commonly used in the elderly. However, clear evidence for an etiological role is most often lacking. This leaves clinicians with little guidance on how to identify drug-related depressions; how to estimate the magnitude of the vulnerability that can be attributed to patient-related, disease-related, and agent-related factors; and how to decide when medications should be withdrawn versus when additional treatments should be offered to help patients tolerate needed treatments. One class of widely discussed agents are the beta-blockers. Here, a recent meta-analysis of research findings has suggested that these agents do not appear to cause depression but may cause fatigue and sexual dysfunction. These findings suggest that controversy about whether these agents cause depression may have sidetracked efforts to determine whether they cause other experiences or symptoms associated with suffering and disability. When subjective experience or behavioral symptoms arise during treatment with medications that may be necessary, behavioral, psychosocial, or psychopharmacological treatments can minimize suffering and disability while helping patients adhere to treatment. Research designed to identify these contexts should focus on the specific agents and contexts rather than on definitions of syndromes imported from younger and healthier patients with psychiatric disorders.

Context-Dependent Mental Disorders

Many psychiatric syndromes vary in their manifestations based on culture and ethnicity and may even be culture bound, such that some types of behaviors and experiences that are considered normal or aberrant in some contexts would not be in others (American Psychiatric Association 2000). Culture may influence how symptoms are expressed and understood. Moreover, symptoms and behaviors that would be considered debilitating in one culture may not be a problem or may even be an advantage in another.

Old age is accompanied by development of medical illness with attendant disability that often results in change in expectations, living environment, and social situation. This may represent a radical contextual change. Within this different context, as within a different culture, new symptoms and behaviors that would at other times of life or circumstance be psychopathological may be normative, even adaptive. Other symptoms that generally result in minor disability or minimal suffering may become quite debilitating. Examples of changes of context include specific medical illnesses or symptoms; changes in roles; impairments and disabilities; losses of significant others or changes in their health and availability; and change of living situation. One of the major issues in psychiatric diagnosis in the elderly is the extent to which it is valid to "import" the disorders that are well defined in younger and healthier adults to the older populations and whether they can account for the burden of mental disorders. An alternative approach would be to determine the extent to which new syndromes and disorders emerge specifically from the contexts of late life.

DYING AS A CONTEXT

Dying represents, on many axes, both an extreme change in context and an experience through which all individuals will proceed. Context clearly interacts with culture, because what is expected of the dying person depends strongly on such factors as the patient's family, ethnicity, and traditions. Yet the context of dying itself may be determinative of psychological and behavioral changes. To consider the dying state allows examination of a context, perhaps one of many, that exposes the limits of current psychiatric nosology.

The leading causes of death in the United States are cancer, stroke, and cardiac disease. The trajectory toward death and awareness of one's impending demise reflect such factors as disease type, education, personality, and social and financial situation. The epidemiology of where people die is changing. Thirty years ago, 70% of individuals in the United States died in hospitals. Currently about 25% die in hospice care, 25% in nursing homes, and 50% in hospitals, including intensive care units (National Hospice and Palliative Care Organization 2003). The role of hospice is particularly important, because entry into hospice requires that no further life-sustaining efforts for the terminal illness will be pursued and is therefore some degree of acknowledgement of one's impending death. Much of hospice care is delivered in patients' homes, although some occurs in inpatient hospice units and skilled nursing care as well. Furthermore, the hospice movement developed out of grassroots efforts that initially resisted medicalization and developed concepts of normative dying that were not influenced by psychiatry.

Some researchers have focused on adapting diagnostic categories, such as major depression, to very ill and dying patients. Diagnostic criteria for major depressive disorder include not only depressed mood or loss of pleasure but also somatic symptoms such as appetite/weight changes, disrupted sleep or hypersomnia, psychomotor changes, or fatigue and loss of energy that may be attributing to both advanced physical illness and mood disorder. Other criteria for depression, such as recurrent thoughts of death, may not be psychopathological and may even be adaptive if the thoughts promote acceptance of one's situation. Some researchers have suggested excluding physical symptoms easily attributable to terminal disease, such as fatigue and appetite disturbance, from the diagnosis of depression. Others defend including these symptoms on the grounds that making the diagnosis more difficult to establish may deny many dying persons an opportunity for treatment (Goy and Ganzini 2003). Endicott (1983) suggested substituting of some physical symptoms with other psychological symptoms such as tearfulness, social withdrawal, pessimism, or lack of reactivity. Despite this, Chochinov et al. (1994) reported that among cancer patients in inpatient hospice, when psychological symptoms are severe, different methods for diagnosing depression still identify the same group as depressed. What remains uncertain is the degree to which different methods of diagnosing depression in these settings improve prediction of disability, poor outcomes, and other forms of measurable distress.

Other palliative care experts have suggested that the psychological experiences of the dying are not effectively captured by DSM-IV-TR categories. For example, Kissane et al. (1998, 2001) have proposed that demoralization is a potential diagnostic entity in nondepressed terminally ill patients with core features of hopelessness, loss of meaning, and existential distress that may be associated with desire for hastened death. Breitbart (2002; Breitbart and Strout 2000) has focused on the essential role of finding meaning and are testing meaning-centered group psychotherapies in a clinical trial in patients with advanced cancer. Chochinov et al. (2002) focused on dignity and proposed that a sense of fractured dignity can be diagnosed, quantified, correlated with decreased quality of life and desire for hastened death, and potentially treated with "dignity conserving interventions." Anxiety states are common, but current DSM-IV-TR categories for anxiety do not appear to be adequately descriptive, specific, reliable, or valid for the types of dread and fear experienced by some dying patients. Other areas of psychological focus may include grief, apathy, fear of disfigurement, changes in the body, loss of role in the family, and fear of abandonment (Goy and Ganzini 2003). How these fit into syndromic conceptualizations are uncertain. Psychiatrists working with these populations informally report that adjustment disorder is the most common diagnosis. Because adjustment disorder fails to adequately describe the syndrome or point to specific therapy, its frequent use should be verified in epidemiological studies of these patients. Thus, current nosology may be inadequate for diagnosing important debilitating psychological syndromes in elderly patients with advanced disease.

Potentially the most common mental disorder among dying patients is delirium, which can be identified in more than 90% of palliative care patients (Fann 2000; Lawlor et al. 2000). Among medically ill patients delirium is associated with dysphoric states; psychotic experiences, including delusions and hallucinations; behavioral difficulties, including agitation and physical aggression; and functional decline. Yet many palliative care providers challenge whether hypoactive or "quiet" deliria are always psychopathological in the dying. For example, Hallenbeck (2003) pointed out that some altered states are pleasant, even ecstatic, and, like dreams, may be normal in the dying. Within the palliative care literature, many patients are described who, although confused and disoriented, have hallucinations with rich and adaptive content. In support, Hallenbeck (2003) proposed that the most common visions among delirious hospice patients are of dead relatives. Farber referred to this as "decathexis" (Farber et al. 2000)—that is, the "letting go" process that is associated with transcendental and spiritual experiences that facilitate leaving life (Goy and Ganzini 2003).

Although agitated delirium is treated aggressively within palliative care settings and hospice, permissive attitudes toward hypoactive delirium lead to underdiagnosis and undertreatment, especially if the patient seems comfortable and peaceful. Other palliative care experts rebut this nihilistic approach, pointing out that visions that are comforting at one moment can be terrifying the next (Breitbart and Strout 2000). Furthermore, because many deliria in hospice patients are reversible with simple measures, quality of life is almost universally improved and autonomy restored among patients who have improved cognition (Casarett and Inouye 2001). Breitbart et al. (2002) showed that among hospitalized cancer patients, half recalled their delirium experience and rated their distress associated with delirium as very high. Patients with hypoactive delirium rated the experience as just as distressing as those with agitated delirium. More research is needed to understand these experiences in dying patients and the conditions under which they should be recognized and treated. Until then we are challenged to find literature to support the universal psychopathological nature of delirium in terminal care.

Concepts of distress, disability, loss of freedom, increased risk of death, and suffering require further definition and validated and reliable measurement in patients with advanced medical illness and resulting functional illness. In 70% of deaths in hospitalized patients and all deaths in hospice patients, decisions are made to not pursue all life-saving therapies (Field and Cassel 1997). As such, death itself as an adverse outcome becomes difficult to defend. A method to measure how mental illness separately contributed to these pernicious outcomes deserves further thought.

OTHER COMMON CONTEXTS

These thoughts on dying persons may be applicable to other contexts within geriatric psychiatry. For example, the context of nursing home care may change the thresholds for considering psychological experiences and behaviors as well as outcomes in these residents as normal or aberrant. When the focus is on pain, sleep, or sexual dysfunction, it may be possible to diagnose the conditions under the relevant sections of DSM. However, with other foci, for example, fatigue, dizziness, dyspnea, and gastrointestinal distress, the approach to identifying appropriate targets for behavioral, psychosocial, or psychopharmacological treatment is less clear cut. Often they may be components of a mood or anxiety disorder, but they can also occur in the absence of other defining symptoms for these syndromes. There may be cases where they can be subsumed under the diagnostic categories of "psychological factors affecting medical conditions." However, there are other cases in which current criteria for diagnosing mental disorders may present barriers to research and treatment.

Geriatric Syndromes and Mental Disorders

Even before terminal states of the diseases of late life, aging can be associated with chronic deterioration and decline that have been conceptualized as "frailty" and "failure to thrive." Recently, investigators in geriatric medicine have described frailty as a "biological syndrome of decreased reserve and resistance to stressors, resulting from cumulative declines across multiple physiological systems, and causing vulnerability to adverse outcomes" (Fried et al. 2001). They proposed an operational definition that requires three or more of the following: unintentional weight loss of at least 10 pounds over the past year, self-reported exhaustion, weakness evaluated by grip strength, slow walking speed, and low physical activity. Exhaustion, weight loss, slowing, and decreased activities are characteristics of depression as well as frailty. In other research, investigators from the same group that worked toward this definition of frailty found strong associations with depression. In regression models, they found that the associations with exhaustion may have been somewhat more robust than those with depression, per se. However, this does not exclude close associations between depression and frailty. It suggests that frailty may be more closely related to the neurovegetative components of depression than to its dysphoric or ideational features.

Other formulations of depression that stress its similarity to this concept of frailty are those related to "vital exhaustion" or "depression without sadness." The parallels between depression and frailty are readily apparent. Depending on the definitions used, it is possible to make a case for each of these conditions being a cause, consequence, or comorbidity of the other. It is also possible to argue for their congruence; within limits, they may be different labels for the same syndrome. Nevertheless, there are significant similarities as well as differences between the concepts of depression and frailty. In this context, it is important to estimate the extent to which frailty can be considered a mental disorder that may be responsive, in part, to behavioral, psychosocial, or psychopharmacological interventions. However, there are dangers that basing these estimates on operational definitions of depression that are imported from other populations could lead to errors. Instead, studies of context-specific pathology and treatment are indicated.

Sickness behavior, like frailty, may cross the boundary between mental and medical disorders. There is increasing evidence that pro-inflammatory cytokines such as interleukin-1β, interleukin-6, tumor necrosis factor–alpha, and interferon can cause a variety of symptoms affecting mood, motivation, energy, sleep, appetite, and pain sensitivity. They can also cause ill-defined symptoms such as malaise. These findings have led to questions about the extent to which the subjective experience and behavioral symptoms associated with acute illness, infection, inflammation, and tissue injury, often called sickness behavior, are mediated by cytokine effects and whether insight into mechanisms may suggest approaches to treatment or palliation for these symptoms, even when the underlying disease is not treatable. In addition, cytokine effects have been discussed as possible mediators of frailty as described earlier, suggesting specific approaches to intervention.

When interferon is used to treat disorders such as hepatitis C or multiple sclerosis, these symptoms can cause significant suffering and distress and can limit patients' ability to tolerate treatment. Emerging evidence suggests that interferon-related depressions can be treated or prevented with antidepressant medications. This raises questions about the relationship between sickness behavior and depression and about the possible benefits of antidepressant treatment for sickness behavior. However, there must be questions about whether the effects of antidepressants and related treatments are limited to depressive symptoms or can have an impact across the spectrum of sickness behaviors. Further advances in this area will require empirical research. Yet it should focus on defining sickness behavior and evaluating it as a target and outcome for interventions.

Mental Disorders as Causes of Medical Morbidity: An Additional Diagnostic Axis

The discussion of the diagnosis of mental disorders in the face of somatic disease has, until this point, focused on the extent to which the clinical context affects the diagnosis of mental illness. There is, however, a need to focus on the complementary path, the manner in which mental disorders affect overall health and the course of specific somatic disorders. There is evidence that psychiatric symptoms and/or disorders may be associated with the onset or course of illnesses such as ischemic heart disease, diabetes, certain cancers, and osteoporosis. Multiple mechanisms have been proposed, including those related to treatment adherence, health behaviors, and physiological effects of mental disorders. The latter may include abnormalities in platelet functioning or heart rate variability as mediators of the impact of depression on cardiac disease and hypercortisolemia as a mediator of effects on bone density.

The goals of psychiatric treatment must include preventing the increased risk of medical illness or the poorer prognosis of established illnesses in those with mental disorders. To accomplish this, it would be helpful to include factors that contribute to these adverse outcomes as a separate diagnostic axis. Doing so would facilitate planning of intervention. It would also support an increased role for mental health professionals in evaluating treatment adherence and health behaviors in their patients and in working with other providers on interventions to improve outcomes. As physiological mechanisms become better established, they should be included as outcomes in the evaluation of treatment effects. Pursuing these principles, the goals of treatment for mental disorders should not be limited to the alleviation of those symptoms that define the conditions. They should also include interventions designed to prevent the health consequences of the mental disorders, as assessed by monitoring of both behavioral and physiological mediators.

Research Agenda

Addressing these concerns may include radically rethinking the types of disorders that might be relevant to patients in these different contexts. To date, most of the emphasis in examining mental disorder in patients with medical illness has been on the prevalence of disorders defined in healthy patients and fitting these syndromes to patients with advanced disease. Qualitative studies, including those using techniques from ethnography and grounded theory, might be useful to develop hypotheses about the emotional states and behavioral problems that are truly distressing among patients in a variety of contexts, including those in nursing homes, those who are very ill or expected to die, and those with frailty and sickness behavior.

Understanding of sources of suffering among persons with advanced medical illness and frailty would be aided by affiliation with professionals who care for persons in other contexts. For example, many concepts of psychologically normative and pathological dying now come from professionals working in hospice and palliative care who have not felt bound by DSM categories. Yet in a 1996 study of 321 Oregon psychiatrists, only 2 worked in a hospice setting, only 15 were affiliated with a nursing home, and 64% had no terminally ill patients in their practice. As such, clinical experiences from which to develop hypotheses may be lacking if we are dependent only on ideas which come from our own field (Ganzini et al. 1996).

Similarly, in the contexts of acute or chronic illness, there may be sources of suffering and disability and opportunities for interventions that we may be missing by relying on definitions of mental disorders that are imported from other populations. Modifying the approach to the definition of mental disorders to facilitate the identification of context-dependent diagnoses could advance care of older individuals living with serious illnesses as well as those dying from them.

References

American Psychiatric Association: Diagnostic and Statistical Manual of Mental Disorders, 4th Edition, Text Revision. Washington, DC, American Psychiatric Association, 2000

Berkman LF, Blumenthal J, Burg M, et al: Effects of treating depression and low perceived social support on clinical events after myocardial infarction: the Enhancing Recovery in Coronary Heart Disease Patients (ENRICHD) Randomized Trial. JAMA 289:3106–3116, 2003

Breitbart W: Spirituality and meaning in supportive care: spirituality- and meaning-centered group psychotherapy interventions in advanced cancer. Support Care Cancer 10:272–280, 2002

Breitbart W, Strout D: Delirium in the terminally ill. Clin Geriatr Med 16:357–372, 2000

Breitbart W, Gibson C, Tremblay A: The delirium experience: delirium recall and delirium-related distress in hospitalized patients with cancer, their spouses/caregivers, and their nurses. Psychosomatics 43:183–194, 2002

Casarett DJ, Inouye SK: Diagnosis and management of delirium near the end of life. Ann Intern Med 135:32–40, 2001

Chochinov HM, Wilson KG, Enns M, et al: Prevalence of depression in the terminally ill: effects of diagnostic criteria and symptom threshold judgments. Am J Psychiatry 151:537–540, 1994

Chochinov HM, Hack T, McClement S, et al: Dignity in the terminally ill: a developing empirical model. Soc Sci Med 54:433–443, 2002

Endicott J: Measurement of depression patients with cancer. Cancer 53:2243–2248, 1983

Fann JR: The epidemiology of delirium: a review of studies and methodological issues. Semin Clin Neuropsychiatry 5:64–74, 2000

Farber S, Egnew TR, Stempel J, et al: End-of-Life Care: AAFP Home Study Self-Assessment (Monograph 250/251). Leawood, KS, American Academy of Family Physicians, 2000

Field MJ, Cassel CK: Approaching Death: Improving Care at the End of Life. Washington, DC, National Academy Press, 1997

Fried LP, Tangen CM, Walston J, et al: Frailty in older adults: evidence for a phenotype. J Gerontol A Biol Sci Med Sci 56:146–156, 2001

Ganzini L, Fenn DS, Lee MA, et al: Attitudes of Oregon psychiatrists toward physician-assisted suicide. Am J Psychiatry 153:1469–1475, 1996

Goy ER, Ganzini L: Delirium, anxiety and depression, in Geriatric Palliative Care. Edited by Morrison RS, Meier DE, Capello C. Oxford, United Kingdom, Oxford University Press, 2003

Hallenbeck JL: Palliative Care Perspectives. Oxford, United Kingdom, Oxford University Press, 2003

Jorge RE, Robinson RG, Arndt S, et al: Mortality and poststroke depression: a placebo-controlled trial of antidepressants. Am J Psychiatry 160:1823–1829, 2003

Kissane DW: Demoralisation: its impact on informed consent and medical care. Med J Aust 175:537–539, 2001

Kissane DW, Street A, Nitschke P: Seven deaths in Darwin: case studies under the Rights of the Terminally Ill Act, Northern Territory, Australia. Lancet 352:1097–1102, 1998

Lawlor PG, Gagnon B, Mancini IL, et al: Occurrence, causes, and outcome of delirium in patients with advanced cancer: a prospective study. Arch Intern Med 160:786–794, 2000

Lesperance F, Frasure-Smith N, Theroux P, et al: The association between major depression and levels of soluble intercellular adhesion molecule 1, interleukin-6, and C-reactive protein in patients with recent acute coronary syndromes. Am J Psychiatry 161:271–277, 2004

Narushima K, Kosier JT, Robinson RG: A reappraisal of poststroke depression, intra- and inter-hemispheric lesion location using meta-analysis. J Neuropsychiatry Clin Neurosci 15:422–430, 2003

National Hospice and Palliative Care Organization: Facts and Figures on Hospice Care in America. Alexandria, VA, National Hospice and Palliative Care Organization, 2003

Robinson RG, Chemerinski E, Jorge R: Pathophysiology of secondary depressions in the elderly. J Geriatr Psychiatry Neurol 12:128–136, 1999

25

USE OF BIOMARKERS IN THE ELDERLY

Current and Future Challenges

Trey Sunderland, M.D.
Raquel E. Gur, M.D., Ph.D.
Steven E. Arnold, M.D.

In geriatric psychiatry, as well as any other specialty, an ideal biomarker should detect a fundamental feature of the underlying pathophysiology of a disease and distinguish that illness from other conditions with an acceptable positive and negative predictive value. Furthermore, the biomarkers should be reliable, relatively noninvasive, simple to perform, and inexpensive. These criteria, outlined by a work group report about the use of biomarkers in Alzheimer's disease (AD; Ronald and Nancy Reagan Research Institute of the Alzheimer's Association and the National Institute on Aging Working Group 1998), are currently not met by any single marker, but they represent the high standards to which the field aspires (Table 25–1).

Biomarkers have been developed in general medicine to diagnose, form prognoses, and monitor disease progression according to criteria similar to that just outlined, but general psychiatry has not frequently participated in this process, perhaps due to the paucity of established pathophysiological mechanisms in psychiatric disorders. Nonetheless, there is great interest in this type of psychiatric research, as was evidenced by the profound reaction following the publication detailing the dexamethasone suppression test in depression years ago (Carroll et al. 1981). Although this testing did not fulfill its initial promise, and clinical symptoms remain the main

TABLE 25–1. Characteristics of an ideal diagnostic marker for Alzheimer's disease (AD)

1. Detects a fundamental feature of AD
2. Validated in autopsy-proven cases of AD
3. Specific for AD compared with other dementias
4. Reliable in many laboratories
5. Noninvasive
6. Simple to perform
7. Inexpensive

markers of disease severity and progression in psychiatry, there has been some positive experience with surrogate markers within geriatric psychiatry.

More than 20 years ago, nortriptyline blood levels were used to predict response and monitor antidepressant therapy when tricyclic antidepressants were the mainstay of depression treatment in geriatric populations (Jarvik et al. 1983; Kragh-Sorensen 1978; Montgomery et al. 1977). These tests might be considered the earliest biomarkers in geriatric psychiatry. Over the past decade, however, the geriatric illness that has seen the most serious growth of potential biomarkers is AD, for which neuropsychological testing has long been the mainstay diagnostic and disease severity marker and autopsy verification the ultimate gold standard (Mirra et al. 1991; Mohs and Cohen 1988; Petersen et al. 1999). At the current time, one could make a case for emerging biomarkers in AD across multiple platforms, including neuropsychological testing, blood tests, genetic markers, cerebrospinal fluid (CSF), and brain imaging. We use this illness as a model for future development of biomarkers in other diseases.

Although neuropsychological tests are not generally considered as classic biomarkers, such tests certainly track the underlying condition and have often been used as dependent variables in drug efficacy trials (Gottwald and Rozanski 1999; Raskind et al. 2000; Rogers et al. 1998). In fact, changes in neuropsychological testing are an integral part of the diagnostic criteria for AD and mild cognitive impairment, a possible prodrome of AD (McKhann et al. 1984; Petersen et al. 1999). Neuropsychological tests that are predictive of AD have been sought for decades without great success, although there are suggestions of some subtle changes that may precede the onset of clinical illness (Snowdon 2003). Many candidate tests have been proposed as early markers (Greenwood et al. 2000; Levy et al. 2004; Rosen et al. 2002). Still, no single test or battery of tests has fulfilled the criteria required of a standardized biomarker.

Rare genetic mutations for AD have also been recognized for many years that account for only 1%–2% of Alzheimer's disease (Tanzi et al. 1987), and there are now multiple known mutations across three separate chromosomes, with others likely to be identified in the future (Tanzi and Bertram 2001). Although these autosomal dominant mutations are fully penetrant, they do not in themselves identify the underlying biology of AD with any temporal accuracy, because the clinical phenotype is expressed only if the subjects live long enough to reach the age of vulnerability. Strictly speaking, these mutations are therefore long-term prognostic biomarkers of AD and not diagnostic biomarkers. They are "trait" variables and not "state" variables. Another most interesting genetic marker is that located on chromosome 19, the apolipoprotein E gene (*APOE*), and the ε4 allele has been found to be strongly associated with AD (Corder et al. 1993). Presence of one or more of the relatively common ε4 alleles is associated with an increased risk of AD and is perhaps the most replicated finding in all of AD research (Cacabelos 2003). In contrast to the rare genetic mutations, however, there is no absolute certainty of developing AD with increasing age, only an increased likelihood. Nevertheless, *APOE* ε4 has become an important predictor of risk; when combined with other markers such as neuropsychological testing, the *APOE* ε4 allele has already proven to be of value in discerning potential subsets of individuals at even greater risk of developing AD (Greenwood et al. 2000; Levy et al. 2004; Rosen et al. 2002). Similarly, combining the risk associated with the *APOE* ε4 allele with neuroimaging measures has produced a potential for further refinement of identifying individuals at greater risk for developing AD (Reiman et al. 1996, 2004; Small et al. 2000).

Some blood tests available at baseline evaluation of individuals have been proposed as markers of risk for AD. Serum homocysteine is an example of such a test, but the association with AD is relatively weak and needs further validation (Seshadri et al. 2002). Vitamin B_{12} and folate are sometimes mentioned as biomarkers of AD, but they are more important as markers of other illnesses and used primarily as markers of exclusion in the evaluation of potential AD cases (Wang et al. 2001). Plasma β-amyloid is very attractive as a potential biomarker because of its natural association with the amyloid plaque and the known pathophysiology of AD (Hardy and Selkoe 2002; Selkoe 2000). However, there is much question concerning the variability of the plasma levels and whether they are significantly related to brain levels and the disease process itself (Fagan et al. 2000); much more validation is needed before the measure can be determined to be an attractive AD biomarker.

CSF is generally considered a more proximal measure of brain activity than plasma. Indeed, CSF levels of β-amyloid, total tau, and phosphotau have been proven reliably altered in AD versus control subjects (Andreasen et al. 1999; Arai et al. 1996; Blennow et al. 2001; Galasko et al. 1998; Hampel et al. 2003; Sunderland et al. 2003). Much more work in this area is needed to establish the usefulness of such biomarkers as a predictive measure of disease development or progression, but there is already evidence that these CSF measures are as accurate (85%–90%) in establishing a diagnosis of mild-to-moderate AD versus control subjects (Blennow 2004; Galasko et al. 1998; Sunderland et al. 2003) as autopsy studies (Lim et al. 1999; Mendez et al. 1992; Mirra et al. 1991; Newell et al. 1999). This degree of accuracy is remarkable given that a CSF measure is a one-time, cross-sectional measure available today clinically, whereas autopsy studies, by definition, require years of longitudinal follow-up to the time of death. However, the diagnostic specificity and sensitivity of these biological measures are not yet well established when the comparison populations are other groups with non-AD dementia, so the use of biomarkers do not have the sensitivity and sensitivity required of routine clinical diagnostic tests. Nonetheless, there is much excitement in this area of research because there has been some suggestion of changes in CSF biological markers in those with mild cognitive impairment (Andreasen and Blennow 2002; Hampel et al. 2004) and even in "at risk" control subjects (Sunderland et al. 2004), but many more longitudinal data are needed to establish the link between these CSF changes and the early development of AD. This is also an area in which the potential power of high-throughput proteomic exploration may be crucial, but the methodological issues of quantification and validation remain temporary obstacles (Dunckley et al. 2005).

Perhaps the best-studied category of biomarkers in AD and geriatric psychiatry in general is that of neuroimaging (Gur and Gur 2002). Starting with regional cerebral blood flow scans and electroencephalographic studies in the 1980s (Ihl et al. 1989), researchers have been searching for imaging correlates of the brain deterioration in Alzheimer's dementia, but there has been only limited success. More recently, structural imaging with magnetic resonance imaging (MRI) has been common, and there are numerous studies of various measures ranging from total brain volume to hippocampal volume that have been proposed as surrogate markers of AD progression (Cohen et al. 2001; de Leon et al. 1996; Fox et al. 1996; Jack et al. 1997). Although there are ongoing studies attempting to establish appropriate evidence for the specificity and sensitivity of these findings in AD populations, much more work is needed (Laakso et al. 2000). For instance, it has not yet been established whether the rates of change are similar at different stages of the illness as well or whether there is a positive predictive value of early hippocampal changes seen in subjects with mild cognitive impairment and those "at risk" for developing AD (Anstey and Maller 2003; Mortimer et al. 2004).

Functional neuroimaging with positron emission tomography also has a relatively long history in AD research, dating back to the 1980s to measures of glucose metabolism (Cutler et al. 1985; Reiman et al. 1996; Small et al. 1996). Functional MRI studies have been conducted more recently, and they show signs of great promise, especially with concurrent cognitive testing (Bookheimer et al. 2000; Devous 2002). Perhaps the most exciting development has been the addition of ligands to functional scanning, especially the markers that have the potential for measuring the β-amyloid or tangle burden (Klunk et al. 2004; Small et al. 2002). Whereas other ligands have been examined for some time (Cohen et al. 1997; Podruchny et al. 2003; Sunderland et al. 1995), the β-amyloid ligand offers an opportunity to investigate pathophysiologically relevant changes both during the course of illness and perhaps even before the clinical symptoms of AD are manifest, if the ligands are sensitive and specific enough. Such studies are currently ongoing. Once more, the possibility of combining risk factors from various modalities (i.e., genetic, CSF, neuropsychological testing, and neuroimaging studies) offers an opportunity to maximize the individual risk factors and predict those that might go on to develop the illness, but this work is still in its infancy.

Implications for Biomarker Research in Geriatric Conditions Other Than Alzheimer's Disease

Clearly, biomarker research in AD is further developed than in any other neuropsychiatric illnesses in the elderly. However, there are also important potential biomarker leads in other illnesses such as Parkinson's disease, Pick's disease, frontotemporal dementia, Lewy body dementia, and various familial tauopathies (Arnold 2004; Ballmaier et al. 2004; Lee et al. 2005; Polymeropoulos et al. 1997; Riemenschneider et al. 2002; Sheline et al. 2003; D. Tsuang et al. 2004; Zhukareva et al. 2004). Establishing biomarkers for other major psychiatric illnesses, such as schizophrenia or depression in general, or geriatric schizophrenia or depression in particular, presents significantly greater challenges than for neurodegenerative dementias. The reasons are multiple and include a lack of any gold standard (i.e., pathognomonic lesion) against which to evaluate the biomarker, marked heterogeneity of the clinical and biological profile, complex genetics, and substantial psychiatric and medical comorbidity.

The extensive neurobiological research on schizophrenia in the past two decades and the recent articulation of the concept of endophenotypes have done much to generate potential biomarkers of the disease. Specific genes recently associated with schizophrenia include those for dysbindin, neuregulin 1, D-amino acid oxidase, catechol-O-methyl transferase, epsin 4, G72, and regulator of G-protein signaling 4 (Arnold et al. 2005; Owen et al. 2005). Although the variations in the nucleotide composition of these genes confer only modest increases in risk for schizophrenia in each case, and thus would not be very useful as biomarkers in themselves, the genes point to physiological pathways that are being examined and may yield clinically relevant tools. Endophenotypic markers pursued include neurocognitive measures, functional and structural MRI, and electrophysiological event-related potentials such as mismatch negativity and the N100 and P300 potentials. In biochemical studies, there have been many proteins measured in serum, blood cells, urine, and CSF in schizophrenia, from neurotransmitters and their metabolites to inflammatory cytokines to markers of oxidative stress. The degree to which any of these will demonstrate utility as clinical diagnostic markers or indicators of clinical severity or treatment responsiveness awaits further work. One novel approach recently took advantage of new microarray platforms to examine gene expression in blood and found distinct gene expression profiles for schizophrenia, bipolar disorder, and nonpsychiatric control groups, with 95%–97% accuracy of diagnosis (M.T. Tsuang et al. 2005). It is not long before similar strategies will be published using proteomic platforms in serum and CSF.

As noted previously, early findings of hypothalamic-pituitary-adrenal axis dysregulation in depression generated great interest in cortisol-related biomarkers for depression, but success has remained limited. Functional neuroimaging abnormalities in depression that have offered potential as biomarkers include globally decreased cerebral blood flow, globally decreased glucose metabolism, or region-specific abnormalities in neurotransmitter-specific ligand receptor binding identified with positron or single photon emission computed tomography. Biochemical studies of CSF have focused on monoamines, neuropeptides, other neurotransmitters, and cytokines, whereas blood cell research has examined various signal transduction pathways (e.g., G-coupled proteins and protein kinase C). Consistent findings from these studies have yet to emerge, so their utility as biomarkers remains unresolved.

With respect to the elderly, there are interesting beginnings of such research in older adults with schizophrenia. Although neuropathological studies in elderly patients with schizophrenia have shown no classic markers of neurodegeneration despite evidence of cognitive decline (Arnold et al. 1998; Harvey et al. 1999), more recent work suggests there may be evidence of oxidative DNA damage in the patients with poor outcome (Nishioka and Arnold 2004). Similarly, there would be great interest in predicting and characterizing the psychiatric complications of neurodegenerative diseases because these complications greatly compound morbidity and may modify the course of AD. Some initial studies have already begun to define genetic risk factors for these disease subtypes (Sweet et al. 2003). Finally, geriatric depression has frequently been linked with cognitive impairment, cardiovascular disease, and neuroimaging abnormalities (Alexopoulos et al. 1997, 2002; Bennett et al. 2004; Cervilla et al. 2004; Krishnan et al. 2004). Although much more work is needed to establish firm links with reliable and reproducible biological markers (Sweet et al. 2003), it is clear that the relationship between cerebrovascular disease and late-life depression is both profound and deleterious clinically (Kales et al. 2005; Veenstra et al. 2005).

In summary, we have presented the preliminary work in AD as an example for future biomarker study in other illnesses, particularly as the pathophysiology becomes better understood and biomarkers analogous to β-amyloid and tau are identified in other geriatric conditions. To anticipate and facilitate this line of research, we offer the following recommendations for the research agenda:

1. Introduce experimental biomarker targets (i.e., neuroimaging ligands when available and molecule-specific bioassays) in large-scale therapeutic studies of AD to broaden the range of outcome variables in such trials while continuing to emphasize the need for autopsy verification of diagnosis.

2. Continue collection of research populations of subjects "at risk" for AD who can be candidates for future prophylactic trials and who can contribute a longitudinal bank of biological specimens (i.e., MRI, positron emission tomography, CSF, blood and genetic samples) for identification and verification of novel biomarkers.
3. Establish similar populations of subjects "at risk" for the development of schizophrenia and depression. Given that the prediction of risk for these illnesses is perhaps less certain than with AD, these studies might be considered examples of "epidemiological neuropathology" of larger groups with longitudinal follow-up. This effort might also include establishing a national brain bank project for future collaborative research.
4. Focus research attention on statistical methods required to optimize sensitivity and specificity of markers when combined across disparate biological areas (i.e., structural or functional imaging, genetics, and CSF markers). This approach could also include multiple nonbiological dimensions (i.e., cognition, behavior, medical comorbidity, and environmental factors) that also influence the outcome of geriatric conditions.

Gaps in Knowledge Regarding Biomarkers in Geriatric Psychiatry

Although the field of biomarker research has advanced considerably in AD, there is still no clear test that fulfills the criteria identified in the consensus report of the Ronald and Nancy Reagan Research Institute of the Alzheimer's Association and the National Institute on Aging Working Group (1998) (Table 25–1). Even if the proposed marker is pathologically relevant, as in the case of β-amyloid or tau, the sensitivity and specificity of any biomarker must be tested against more than just a control population, and the differential diagnostic approach with biomarkers has only just begun with any of the aforementioned biomarkers (Andreasen et al. 2001; Arai 1996; Blennow 2004; Hampel et al. 2003; Sunderland et al. 2003). Once this differential diagnostic approach is better delineated, then these biomarkers could be applied to "at risk" populations to evaluate the potential prognostic value of these markers. This second level of testing with biomarkers is even more complicated than that previously described, because the prognostic value of these biomarkers will be tested with longitudinal follow-up of individuals at risk for dementia who have not yet developed the illness.

The true value of these prognostic markers will be better gauged after the conversion rate of those with the biomarkers are compared with that of those without. In preparation for that development, the ethical implications of such prognostic markers should be considered, especially given the current lack of preventative therapeutic strategies. How this information is handled would depend on the state of treatment options at the time. In the meantime, there are other valuable uses of biomarkers to be tested. For instance, biomarkers of the underlying pathophysiology of an illness such as AD could be used as a target for therapeutic strategies. This approach is already being tested with brain imaging outcome measures, but the strategy is still in its infancy with AD treatment trials. Ultimately, the reduction of "state-dependent" prognostic biomarkers and the prevention of illness in those at risk will be the true test of the usefulness of biomarkers.

References

Alexopoulos GS, Meyers BS, Young RC, et al: "Vascular depression" hypothesis. Arch Gen Psychiatry 54:915–922, 1997

Alexopoulos GS, Kiosses DN, Choi SJ, et al: Frontal white matter microstructure and treatment response of late-life depression: a preliminary study. Am J Psychiatry 159:1929–1932, 2002

Andreasen N, Blennow K: Beta-amyloid (Abeta) protein in cerebrospinal fluid as a biomarker for Alzheimer's disease. Peptides 23:1205–1214, 2002

Andreasen N, Minthon L, Clarberg A, et al: Sensitivity, specificity, and stability of CSF-tau in AD in a community- based patient sample. Neurology 53:1488–1494, 1999

Andreasen N, Minthon L, Davidsson P, et al: Evaluation of CSF-tau and CSF-Abeta42 as diagnostic markers for Alzheimer disease in clinical practice. Arch Neurol 58:373–379, 2001

Anstey KJ, Maller JJ: The role of volumetric MRI in understanding mild cognitive impairment and similar classifications. Aging Ment Health 7:238–250, 2003

Arai H: Biological markers for the clinical diagnosis of Alzheimer's disease. Tohoku J Exp Med 179:65–79, 1996

Arai H, Terajima M, Miura M, et al.: Tau in cerebrospinal fluid: a potential diagnostic marker in Alzheimer's disease. Ann Neurol 38:649–652, 1996

Arnold SE: Bedside to bench and back again: Translational neuroscience research in geriatric psychiatry. Am J Geriatr Psychiatry 12:122–125, 2004

Arnold SE, Trojanowski JQ, Gur RE, et al: Absence of neurodegeneration and neural injury in the cerebral cortex in a sample of elderly patients with schizophrenia. Arch Gen Psychiatry 55:225–232, 1998

Arnold SE, Talbot K, Hahn CG: Neurodevelopment, neuroplasticity, and new genes for schizophrenia. Prog Brain Res 147:319–345, 2005

Ballmaier M, Sowell ER, Thompson PM, et al: Mapping brain size and cortical gray matter changes in elderly depression. Biol Psychiatry 55:382–389, 2004

Bennett DA, Wilson RC, Schneider JA,: Cerebral infarctions and the relationship of depression symptoms to level of cognitive functioning in older persons. Am J Geriatr Psychiatry 12:211–219, 2004

Blennow K: Cerebrospinal fluid protein biomarkers for Alzheimer's disease. NeuroRx 1:213–225, 2004

Blennow K, Vanmechelen E, Hampel H: CSF total tau, Abeta42 and phosphorylated tau protein as biomarkers for Alzheimer's disease. Mol Neurobiol 24:87–97, 2001

Bookheimer SY, Strojwas MH, Cohen MS, et al: Patterns of brain activation in people at risk for Alzheimer's disease. N Engl J Med 343:450–456, 2000

Cacabelos R: The application of functional genomics to Alzheimer's disease. Pharmacogenomics 4:597–621, 2003

Carroll BJ, Feinberg M, Greden JF, et al: A specific laboratory test for the diagnosis of melancholia: standardization, validation, and clinical utility. Arch Gen Psychiatry 38:15–22, 1981

Cervilla J, Prince M, Joels S, et al: Genes related to vascular disease (APOE, VDRL-R, DCP-1) and other vascular factors in late-life depression. Am J Geriatr Psychiatry 12:202–210, 2004

Cohen RM, Andreason PJ, Doudet DJ, et al: Opiate receptor avidity and cerebral blood flow in Alzheimer's disease. J Neurol Sci 148:171–180, 1997

Cohen RM, Small C, Lalonde F, et al: Effect of apolipoprotein E genotype on hippocampal volume loss in aging healthy women. Neurology 57:2223–2228, 2001

Corder EH, Saunders AM, Strittmatter WJ, et al: Gene dose of apolipoprotein E type 4 allele and the risk of Alzheimer's disease in late onset families. Science 261:921–923, 1993

Cutler NR, Haxby JV, Duara R, et al: Brain metabolism as measured with positron emission tomography: serial assessment in a patient with familial Alzheimer's disease. Neurology 35:1556–1561, 1985

de Leon MJ, Convit A, George AE, et al: In vivo structural studies of the hippocampus in normal aging and in incipient Alzheimer's disease. Ann NY Acad Sci 777:1–13, 1996

Devous MD Sr: Functional brain imaging in the dementias: role in early detection, differential diagnosis, and longitudinal studies. Eur J Nucl Med Mol Imaging 29:1685–1696, 2002

Dunckley T, Coon KD, Stephan DA: Discovery and development of biomarkers of neurological disease. Drug Discov Today 10:326–334, 2005

Fagan AM, Younkin LH, Morris JC, et al: Differences in the Abeta40/Abeta42 ratio associated with cerebrospinal fluid lipoproteins as a function of apolipoprotein E genotype. Ann Neurol 48:201–210, 2000

Fox NC, Warrington EK, Stevens JM, et al: Atrophy of the hippocampal formation in early familial Alzheimer's disease: a longitudinal MRI study of at-risk members of a family with an amyloid precursor protein 717Val-Gly mutation. Ann NY Acad Sci 777:226–232, 1996

Galasko D, Chang L, Motter R, et al: High cerebrospinal fluid tau and low amyloid beta42 levels in the clinical diagnosis of Alzheimer disease and relation to apolipoprotein E genotype. Arch Neurol 55:937–945, 1998

Gottwald MD, Rozanski RI: Rivastigmine, a brain-region selective acetylcholinesterase inhibitor for treating Alzheimer's disease: review and current status. Expert Opin Investig Drugs 8:1673–1682, 1999

Greenwood P, Sunderland T, Friz J,et al: Genetics and visual attention: selective deficits in healthy adult carriers of the E4 allele of the apolipoprotein E gene. Proc Natl Acad Sci USA 97:11661–11666, 2000

Gur RC, Gur RE: Neuroimaging applications in elderly patients. Am J Geriatr Psychiatry 10:5–11, 2002

Hampel H, Goernitz A, Buerger K: Advances in the development of biomarkers for Alzheimer's disease: from CSF total tau and Abeta(1–42) proteins to phosphorylated tau protein. Brain Res Bull 61:243–253, 2003

Hampel H, Teipel SJ, Fuchsberger T, et al: Value of CSF beta-amyloid(1–42) and tau as predictors of Alzheimer's disease in patients with mild cognitive impairment. Mol Psychiatry 9:705–710, 2004

Hardy J, Selkoe DJ: The amyloid hypothesis of Alzheimer's disease: progress and problems on the road to therapeutics. Science 297:353–356, 2002

Harvey PD, Silverman JM, Mohs RC, et al: Cognitive decline in late-life schizophrenia: a longitudinal study of geriatric chronically hospitalized patients. Biol Psychiatry 45:32–40, 1999

Ihl R, Eilles C, Frlich L, et al: Electrical brain activity and cerebral blood flow in dementia of the Alzheimer type. Psychiatry Res 29:449–452, 1989

Jack CR Jr, Petersen RC, Xu YC, et al: Medial temporal atrophy on MRI in normal aging and very mild Alzheimer's disease. Neurology 49:786–794, 1997

Jarvik LF, Read SL, Mintz J, et al: Pretreatment orthostatic hypotension in geriatric depression: predictor of response to imipramine and doxepin. J Clin Psychopharmacol 3:368–372, 1983

Kales HC, Maixner DF, Mellow AM: Cerebrovascular disease and late-life depression. Am J Geriatr Psychiatry 13:88–98, 2005

Klunk WE, Engler H, Nordberg A, et al: Imaging brain amyloid in Alzheimer's disease with Pittsburgh Compound-B. Ann Neurol 55:306–319, 2004

Kragh-Sorensen P: Correlation between plasma levels of nortriptyline and clinical effects. Commun Psychopharmacol 2:451–456, 1998

Krishnan KR, Taylor WD, McQuoid DR, et al: Clinical characteristics of magnetic resonance imaging-defined subcortical ischemic depression. Biol Psychiatry 55:390–397, 2004

Laakso MP, Lehtovirta M, Partanen K, et al: Hippocampus in Alzheimer's disease: a 3-year follow-up MRI study. Biol Psychiatry 47:557–561, 2000

Lee VM, Kenyon TK, Trojanowski JQ: Transgenic animal models of tauopathies. Biochim Biophys Acta 1739:251–259, 2005

Levy J, Bergeson JL, Putnam KT, et al.: Context-specific memory and apolipoprotein E (ApoE) E4: Cognitive evidence from the NIMH prospective study of risk for Alzheimer's disease. J Int Neuropsychol Soc 10:362–370, 2004

Lim A, Tsuang D, Kukull W, et al: Clinico-neuropathological correlation of Alzheimer's disease in a community-based case series. J Am Geriatr Soc 47:564–569, 1999

McKhann G, Drachman D, Folstein M, et al: Clinical diagnosis of Alzheimer's disease: report of the NINCDS-ADRDA work group under the auspices of Department of Health and Human Services Task Force on Alzheimer's Disease. Neurology 34:939–944, 1984

Mendez MF, Mastri AR, Sung JH, et al: Clinically diagnosed Alzheimer disease: neuropathologic findings in 650 cases. Alzheimer Dis Assoc Disord 6:35–43, 1992

Mirra SS, Heyman A, McKeel D, et al: The Consortium to Establish a Registry for Alzheimer's Disease (CERAD), part II: standardization of the neuropathologic assessment of Alzheimer's disease. Neurology 41:479–486, 1991

Mohs RC, Cohen L: Alzheimer's Disease Assessment Scale (ADAS). Psychopharmacol Bull 24:627–628, 1988

Montgomery SA, Braithwaite RA, Crammer JL: Routine nortriptyline levels in treatment of depression. Br Med J 2:166–167, 1977

Mortimer JA, Gosche KM, Riley KP, et al: Delayed recall, hippocampal volume and Alzheimer neuropathology: findings from the Nun Study. Neurology 62:428–432, 2004

Newell KL, Hyman BT, Growdon JH, et al: Application of the National Institute on Aging (NIA)–Reagan Institute criteria for the neuropathologic diagnosis of Alzheimer disease. J Neuropathol Exp Neurol 58:1147–1155, 1999

Nishioka N, Arnold SE: Evidence of oxidative DNA damage in the hippocampus of elderly patients with chronic schizophrenia. Am J Geriatr Psychiatry 12:167–175, 2004

Owen MJ, O'Donovan MC, Harrison PJ: Schizophrenia: a genetic disorder of the synapse? Br Med J 330:158–159, 2005

Petersen RC, Smith GE, Waring SC, et al: Mild cognitive impairment: clinical characterization and outcome. Arch Neurol 56:303–308, 1999

Podruchny TA, Connolly C, Bokde A, et al: In vivo muscarinic 2 receptor imaging in cognitively normal young and older volunteers. Synapse 48:39–44, 2003

Polymeropoulos MH, Lavedan C, Leroy E, et al: Mutation in the alpha-synuclein gene identified in families with Parkinson's disease. Science 276:2045–2047, 1997

Raskind MA, Peskind ER, Wessel T, et al: Galantamine in AD: A 6-month randomized, placebo-controlled trial with a 6-month extension. The Galantamine USA-1 Study Group. Neurology 54:2261–2268, 2000

Reiman EM, Caselli RJ, Yun LS, et al: Preclinical evidence of Alzheimer's disease in persons homozygous for the epsilon 4 allele for apolipoprotein E (see comments). N Engl J Med 334:752–758, 1996

Reiman EM, Chen K, Alexander GE, et al: Functional brain abnormalities in young adults at genetic risk for late-onset Alzheimer's dementia. Proc Natl Acad Sci USA 101:284–289, 2004

Riemenschneider M, Lautenschlager N, Wagenpfeil S, et al: Cerebrospinal fluid tau and beta-amyloid 42 proteins identify Alzheimer disease in subjects with mild cognitive impairment. Arch Neurol 59:1729–1734, 2002

Rogers SL, Farlow MR, Doody RS, et al: A 24-week, double-blind, placebo-controlled trial of donepezil in patients with Alzheimer's disease. Donepezil Study Group. Neurology 50:136–145, 1998

Ronald and Nancy Reagan Research Institute of the Alzheimer's Association and the National Institute on Aging Working Group: Consensus report of the working group on "molecular and biochemical markers of Alzheimer's disease." The Ronald and Nancy Reagan Research Institute of the Alzheimer's Association and the National Institute on Aging Working Group. Neurobiol Aging 19:109–116, 1998

Rosen VM, Bergeson JL, Putnam K, et al: Working memory and apolipoprotein E: what's the connection? Neuropsychologia 40:2226–2233, 2002

Selkoe DJ: The origins of Alzheimer disease: a is for amyloid. JAMA 283:1615–1617, 2000

Seshadri S, Beiser A, Selhub J, et al: Plasma homocysteine as a risk factor for dementia and Alzheimer's disease. N Engl J Med 346:476–483, 2002

Sheline YI, Gado MH, Kraemer HC: Untreated depression and hippocampal volume loss. Am J Psychiatry 160:1516–1518, 2003

Small GW, Komo S, La Rue A, et al: Early detection of Alzheimer's disease by combining apolipoprotein E and neuroimaging. Ann NY Acad Sci 802:70–78, 1996

Small GW, Ercoli LM, Silverman DHS, et al: Cerebral metabolic and cognitive decline in persons at genetic risk for Alzheimer's disease. Proc Natl Acad Sci USA 97:6037–6042, 2000

Small GW, Agdeppa ED, Kepe V, et al: In vivo brain imaging of tangle burden in humans. J Mol Neurosci 19:323–327, 2002

Snowdon DA: Healthy aging and dementia: findings from the Nun Study. Ann Intern Med 139:450–454, 2003

Sunderland T, Esposito G, Molchan SE, et al: Differential cholinergic regulation in Alzheimer's patients compared to controls following chronic blockade with scopolamine: a SPECT study. Psychopharmacology (Berl) 121:231–241, 1995

Sunderland T, Linker G, Mirza N, et al: Decreased beta-amyloid1–42 and increased tau levels in cerebrospinal fluid of patients with Alzheimer disease. JAMA 289:2094–2103, 2003

Sunderland T, Mirza N, Putnam KT, et al: Cerebrospinal fluid beta-amyloid1–42 and tau in control subjects at risk for Alzheimer's disease: the effect of APOE epsilon4 allele. Biol Psychiatry 56:670–676, 2004

Sweet RA, Nimgaonkar VL, Devlin B, et al: Psychotic symptoms in Alzheimer disease: evidence for a distinct phenotype. Mol Psychiatry 8:383–392, 2003

Tanzi RE, Bertram L: New frontiers in Alzheimer's disease genetics. Neuron 32:181–184, 2001

Tanzi RE, St George-Hyslop PH, Haines JL, et al: The genetic defect in familial Alzheimer's disease is not tightly linked to the amyloid beta-protein gene. Nature 329:156–157, 1987

Tsuang D, DiGiacomo L, Bird TD: The familial occurrence of dementia with Lewy bodies. Am J Geriatr Psychiatry 12:179–188, 2004

Tsuang MT, Nossova N, Yager T, et al: Assessing the validity of blood-based gene expression profiles for the classification of schizophrenia and bipolar disorder: a preliminary report. Am J Med Genet B Neuropsychiatr Genet 133:1–5, 2005

Veenstra TD, Conrads TP, Hood BL: Biomarkers: Mining the biofluid proteome. Mol Cell Proteomics 4:409–418, 2005

Wang HX, Wahlin A, Basun H, et al: Vitamin B(12) and folate in relation to the development of Alzheimer's disease. Neurology 56:1188–1194, 2001

Zhukareva V, Trojanowski JQ, Lee VM: Assessment of pathological tau proteins in frontotemporal dementias: qualitative and quantitative approaches. Am J Geriatr Psychiatry 12:136–145, 2004

26

IMPACT OF PSYCHOSOCIAL FACTORS ON LATE-LIFE DEPRESSION

Patricia A. Areán, Ph.D.
Charles F. Reynolds III, M.D.

Mental illness in late life results from many contributing factors, including biological, psychosocial, and environmental. These factors all influence the course of mental illness from onset to maintenance of the illness and finally to offset, or end of the illness. As an example, depression in late life is often a function of age-related biological changes, medical illness, new and unexpected life events, and history of mental illness. No one factor has been found to be more important than another. In fact, several researchers now believe that discovery of the best treatments for late-life depression will come from a solid understanding of how all these factors affect mental illness. Whereas the valence of biological risk factors is stronger in some mental illnesses than others, the addition of psychosocial stress can influence the course and outcome of even biologically loaded illnesses. As an example, psychotic symptoms have been found to increase in intensity and duration following a neg-

Supported in part by the Intervention Research Center for Late Life Mood Disorders (P30 MH52247), the John A. Hartford Center of Excellence in Geriatric Psychiatry, and Project EXPORT at the Center for Minority Health, Graduate School of Public Health (P60 MD00020702) at the University of Pittsburgh; and by the University of California, San Francisco, Center for Aging in Diverse Communities (P30 AG5272).

ative psychological event (Morrison et al. 2004). Our purpose here is to discuss the impact of psychosocial risk factors on the onset, maintenance, and offset of mental illness in late life. Because the majority of research in the geriatric literature has focused on depression, our main focus is on this disorder. In particular, we review the common psychosocial risk factors associated with depression and whether they can be modified to affect onset, offset, and maintenance. Finally, we provide suggestions for future research.

Common Psychosocial Risk Factors in Late-Life Depression

Psychosocial risk factors for depression in later life consist of demographic variables such as socioeconomic status, negative life events, and other events characterized by loss and/or disability. These variables are often intertwined; rarely do older people have just one risk factor. The impact of these risk factors on late-life functioning will be in large part determined by the presence of other psychosocial variables, such as social support and coping skill. Furthermore, the undesirability, uncontrollability, magnitude, and duration of these psychosocial events all influence whether an older adult will become depressed in the face of these events. Knowing not only the common risk factors for a mental illness but also the magnitude, perceived controllability, and available external and interpersonal resources available to the older person exposed to a risk factor is important in identifying who is at most risk for developing a late-life mental illness; such information also can help identify the degree to which the person is likely to respond to traditional treatments. In this section we first discuss what the common psychosocial risk factors are for depression and then discuss how they relate to one another in the onset, maintenance, and offset of depression in later life.

The most important and best-studied risk factors for new-onset and recurrent depression in later life are bereavement, caregiver strain, social isolation, disability from medical illness, and need for rehabilitation (Bruce 2002). Aging often involves the loss of important people from one's life and the loss of societal roles and social goals. According to Bruce (2002), the degree to which these negative life events become salient risk factors for late-life depression depends upon how much these events are seen as undesirable or uncontrollable, how disruptive the events are, and how long the person must endure them. Although some studies suggest that the actual number and duration of stressful life events may be related to new onset or maintenance of depression (Brilman and Ormel 2001; Chen et al. 2002), the findings tend not to be consistent across studies (Bruce 2002).

The onset of medical illness also appears to contribute to the onset of depression in older adults. Most research on medical burden and disability in late life point to an increased risk for depression (Geerlings et al. 2000; Mazure and Maciejewski 2003). The increased risk for depression could be due as much to biological factors as to psychosocial factors. Recent research suggests, however, that even if medical burden increases depression risk via biological issues, psychological factors mediate the impact medical burden will have on the onset of depression. In a longitudinal study of older adults who underwent elective hip replacement surgery, older patients who had poor self-efficacy related to their ability to handle recovery from hip replacement surgery were at much greater risk of becoming significantly depressed 6 weeks after surgery than those who had greater self-efficacy (Kurlowicz 1998).

Loss of a loved one is one of the most significant risk factors for depression in late life (Bruce et al. 1990). The association between depression and loss is clouded by overlapping presentation of normal grief and depression, but recent research into what is termed "traumatic" or "complicated" grief indicates that how one copes with the death of a loved one, how traumatic or unexpected the death is, and the degree to which the death results in social isolation may be the linking feature between loss and new-onset depression.

Another potential, but less studied, psychosocial risk factor for mental illness in late life is exposure to a traumatic event. Although we are all exposed to traumatic events via the media and literature, exposure to a traumatic event is typically problematic when the event evokes intense fear, helplessness, or horror in the exposed person (American Psychiatric Association 2000). The literature on the prevalence of trauma exposure in older adults is very limited (Averill and Beck 2000; Flint 1994). Most of the information we have on exposure to traumatic events in older adults is from the literature on combat veterans and Holocaust survivors. Although we know that unresolved trauma in these populations does have an impact on mental health functioning (Averill and Beck 2000), we know very little about what other types of individuals are at greatest risk for trauma exposure and the sequelae associated with trauma exposure. We can speculate, however, that older, low-income elderly persons may be a potential group who are at risk for this exposure. Despite the declining crime rates in the United States, low-income older adults living in urban centers are still at great risk of exposure to crime. Although older adults as a group are less likely to be the *victims* of crime, their lifetime *exposure* may be quite significant. In one study on risk of trauma exposure, 67% of people living in urban centers had experienced a lifetime trauma, such as tragic death, sexual assault, or motor vehicle accident (Norris 1992). Older African Americans are victimized at twice the rate of older whites. Older, low-income elderly persons are disproportionately exposed to household crime. The rate for low-income elderly is 154 per 1,000, whereas the rate for household crime in higher income elderly populations is 70 per 1,000 (Norris 1992). According to two studies in two urban settings in the San Francisco Bay Area, between 20% and 52% of older adults seen for mental health treatment had been exposed to traumatic experiences in their lifetime, many of which involved exposure to violence (Cook et al. 2001). Other studies suggest that for low-income elderly, fear of victimization is an even greater problem than actual victimization (Johnson-Dalzine et al. 1996). Fear of victimization often forces individuals to make behavioral adjustments in their lifestyles and coping, such as increased avoidance of outside activities. As stated before, increased social isolation is a risk factor for depression in older adults. Thus, fear of victimization may be related to onset of late-life mental illness through the behavioral sequelae of fear.

This discussion points out another risk factor in developing mental illness in late life: socioeconomic status. Lower income is related to poorer access to health and mental health services. Poor access to care influences the diagnosis and treatment of depression, because patients are less likely to be seen by providers for healthcare needs on a regular basis and thus are unlikely to be screened for depressive disorders. Even if screening were to take place, mental health resources that could either prevent a severe episode of depression or appropriately treat an existing episode are very scarce, and access is difficult. As an example, older African Americans with depression represent a worst-case scenario with respect to disparities in mental healthcare access and outcomes. Although progress in biomedical research has been dramatic in the past 20 years, it has not narrowed the gap in health status between minority and majority groups (Charney et al. 2003). Whereas impediments to good depression outcomes exist for all patients, they may be more salient for older patients and represent even larger barriers for older black patients. Predominantly, older patients receive mental healthcare from their primary care physicians, and they are often reluctant to accept referral to mental health specialists (Miranda et al. 2003) because of logistic (e.g., transportation, financial disincentives) and personal factors (e.g., personal preferences, stigma) (Cooper et al. 2003). Their depression is less likely to be identified and formally diagnosed (Brown et al. 1995; Cooper-Patrick et al. 1999; Harman et al. 2001), confirming a well-documented bias in clinical judgment (Neighbors et al. 1989). Even when depression is diagnosed, treatment may differ. Research findings suggest that there is less patient participation in medical decision making when the patient and clinician differ in cultural backgrounds (Cooper-Patrick et al. 1999).

Decreased social support in the form of emotional support is another risk factor for depression in older adults. In general, the concept of social support is a complex and multifaceted one. It is important to note that it is not the absolute number of people in one's lives that serves as a protective factor against depression onset, but the type of support received regarding more emotional matters. According to Antonucci (1991) and Carstensen (1991), older adults naturally tighten their social networks, making them smaller over time. This socio-emotional selectivity represents a kind of natural selection as one ages; older people, faced with the end of their lives and hoping to make their existences less complicated, start to spend more time with people who are like-minded and to avoid people who are not as enjoyable to be around. Thus, as the social network begins to decrease, the quality of social interaction and emotional support increases. Once that social network begins to dwindle over time, and there are fewer and fewer people to provide emotional support, the risk of depression onset is likely to increase (Bruce and Hoff 1994). According to Bruce, research on social support as a protective factor against depression onset is still needed, because many studies on this topic have yielded different outcomes depending on how social support is defined and which aspect of social support is being studied (Bruce and Hoff 1994).

Finally, coping style, or psychological resilience, is related to the onset and maintenance of depression in late life. Although there was considerable research in the late 1980s and early 1990s on the psychological variables associated with mental health risk in older adults, that research has virtually stalled, even though several questions along this line still need to be answered. Research on active versus passive coping in older adults shows that older people who take a more passive stance in solving everyday problems tend to be more vulnerable to depression and anxiety. *Active coping* is defined as any strategy that directly addresses solving or adjusting to a new problem. This includes the spectrum of actively mobilizing resources in the community to solve problems to relying on prayer to adjust to a stressor. For instance. Denney (1995) found that using problem-solving skills to deal with life strain is related to better psychological adjustment in late life, and Koenig et al. (1997) found that spirituality and being actively involved in spiritual endeavors is also related to better psychological well-being in later life. Passive coping is characterized by avoidant-type behaviors, such as the use of distraction techniques, leaving solutions to problems in the hands of others, and rumination on a problem. These strategies are consistently related to depression in both older and younger adults.

In summary, a number of psychosocial variables correlate with late-life depression. Loss, trauma, social isolation, coping style, socioeconomics, gender, and ethnicity are all related to late-life depression. How exactly these risk factors intermingle to contribute to the onset and maintenance of depression is the subject of the next section.

Are Psychosocial Risk Factors Modifiable?

Given that not everyone who loses a spouse, is poor, or experiences a medical problem becomes depressed, there has been much speculation on the moderating effects of other variables on psychosocial risk factors. Knowing what variables influence the impact of a risk factor on the onset of mental illness is important in order to develop interventions aimed at preventing the onset or maintenance of a disorder. According to the existing research, the impact that a negative life event or negative living situation will have on the onset of depression in late life has to do with several psychological and socioeconomic factors. These include psychological resilience, strength of social support, and past psychiatric history. As a concrete example, an older person with a recent medical diagnosis may be more likely to become suicidal if he or she also has a previous psychiatric history, feelings of hopelessness regarding the illness, avoidant coping style, and poor social support (Conwell et al. 2002).

Psychological resilience is a variable that has been found to influence the negative effects of stress in older adults (Wagnild and Young 1993). Wagnild (2003) defines *psychological resilience* as consisting of five characteristics, *equanimity* (a balanced view of life), *meaningfulness* (a sense of purpose in life), *perseverance* (ability to function even in the face of failures), *existential aloneness* (acceptance of one's life) and *self-reliance* (self efficacy). Each of these variables is potentially modifiable through behavioral intervention and thus could be addressed either through preventative or acute treatment. For instance, cognitive-behavioral therapies specifically address people's beliefs about the world (equanimity), their lives (meaningfulness), and their abilities to function in the world despite adversity (perseverance) through cognitive restructuring activities. In addition, cognitive-behavioral interventions also teach people skills to cope with adversity, which often leads to improved self-reliance.

The impact of social support on the onset and maintenance of depression is less clear. Some studies have found that the quality of social support can have a protective influence on life stress (Fratiglioni et al. 2000), but others have shown that social support can be affected by depression (Gurung et al. 2003). There is some evidence to suggest that the individuals in a person's social networks have specific roles in moderating the impact of negative life events, and the loss of protective people in a social network can result in particularly devastating results. The impact that this loss would have may be moderated through interventions designed to mitigate bereavement-related depression; for example, Reynolds et al. (1999b) demonstrated in a randomized, double-blind, placebo-controlled study that the highest rates for remission from bereavement-related major depression followed the use of combined antidepressant medication (nortriptyline) and interpersonal psychotherapy. A more recent open pilot study by Shear et al. (2001) suggested that traumatic grief psychotherapy may be particularly helpful for people living with traumatic or complicated grief.

Past psychiatric history is another moderator of negative life events (and also is considered to be a biological risk factor for mental illness). Those who have had a past history of depression, abuse, or anxiety tend to be at greater risk for new episodes in later life. Although past history itself cannot be changed, how a provider or older person uses that information to prevent new episodes can be a point of mediation. Relapse prevention interventions for depression show some promise in offsetting the recurrence of depression in older populations (Reynolds et al. 1999a), however, these interventions tend to address relapse prevention immediately after treatment. There is little research on relapse prevention interventions in the face of new life events. There is some preliminary research indicating that interventions aimed at increasing coping skills after recent diagnoses of chronic illnesses can reduce initial distress reactions (Lorig et al. 2001; Nezu et al. 2003). More research is needed to determine whether these types of interventions could be potentially helpful in preventing depression recurrence in older adults who have a history of depression.

Socioeconomic status, in and of itself, is difficult to modify through psychiatric intervention. However, the sequelae of poverty and social strain may be modifiable through case-management types of interventions. One study on older, poverty-level adults finds that the addition of case-management services addressing housing, legal, financial, and entitlement issues to psychotherapy results in significant improvement in depression outcomes—and in some cases with milder depression, case management alone is sufficient to decrease depression symptoms (Areán et al. 2005).

Suggested Agenda for Research on Psychosocial Risk Factors of Late-Life Mental Illness

As can be seen from our review here, there has been considerable epidemiological research on psychosocial risk factors and their impact on depression in older adults. Although some areas, such as social support and resiliency, still require further study, we think that the field is now ready to move toward an integrative model of mental health risk, one that incorporates biological and psychosocial factors into better understanding the onset and maintenance of mental illness. As Inui (2003) noted, the field will not truly understand mental health in late life until it recognizes the complexities and interrelatedness of biological and psychosocial variables in mental health. Mental health is determined as much by biology as by the psychosocial context of the older adult, and until we are able to understand how biology interacts with psychology and societal factors, we will be unable to develop assessment tools and interventions that can thoroughly address the mental health needs of older adults. As an example, recent work by Caspi et al. (2003) underscores the importance of biological variables, such as the serotonin transporter promoter polymorphism, in vulnerability to depression following adverse life events. Work such as this can inform methods for detecting patients at risk for mental illness and for classifying patients based on the biological and psychosocial features of their disorder. This type of approach may in turn inform treatment choice. In the following sections we discuss the role psychosocial variables may have in these arenas.

DETECTING AT-RISK PATIENTS

More prospective research is needed to determine the degree to which certain psychosocial factors truly influence the impact of life events on mental health. In particular, research to determine how reliably psychosocial risk factors can be used as a screening tool for the occurrence of a potential depressive episode is needed. A particularly important research focus for clinicians trying to identify older adults at risk for the onset of mental illness is to investigate the effect that previous trauma exposure has on the development of mental illness following a new traumatic medical event such as a heart attack. Studies have shown that people with previous traumatic exposure are at risk for a new mental illness when they are exposed to another traumatic experience (Cook et al. 2001). If we were to find that past traumatic experience is a predictor of developing anxiety after a cardiac event, for example, cardiologists and the patient's primary care providers could easily assess this risk factor and then closely monitor at-risk patients for the development of anxiety.

In addition, research on reliable measures of psychosocial risk factors for depression is needed to facilitate risk assessment in older adults. Although measures of psychological resiliency exist, they tend to be lengthy and too complex to use in everyday practice. Life event interviews are equally cumbersome, and although useful as research tools, they have equivocal value as clinical tools. Quick, easy, and reliable risk assessment measures need to be developed to facilitate early detection of mental illness.

The research on risk factors associated with late-life depression in particular suggests that there may be different etiologies for depressive disorder that could act as qualifiers for treatment decision making and even suggests that there may be subclassifications of late-life mental illness. For instance, bereavement-related depression may be a risk factor for traumatic grief, also called "complicated grief," a debilitating condition in which the reaction to the loss is the primary problem (Shear et al. 2001). The condition is characterized by the persistence of the sense of disbelief, yearning, longing, and pining for the deceased and preoccupation with the person who died, lasting more than 6 months after the loss. Other prominent symptoms include intrusive images related to the death, avoidance of reminders of the loss, recurrent intense pangs of grief, and difficulty coping with daily life and engaging with others. Individuals who report an overabundance of these symptoms on the Inventory of Complicated Grief (Prigerson et al. 1999) are at risk for myriad physical and mental health problems, including new-onset cardiovascular illness, cancer, and depression (Prigerson et al. 1997), and are at increased risk for suicidality (Szanto et al. 1998). A subcategory in our diagnostic nomenclature would help providers monitor patients who have experienced a loss and refer at-risk patients for grief-related treatment, because it appears that the symptoms are relatively refractory to standard depression treatment.

Although a subcategory of "depression due to socioeconomic stress" is unlikely to be included in any iteration of our psychiatric nosology, the degree to which elderly persons living at poverty level experience mental illness in the face of significant psychosocial stress is important to consider when making treatment decisions. Depression and anxiety in overly stressful environments with little hope of change is understandable but nonetheless should be treated. The first-line treatment for low-income elderly persons with depression, for instance, may not be antidepressant medication alone but rather clinical case management in combination with some active intervention to address the immediate psychosocial needs of this population (Areán et al. 2005). Recent research suggests that simply increasing access to depression interventions—medication or psychotherapy—in minority older adults, who tend to be disproportionately low-income, results in treatment outcomes as good as those found in non-minority older adults (Areán et al. 2005).

There is a growing literature indicating that certain presentations of late-life depression suggest underlying pathologies related to poor or unstable response to first-line antidepressant medication. In particular, older patients with an apathetic presentation and significant executive dysfunction tend to respond poorly to antidepressant medication but have a good response to selected psychotherapies that address the behavioral sequelae of the dysfunction (Alexopoulos et al. 2002, 2003). Although the depression is not a result of psychosocial risks, certain populations may be at risk for depression with executive dysfunction. Low-income older adults tend to have several risk factors for cognitive impairments, including substandard early educational opportunities, higher rates of substance abuse histories, poorer overall health, and exposure to violent crime and accidents (Krawitz and Watson 1997). Once again, we call for more research into the prevalence of comorbidities of this nature in older, low-income populations. Research of this nature would offer providers an opportunity to selectively screen patients with psychosocial risk factors that could presage treatment-resistant presentations of depression and thus refer these patients to appropriate treatments.

There is no doubt that socioeconomic status influences health and mental health. The increased risk for mortality and morbidity in this group underscores the importance of studying what specific psychosocial factors influence the presence of mental illness and increased mortality (Isaacs and Schroeder 2004). Future research should consider the utility of including socioeconomic and ethnic variables in the detection of mental illness and treatment selection for this particularly vulnerable group of people.

PREDICTING ONSET, MAINTENANCE, AND OFFSET OF LATE-LIFE MENTAL ILLNESS

Another area in need of investigation is the impact of psychosocial variables on the onset, maintenance, and offset of other mental disorders. For instance, we know very little about what factors contribute to the onset and maintenance of anxiety disorders and substance abuse. Although the onset of disorders such as Alzheimer's disease and psychotic disorders may be less influenced by psychosocial variables, certainly their maintenance and severity could be affected by psychosocial variables. For instance, early detection of Alzheimer's disease may be important in forestalling the disabilities associated with cognitive impairments over time. Studies have shown that the use of cognitive enhancers early in the course of the disease can slow the progress of the disabilities associated with it (Wilkinson et al. 2004). The timing of disease identification can be influenced by several psychosocial factors, such as access to a healthcare provider who can make a diagnosis, stigma concerns that can influence family willingness to detect a problem, and coping style, which determines how active a person will be in attending to his or her health. Likewise, the degree to which psychotic symptoms are controlled may be in large part determined by the quality of social support in the older psychotic person's life; there is some indication that social support influences medication adherence and therefore could be an important factor in adherence to psychotropic medication in older people.

TREATING LATE-LIFE DEPRESSION: SELECTION OF TREATMENT BASED ON PSYCHOSOCIAL RISK FACTORS FOR TREATMENT RESPONSE

Because less than 50% of elderly depressed patients achieve remission and recovery in response to first-line antidepressant pharmacotherapy, the majority of patients, especially in primary care, may be left with residual symptoms and functional impairment, putting them at risk for chronic, relapsing illness; increasing incapacity; nonadherence to other medical treatments; suicide; and family caregiver burden. The recently completed Improving Mood—Promoting Access to Collaborative Treatment (IMPACT; Unutzer et al. 2002) and Prevention of Suicide in Primary Care Elderly: Collaborative Trial (PROSPECT; Bruce et al. 2004) studies have demonstrated the efficacy of collaborative depression care management in primary care settings for bringing about greater reductions in depressive symptoms and suicidal ideation in elderly patients with major depression, relative to usual care. Nevertheless, the interventions in both studies left a considerable burden of residual depressive symptoms, underscoring the need for further efficacy research to determine how to bring more patients to full remission and recovery. An important hypothesis, yet to be tested, is whether certain psychosocial risk factors are related to partial response to traditional treatment and, if so, whether these profiles can be used to select more appropriate treatments. As discussed earlier, there is evidence that certain neurocognitive presentations are related to poor response to antidepressant medication but better response to targeted psychotherapies. The same may be true of patients with particular profiles of depression. Bereavement is one example of a psychosocial profile that could indicate a different treatment decision than what is typically recommended.

Bereavement is a universal life event that, more than any other, is a risk factor for the onset of depression and other mental health sequelae, including traumatic grief and suicide. Nearly 1 million Americans each year experience bereavement-related depression. Such depression is as pernicious as any nonbereavement major depression in its persistence and association with diminished quality of life, poor general health, increased suicidality, and increased substance abuse. Major depression within the first 6 months after a loss is often left untreated because of the misconception that depression is often a normal manifestation of grief and will remit spontaneously. Some even think that treatment of depression could impede normal grief work. Data from controlled trials are sorely needed to improve the evidence base for treating bereavement-related depression and to guide clinicians who now struggle to understand whether, how, and how long to treat depression associated with the unavoidable and universal stress of bereavement.

Similarly, further research is needed to assess the efficacy of psychotherapeutic approaches to suicidality in late-life depression and to address the question of how psychosocial risk factors contribute to suicidality. Based upon a consideration of psychosocial risk factors for suicide, we believe that psychosocial interventions designed to reduce risk for suicide in later life will need to focus on optimizing relationships with significant others (because social isolation increases the risk for suicide); improving compliance with medication management, especially for depression (because depression is also a major risk factor); sustaining abstinence from alcohol; reducing hopelessness; improving social problem solving; and improving self-esteem. Recent research has shown that collaborative care management of depression in elderly primary care patients reduces two of the major risk factors for suicide in later life (depression and suicidal ideation; Bruce et al. 2004). However, the presence of suicidal ideation is associated with prolonged time to response and diminished likelihood of response (Szanto et al. 2003), necessitating further careful assessment and treatment development for suicidal elderly persons.

Research is also needed to assess the use of psychosocial interventions for elderly patients who respond with sadness, loneliness, or insomnia to the vicissitudes of later life, such as bereavement, caregiving, and onset of new medical illness and its associated disability and loss of autonomy. These elderly are at high risk for developing mental illnesses such as depression. Early intervention may serve to bolster their psychological resilience and continued engagement in life ("successful aging").

In summary, more research is needed in three pertinent areas. First, a better understanding is needed of how psychosocial events intermingle with other medical and biological risk factors in the development of late-life depression. Second, methods for using psychosocial assessments—tools that have both ecological validity and clinical functionality—are needed to identify older adults at risk of developing late-life depression in the face of a life event. Third, research on the use of psychosocial factors in treatment response is needed to assist clinicians in both diagnostic classification and treatment selection. More research is needed to determine if certain psychosocial profiles are related to response to different treatments, so that clinicians can be more efficient in selecting treatment.

References

Alexopoulos G, Borson S, Cuthbert B, et al: Assessment of late-life depression. Biol Psychiatry 52:164–174, 2002

Alexopoulos GS, Raue P, Areán PA: Problem-solving therapy versus supportive therapy in geriatric major depression with executive dysfunction. Am J Geriatr Psychiatry 11:46–52, 2003

American Psychiatric Association: Diagnostic and Statistical Manual of Mental Disorders, 4th Edition, Text Revision. Washington, DC, American Psychiatric Association, 2000

Antonucci TC: Attachment, social support, and coping with negative life events in mature adulthood, in Life Span Developmental Psychology: Perspectives on Stress and Coping. Edited by Cummings EM, Greene AL, Karraker K. Hillsdale, NJ, Erlbaum, 1991, pp 261–276

Areán PA, Gum A, McCulloch CE, et al: Treatment of depression in low-income older adults. Psychol Aging 20:601–609, 2005

Averill PM, Beck JG: Posttraumatic stress disorder in older adults: a conceptual review. J Anxiety Disord 14:133–156, 2000

Brilman EI, Ormel J: Life events, difficulties and onset of depressive episodes in later life. Psychol Med 31:859–869, 2001

Brown DR, Ahmed F, Gary LE, et al: Major depression in a community sample of African Americans. Am J Psychiatry 152:373–378, 1995

Bruce ML: Psychosocial risk factors for depressive disorders in late life. Biol Psychiatry 52:175–184, 2002

Bruce ML, Hoff RA: Social and physical health risk factors for first-onset major depressive disorder in a community sample. Soc Psychiatry Psychiatr Epidemiol 29:165–171, 1994

Bruce ML, Kim K, Leaf PJ, et al: Depressive episodes and dysphoria resulting from conjugal bereavement in a prospective community sample. Am J Psychiatry 147:608–611, 1990

Bruce ML, Ten Have TR, Reynolds CF, et al: Reducing suicidal ideation and depressive symptoms in depressed older primary care patients: a randomized controlled trial. JAMA 291:1081–1090, 2004

Carstensen LL: Socioemotional and selectivity theory: social activity in life-span context. Annu Rev Gerontol Geriatr 11:195–217, 1991

Caspi A, Sugden K, Moffitt TE, et al: Influence of life stress on depression: moderation by a polymorphism in the 5-HTT gene. Science 301:386–389, 2003

Charney DS, Reynolds CF, Lewis L, et al: Depression and bipolar support alliance consensus statement on the unmet needs in diagnosis and treatment of mood disorders in late life. Arch Gen Psychiatry 60:664–672, 2003

Chen LS, Eaton WW, Gallo JJ: Empirical examination of current depression categories in a population-based study: symptoms, course, and risk factors. Am J Psychiatry 157:573–580, 2002

Conwell Y, Duberstein PR, Caine ED: Risk factors for suicide in later life. Biol Psychiatry 52:193–204, 2002

Cook JM, Areán PA, Schnurr PP: Symptom differences between older depressed primary care patients with and without history of trauma. Int J Psychiatry Med 31:401–414, 2001

Cooper LA, Roter DL, Johnson RL, et al: Patient-centered communication, ratings of care, and concordance of patient and physician race. Ann Intern Med 139:907–915, 2003

Cooper-Patrick L, Gallo JJ, Powe NR, et al: Mental health service utilization by African Americans and Whites: the Baltimore Epidemiologic Catchment Area Follow-Up. Med Care 37:1034–1045, 1999

Denney NW: Critical thinking during the adult years: has the developmental function changed over the last four decades? Exp Aging Res 21:191–207, 1995

Flint AJ: Epidemiology and comorbidity of anxiety disorders in the elderly. Am J Psychiatry 151:640–649, 1994

Fratiglioni L, Wang HX, Ericsson K, et al: Influence of social network on occurrence of dementia: a community-based longitudinal study. Lancet 355:1315–1319, 2000

Geerlings SW, Beekman AT, Deeg DJ, et al: Physical health and the onset and persistence of depression in older adults: an eight-wave prospective community-based study. Psychol Med 30:369–380, 2000

Gurung RA, Taylor SE, Seeman TE: Accounting for changes in social support among married older adults: insights from the MacArthur Studies of Successful Aging. Psychol Aging 18:487–496, 2003

Harman JS, Schulberg HC, Mulsant BH, et al: Effect of patient and visit characteristics on diagnosis of depression in primary care. J Fam Pract 50:1068, 2001

Inui TS: The need for an integrated biopsychosocial approach to research on successful aging. Ann Intern Med 139:391–394, 2003

Isaacs SD, Schroeder SA: Class: the ignored determinant of the nation's health. N Engl J Med 351:1137–1142, 2004

Johnson-Dalzine P, Dalzine L, Martin-Stanley CH: Fear of criminal violence and the African American elderly: assessment of a crime prevention strategy. J Negro Educ 65:462–469, 1996

Krawitz R, Watson C: Gender, race and poverty: bringing the sociopolitical into psychotherapy. Aust N Z J Psychiatry 31:474–479, 1997

Koenig HG, Weiner DK, Peterson BL, et al: Religious coping in the nursing home: a biopsychosocial model. Int J Psychiatry Med 27:365–376, 1997

Kurlowicz LH: Perceived self-efficacy, functional ability, and depressive symptoms in older elective surgery patients. Nurs Res 47:219–226, 1998

Lorig KR, Sobel DS, Ritter PL, et al: Effect of a self-management program on patients with chronic disease. Eff Clin Pract 4:256–262, 2001

Mazure CM, Maciejewski PK: A model of risk for major depression: effects of life stress and cognitive style vary by age. Depress Anxiety 17:26–33, 2003

Miranda J, Chung JY, Green BL, et al: Treating depression in predominantly low-income young minority women: a randomized controlled trial. JAMA 290:57–65, 2003

Morrison AP, Nothard S, Bowe SE, et al: Interpretations of voices in patients with hallucinations and non-patient controls: a comparison and predictors of distress in patients. Behav Res Ther 42:1315–1323, 2004

Neighbors HW, Jackson JS, Campbell L, et al: Influence of racial factors on psychiatric diagnosis: a review and suggestions for research. Community Ment Health J 25:301–311, 1989

Nezu AM, Nezu CM, Felgoise SH: Project Genesis: assessing the efficacy of problem-solving therapy for distressed adult cancer patients. J Consult Clin Psychol 71:1036–1048, 2003

Norris FH: Epidemiology of trauma: frequency and impact of different potentially traumatic events on different demographic groups. J Consult Clin Psychol 60:409–418, 1992

Prigerson HG, Bierhals AJ, Kasl SV, et al: Traumatic grief as a risk factor for mental and physical morbidity. Am J Psychiatry 154:616–623, 1997

Prigerson HG, Shear MK, Jacobs SC, et al: Consensus criteria for traumatic grief. Br J Psychiatry 174:67–73, 1999

Reynolds CF, Frank E, Perel JM, et al: Nortriptyline and interpersonal psychotherapy as maintenance therapies for recurrent major depression: a randomized controlled trial in patients older than 59 years. JAMA 281:39–45, 1999a

Reynolds CF, Miller MD, Pasternak RE, et al: Treatment of bereavement-related major depressive episodes in later life: a controlled study of acute and continuation treatment with nortriptyline and interpersonal psychotherapy. Am J Psychiatry 156:202–208 1999b

Shear MK, Frank E, Foa EB, et al: Traumatic grief therapy: a pilot study. Am J Psychiatry 158:1506–1508, 2001

Szanto K, Reynolds CF, Conwell Y, et al: High levels of hopelessness persist in geriatric patients with remitted depression and a history of suicide attempt. J Am Geriatr Soc 46:1401–1406, 1998

Szanto K, Mulsant BH, Houck P, et al: Occurrence and course of suicidality during short-term treatment of late-life depression. Arch Gen Psychiatry 60:610–617, 2003

Unutzer J, Katon W, Callahan CM, et al: Collaborative care management of late-life depression in the primary care setting: a randomized controlled trial. JAMA 288:2836–2845, 2002

Wagnild G: Resilience and successful aging: comparison among low and high income older adults. J Gerontol Nurs 29:42–49, 2003

Wagnild GM, Young HM: Development and psychometric evaluation of the Resilience Scale. J Nurs Meas 1:165–178, 1993

Wilkinson DG, Francis PT, Schwam E, et al: Cholinesterase inhibitors used in the treatment of Alzheimer's disease: the relationship between pharmacological effects and clinical efficacy. Drugs Aging 21:453–478, 2004

INDEX

Page numbers printed in **boldface** *type refer to tables or figures.*

ACTH. *See* Adrenocorticotropic hormone
AD. *See* Alzheimer's disease
ADHD. *See* Attention-deficit/hyperactivity disorder
Adjustment disorder, sex/gender ratio, **25**
Adolescents. *See also* Children; Puberty
  sex/gender disorder ratios, 23
Adrenocorticotropic hormone (ACTH), 51
Age. *See also* Adolescents; Children; Elderly
  aging-related diagnostic variations, 273–288
  diagnosis of psychopathology in infants, toddlers, and preschool children, 145–150
  validation of age-adjusted criteria for depression, 192–196
Aggression, **251–252**
Agoraphobia
  sex/gender ratio, 25
  use of services for treatment by sex, 118
Alcohol use, **13**
  brain sensitivity to, 55
  lifetime prevalence by sex, compared, 37
  sex differences in the effects of, 55
  sex/gender ratio, 24
  use of services for treatment by sex, 120
Alzheimer's disease (AD)
  biomarkers for, 317–321
  characteristics of diagnostic marker for, **318**
  in the elderly, 280
  sex/gender ratio, 24
American Academy of Child and Adolescent Psychiatry's Task Force for Research Diagnostic Criteria: Infants and Preschool, 229
American Academy of Sleep Medicine, 216
American Psychiatric Institute for Research and Education (APIRE), xvii
γ-Aminobutyric acid (GABA), 50, 86
Amnestic disorders, sex/gender ratio, **24**
Amphetamine use, sex/gender ratio, **24**
Amygdalar dysfunction, 295–296
Andropause, 105
Anhedonia, 193
Anorexia nervosa, 69–70
  prevalence in men and women, 115–116
  sex/gender ratio, **26**
  use of services for treatment by sex, 119
Antisocial personality disorder
  sex/gender disorder, **27**
  use of services for treatment by sex, 119

Anxiety disorders
diagnosis in infants, toddlers, and preschool children, 201–214
advances in developmental science, 208–210
generating a developmentally informed phenotype, 210–211
state of the science, 201–208, **203–205**
in the elderly, 281
lifetime prevalence by sex, compared, **37**
pathological, 210
sex and gender by year, 8–10, **9**
sex/gender ratio, **25**
sociocultural factors and, 66–69
studies in children less than 5 years of age, **203–205**
use of services for treatment by sex, 118
APIRE. *See* American Psychiatric Institute for Research and Education
Asperger's disorder, sex/gender ratio, **23**
Assigned sex, 85
Attention-deficit/hyperactivity disorder (ADHD), 86. *See also* Oppositional defiant disorder
diagnostic criteria in infants, toddlers, and preschool children, 149
out-of-home setting, 178–179
in preschool children, 192, 243–257
sex/gender ratio, **23**
sleep disorders and, 220
Autism, 86
advances in developmental science, 262–264
definition in DSM-IV-TR, 260
diagnosis in infants and young children, 259–270
diagnostic criteria according to DSM-IV-TR, 260–262
generating a developmentally informed phenotype, 264–267
neurobiological basis of, 264
screening procedures, 263
sex/gender ratio, **23**
state of the science, 259–262
Autism Diagnostic Interview—Revised, 183
Autism Diagnostic Observation Schedule—Generic, 183
Autistic disorder. *See* Autism
Avoidant personality disorder
prevalence of DSM-IV by sex, **38**
sex/gender ratio, **28**
studies in children less than 5 years of age, 203–205

Behavior. *See also* Disruptive behavior disorders
cognitive-behavior therapy, 121
comparison studies of neurobiology and, 57
gender and, 8
in infants, toddlers, and preschool children, 145–150
inhibition, 208–210
patterns, 249–250
preschool disruptive behavior disorders, **251–252**
research review of sleep disorders, **218–220**
sex/gender differences in childhood behavior and psychopathology, 85–86
sickness, 312
socially aberrant, 169–170
treatment-seeking, 117, 118–120
Bereavement, 330, 338–339
Biomarkers, in the elderly, 317–328
for Alzheimer's disease, **318**
gaps in knowledge in geriatric psychiatry, 323–324

in geriatric conditions other than
Alzheimer's disease, 321–323
history of, 318
research, 321–323
Bipolar disorder
case descriptions, 196
course of, 116
data on sex differences, 43
lifetime prevalence by sex, compared, **37**, 39
preliminary findings and ongoing investigations, 197–198
in preschool children, 196–198, 198–199
prevalence in men and women, 114
sex and gender by year, 8–10, **9**
sex/gender ratio, **25**
use of services for treatment by sex, 118, 119
Blood tests, as biomarkers, 319
Body dysmorphic disorder, sex/gender ratio, **25**
Borderline personality disorder, sex/gender ratio, **27**
Brain
diseases, 296
pain stimulus and, 55
sensitivity to alcohol, 55
sex differences in, 49–50
neurochemistry, 50–51
Breathing-related sleep disorder, sex/gender ratio, **26**
Bulimia nervosa, 69–70
prevalence in men and women, 115–116
sex/gender ratio, 26

Caffeine use, sex/gender ratio, **24**
Canada
diagnoses of psychiatric disorders assessment, **35**
lifetime prevalence of major depression and bipolar disorder, by sex, compared, **39**
lifetime prevalence of panic disorder, social phobia, and obsessive-compulsive disorder by sex, compared, 40
Cancer, **13**
Cannabis use, sex/gender ratio, **24**
Cardiovascular disease, **13**
in women, 11–12
CATEGO diagnostic system, 177
Center for Epidemiologic Studies Depression Scale (CES-D), 276
Centers for Disease Control, 91
Central nervous system (CNS)
degenerative, 13
late-life depression and, 291–292
Cerebrospinal fluid (CSF), as biomarkers, 319–320
CES-D. *See* Center for Epidemiologic Studies Depression Scale
Child abuse, 91–92
Child and Adolescent Psychiatric Assessment, 202
Child Behavior Checklist, 181, 182, 195
Childhood. *See also* Adolescents; Puberty
adversity, 94
developmental perspective on trauma, 81–100
development over the life span and its relation to psychopathology, 85–89
dimensions of sex/gender, 83–85
gaps in the literature and research recommendations, 93–95
importance of perspective, 81–82
sex/gender as a multidimensional developmental construct, 82–83
sex vs. gender, 82
diagnosis of psychopathology in infants, toddlers, and preschool children, 145–150
DSM-IV-TR diagnostic criteria for feeding disorder, **228**

Childhood *(continued)*
mental disorders in, xvii
role of gender in childhood trauma and risk for adult psychopathology, 89–92
sex differences in the neurobiological response to childhood adversity, 92–93
sex/gender disorder ratios, **23**
sexual development in, 86–87
temperament, 180
Children. *See also* Adolescents; Puberty
age at sex differences, 41
classification of feeding disorders of infancy and early childhood, 227–242
classification of sleep disorders in infants and toddlers, 215–226
diagnosis of anxiety disorders in infants, toddlers, and preschool children, 201–214
diagnosis of autism in infants and young children, 259–270
diagnosis of psychopathology, 145–150
disruptive behavior disorders and ADHD in preschool children, 243–257
institutionalized/post-institutionalized studies, 165–166
maltreated, 164–165
measurement of psychopathology in children under the age of 6, 177–189
nosology of mood disorders in preschool children, 191–200
reactive attachment disorder in, 163–176
research for posttraumatic stress disorder in infants, toddlers, and preschool children, 151–162
Children's Sleep Habit Questionnaire, 221
Chromosomal sex, 83
Chronic obstructive pulmonary disease (COPD), **13**
Circadian rhythm sleep disorder, sex/gender ratio, **26**
CNS. *See* Central nervous system
Cocaine use, sex/gender ratio, **24**
Cognitive-behavior therapy, 121
Cognitive impairment, use of services for treatment by sex, **119**
Color blindness, 51
Communication disorders, sex/gender ratio, **23**
Compulsive personality disorder, sex/gender ratio, **28**
Conduct disorder
diagnostic criteria, 128–129, 132–133
sex/gender ratio, 23
Congenital adrenal hyperplasia, 58
Conversion disorder, sex/gender ratio, **25**
COPD. *See* Chronic obstructive pulmonary disease
Coping style, 333
Corticotropin-releasing hormone (CRH), 49
Cortisol, 192
Creutzfeldt-Jakob disease, sex/gender ratio, **24**
CRH. *See* Corticotropin-releasing hormone
Cross-National Collaborative Group, 34, **35**
CSF. *See* Cerebrospinal fluid
Culture
assessment strategy development, 74
definition, 65
eating disorders and, 70
influences on sex differences, 41–42
personality, personality disorders, gender and, 70–73
work-related values, 68
Cyclothymic disorder, sex/gender ratio, **25**

DALYs. *See* Disability-adjusted life years
DBDs. *See* Disruptive behavior disorders
Death. *See also* Suicide
of a loved one, 331
psychiatric disorders and, 308–310
"Decathexis," 310
Delirium
in the elderly, 309–310
sex/gender ratios, 24
Delusional disorder, sex/gender disorder, **25**
Dementia, xvii, **13**
sex/gender ratio, 24
Dependent personality disorder
diagnostic criteria, 129, 133
prevalence of DSM-IV by sex, **38**
sex/gender ratio, 28
Depersonalization, sex/gender ratio, **25**
Depression, **13**
biological correlates of, 193
continuity of established nosology in young children, 193
convergent validity, 194–195
depressive subtypes, 193–194
disease burden, **14**
due to Alzheimer's disease, 278
in the elderly, xvii, 276–278
episode duration, 195
familial aggregation and impairment, 194
geriatric, 293–298
history of recognition of depressive manifestations in early childhood, 191–192
illness and, 330–331
late-life, 289–304
impact of psychosocial factors on, 329–342
treating, 338–339
limitations of data and ongoing data collection, 195
minor, 276–277
phenomenology, 193
postpartum onset, 103–104, 106–107
predisposition to, 297
in preschool children, 191–196
psychotic, 278
sex and gender by year, 8–10, **9**
social support and, 334
sociocultural factors and, 66–69
standard symptom measures, 109
validation of age-adjusted criteria for, 192–196
validation of depressive disorders in early childhood, 195–196
vascular, 278
without sadness, 277
in women, 12
Developing countries, research on eating behavior and attitudes in, 75
Developmental coordination disorder, sex/gender ratio, **23**
Developmental neuroscience, advances in, 156–159, **158**
Diabetes, **13**
Diagnostic Classification: 0–3, 182, 207–208
Diagnostic criteria, gender and, 127–137
aging-related diagnostic variations, 273–288
biases, 128
gender differences in clinical features or symptoms, 129–130
gender-neutral diagnostic criteria, 127–129
gender-related modifiers or specifiers, 130–131
gender-specific diagnostic criteria, 131–133
gender-specific disorders, 133–134
gender-specific thresholds for diagnosis, 131
lack of self-reports of symptoms, 178
resolve of issues, 134–135
sensitivity, 178
validity, 178

Diagnostic Interview Schedule for Children–DSM-IV, 182–183
Diagnostic Interview Schedule for Children–IV—Young Child, 195
Disabilities, 330
Disability-adjusted life years (DALYs), **14**
Disruptive Behavior Diagnostic Observation Schedule, 253
Disruptive behavior disorders (DBDs). *See also* Behavior
- clinical criteria, 247
- developmentally informed nosology, **251–252**
- distinctions between disorders and subtypes, 249–250
- duration criteria, 247
- generating a developmentally informed nosology, 250–254, **251–252**
- in preschool children, 243–257
- state of the science, 245–250
- symptom constellations, 245–247
- symptom definition, 247–249

Dissociative amnesia, sex/gender ratio, **25**
Dissociative disorders, 22
- sex/gender ratio, 25

Dissociative fugue, sex/gender ratio, **25**
Dissociative identity disorder, sex/gender ratio, **25**
Domestic violence, 67. *See also* Marital status
Dopamine, 298
Drugs
- sex differences in the effects of, 55
- use of services for treatment by sex, 120

DSM
- approach to gender, 19–29
- objections to DSM-style diagnoses in younger children, 179–182
- research agenda for psychiatric disorders, 41–43

DSM-I, approach to gender, 19–20
DSM-II, approach to gender, 19–20
DSM-III, late-life depression, 290
DSM-III-R, approach to gender, 21–22
DSM-IV
- approach to gender, 21–22, **38**
- definition of reactive attachment disorder, 168–170
- nosology for posttraumatic stress disorder, 152–154, **154**
- rates of posttraumatic stress disorder by DSM-IV criteria compared with alternative criteria of preschool children, 154

DSM-IV-TR
- approach to gender, 22–28, **23–28**
- definition of autism, 260
- diagnostic criteria for autism, 260–262
- diagnostic criteria for feeding disorder of infancy or early childhood, **228**
- gender differences in clinical features, 129–130
- gender-neutral diagnostic criteria, 127–129
- gender-related modifiers or specifiers, 130–131
- gender-specific diagnostic criteria, 131–133
- gender-specific disorders, 134
- measurement of psychopathology in children under the age of 6, 184–185

DSM-V. *See also* Psychiatric disorders
- research agenda, 41–43
  - on bipolar disorders, 43
  - contribution of race, ethnicity, socioeconomic, sociodemographic, and other risk factors to sex differences in psychiatric disorders, 42
  - coverage of psychiatric disorders assessed, 42–43

cross-cultural epidemiological studies, 41–42
design and analysis, 41
on identification of gender-biased diagnostic criteria, 43
impact of social and cultural traumatic events on gender differences, 42
longitudinal surveys of children and adolescents, 41
on personality disorders, 43
Duchenne muscular dystrophy, 51
Dyspareunia, sex/gender ratio, **27**
Dyssomnia
sleep onset, in toddlers and preschoolers, **223**
in toddlers and preschoolers, 222
Dysthymic disorder
in the elderly, 277
lifetime prevalence by sex, compared, **37**
sex/gender ratio, **25**
use of services for treatment by sex, 119

Eating disorders
cultural aspects of, 69–70
definition, 70
immigration and, 70
prevalence in men and women, 115–116
risk factors for development of, 75
sex/gender ratio, 23, 26
ECA. *See* Epidemiologic Catchment Area Study
Elderly
age-related research agenda, 282–284
epidemiology, 282
etiology, 283
pathophysiology, 283
symptomatology, 282–283
treatment, 283–284
aging-related diagnostic variations, 273–288
causes of diagnostic confusion, 274–275
physical and psychiatric comorbidity, 274–275
subthreshold presentations, 275
true age-related differences, 274
underreporting of symptoms, 275
variation through time of onset, 275
depression in, xvii
diagnosing psychiatric disorders in medically ill patients, 305–315
disorders associated with diagnostic confusion, 276–282
anxiety disorders, 281
late-onset schizoaffective disorder, 280
mood disorders, 276–278
psychosis of Alzheimer's disease, 280
schizophrenia, 278–280
substance use disorders, 281–282
late-life depression, 289–304
impact of psyhosocial factors on, 329–342
use of biomarkers in, 317–328
Elimination disorders, sex/gender ratio, **23**
Emotional support, 332–333
Encopresis, sex/gender ratio, **23**
Endophenotypic markers, 321–322
Enuresis, sex/gender ratio, **23**
Environment
gender and, 8
genes and, 13
importance of neurobiological/environmental interactions, 73–74
women's vs. men's exposure to, 8

Epidemiologic Catchment Area (ECA) Study, 32–33, 117, **32**
 lifetime prevalence of psychiatric disorders by sex, compared, **37**
 sex differences in psychiatric disorders assessment, 34, 36, 37, 38
Erectile disorder, **27**
Estradiol, 49
Estrogen, 54
Ethnicity, 42
Exercise. *See* Physical activity
Exhibitionism, sex/gender ratio, **27**
Expressive language disorder, sex/gender ratio, **23**

Factitious disorder, sex/gender ratio, **25**
Feeding disorders
 advances in understanding, 228–229
 associated with a concurrent medical condition, 237
  proposed diagnostic criteria, 237
  research findings, 237
 associated with lack of parent–infant reciprocity, 232–233
  proposed diagnostic criteria, 232
  research findings, 232–233
 Chatoor classification and previously cited terminology, 230–231
 classification of feeding disorders of infancy and early childhood, 227–242
 comorbidity between subtypes, 237–238
 DSM-IV-TR diagnostic criteria of infancy or early childhood, 228
 generating developmentally informed phenotypes, 229, 232–237
 sex/gender ratio, 23
 state of the science, 227–228, 230–231, 228
 of state regulation, 229, 232
  proposed diagnostic criteria, 229
  research findings, 232
 subtypes, 229, 232–237
 validating diagnoses, 238–239
Fetal alcohol syndrome, 169

Fetishism, sex/gender ratio, 27
Food. *See* Feeding disorders
Food neophobia. *See* Feeding disorders
Fragile X syndrome, 51
France
 diagnoses of psychiatric disorders assessment, **35**
 lifetime prevalence of major depression and bipolar disorder, by sex, compared, **39**
 lifetime prevalence of panic disorder, social phobia, and obsessive-compulsive disorder by sex, compared, 40
Frontostriatal dysfunction, 293–295
Frotteurism, sex/gender ratio, **27**
Functional dysphagia. *See* Feeding disorders
Functional magnetic resonance imaging, 49

GABA. *See* γ-Aminobutyric acid
GABAergic neurotransmission, 55
GAD. *See* Generalized anxiety disorder
Gambling. *See* Pathological gambling
Gender. *See also* Sex/gender
 acute/chronic stress and, 58
 comparison studies of neurobiology and behavior, 57
 definition, 10
 diagnostic criteria, 127–137
  biases, 128
  gender differences in clinical features or symptoms, 129–130
  gender-neutral diagnostic criteria, 127–129
  gender-related modifiers or specifiers, 130–131

gender-specific diagnostic criteria, 131–133
gender-specific disorders, 133–134
gender-specific thresholds for diagnosis, 131
resolve of issues, 134–135
experimental design development, 56–57
research, 141–142
sex vs. gender in childhood development, 82
sociocultural factors and, 70–73
specificity of differences, 59
Gender identity, sex/gender ratio, **27**
Generalized anxiety disorder (GAD)
diagnosis in infants, toddlers, and preschool children, 207
lifetime prevalence by sex, compared, 37
sex/gender ratio, 25
studies in children less than 5 years of age, 203–205
Genes. *See also* Sensory food aversions
as biomarkers, 319
environment interaction and, 13
as factor in diagnosis of anxiety disorders in infants, toddlers, and preschool children, 208
genetic sex, 83–84
parent-of-origin effects, 52
sex differences in genetic vulnerability, 51–52
sex-specific traits, 52
X-linked traits, 51
Y-linked traits, 52
Genital sex, 84–85
Geriatric depression, 293–298. *See also* Late-life depression
amygdalar dysfunction, 295–296
etiology, 297
frontostriatal dysfunction, 293–295
hippocampal dysfunction, 296
mechanisms of the depressive syndrome, 296–297
treatment implications, 297–298
Geriatric syndromes, 311–312
Germany
diagnoses of psychiatric disorders assessment, 35
lifetime prevalence of major depression and bipolar disorder, by sex, compared, 39
lifetime prevalence of panic disorder, social phobia, and obsessive-compulsive disorder by sex, compared, 40
Global Burden of Disease study, 12, **14**
Gonadal sex, 84
Gonadal steroids, regulation, 58
G6PD deficiency, 51

Hallucinogen use, sex/gender ratio, **24**
Hamilton Depression Rating Scale, 109
Harrison's Principles of Internal Medicine, 290
Head trauma, sex/gender ratio, **24**
Health research, gender differences and, 11–12
Heart attack, symptoms, 12
Hemophilia, 51
Hippocampal dysfunction, 296
Histrionic personality disorder
prevalence of DSM-IV by sex, **38**
sex/gender ratio, 27
HIV, sex/gender ratio, **24**
Hobbies, gender and, 8
Hospice, role of, 308
HPA. *See* Hypothalamic-pituitary-adrenal axis function
HPG. *See* Hypothalamic-pituitary-gonadal axis
Huntington's disease, sex/gender ratio, **24**
Hypersomnia, sex/gender ratio, **26**
Hypochondriasis, sex/gender ratio, **25**

Hypomania, lifetime prevalence by sex, compared, **37**
Hypothalamic-pituitary-adrenal (HPA) axis function, 67, 86, 92
as biomarker, 322
in preschool children, 192
Hypothalamic-pituitary-gonadal (HPG) axis, 86

Illness
clinical validators of diagnoses, 113–125
course of, 116
diagnosing psychiatric disorders in medically ill elderly patients, 305–315
disability from, 330
importance of sex/gender in nonpsychiatric illness, 11–12
mental disorders as causes of medical morbidity, 312–313
onset of depression and, 330–331
phenomenology, 114–116
predictive validity evaluation, 108
research agenda for clinical validators of diagnoses, 121–122
sex differences in physiology and vulnerability to, 54–55
treatment response, 117, 121
treatment-seeking behavior, 117, 118–120
Immigration, eating disorders and, 70
IMPACT. *See* Improving Mood—Promoting Access to Collaborative Treatment
Impairment, 183–184
Improving Mood—Promoting Access to Collaborative Treatment (IMPACT), 338
Impulse-control disorders, sex/gender ratio, **27**
Individualism, 68
Infancy. *See also* Toddlers
classification of feeding disorders in, 227–242
classification of sleep disorders in, 215–226
diagnosis of anxiety disorders in, 201–214
diagnosis of autism and related disorders, 259–270
diagnosis of psychopathology, 145–150
DSM-IV-TR diagnostic criteria for feeding disorder, **228**
failure to thrive. See Feeding disorders
research for posttraumatic stress disorder, 151–162
sex/gender disorder ratios, 23
Infant and Young Child Diagnostic Work Group, 145–146
Infantile anorexia, 233–235
proposed diagnostic criteria, 233
research findings, 233–235
Infant-Toddler Social and Emotional Assessment, 182
Inhalant use, sex/gender ratio, **24**
Inhibition, 208–210
Insomnia. *See also* Sleep disorders
sex/gender ratio, 26
Institute of Medicine (IOM), 7, 140, 142
recommendations, 7–8
International Consortium of Psychiatric Epidemiology, 34
IOM. *See* Institute of Medicine
Irritable bowel syndrome, 55
Ischemic heart disease, **13**
SOX9, 49
SRY, 49
Italy
diagnoses of psychiatric disorders assessment, **35**
lifetime prevalence of major depression and bipolar disorder, by sex, compared, **39**

lifetime prevalence of panic disorder, social phobia, and obsessive-compulsive disorder by sex, compared, 40

Kiddie Schedule for Affective Disorders and Schizophrenia, 182–183
Kleptomania, sex/gender ratio, **27**
Klinefelter syndrome, 83
Korea
diagnoses of psychiatric disorders assessment, **35**
lifetime prevalence of major depression and bipolar disorder, by sex, compared, **39**
lifetime prevalence of panic disorder, social phobia, and obsessive-compulsive disorder by sex, compared, 40

Late-life depression, 289–304. *See also* Geriatric depression
DSM-III and, 290
impact of psychosocial factors on, 329–342
implications for geriatric psychiatric syndromes other than depression, 298–299
medical classification, 290–292, **292**
model, **292**
psychosocial risk factors, 330–333
research, 299–300, 336
research on psychosocial risk factors of late-life mental illness, 335–339
detection of at-risk patients, 335–337
prediction of onset, maintenance, and offset of late-life mental illness, 337–338
treating late-life depression, 338–339
Late luteal-phase dysphoric disorder (LLPDD), 21–22
Late paraphrenia, 279
Learning disorders, sex/gender ratio, **23**
Lebanon
diagnoses of psychiatric disorders assessment, **35**
lifetime prevalence of major depression and bipolar disorder, by sex, compared, **39**
lifetime prevalence of panic disorder, social phobia, and obsessive-compulsive disorder by sex, compared, 40
Lewy body dementia, 298–299
LHRH. *See* Luteinizing hormone releasing hormone
Life span
approach in psychiatry, 105–107
lifelong implications of pregnancy, 107–108
Lifestyle, gender and, 8
LLPDD. *See* Late luteal-phase dysphoric disorder; Premenstrual dysphoric disorder
Luteinizing hormone releasing hormone (LHRH), 86

Magnetic resonance imaging (MRI), as biomarker, 320
Major depressive disorder (MDD)
lifetime prevalence by sex, compared, **37, 39**
in preschool children, 192
prevalence in men and women, 114–115
sex/gender ratio, **25**
use of services for treatment by sex, 118
Malnutrition, 239. *See also* Feeding disorders
Mania
case descriptions, 196
developmental issues, 197

Mania *(continued)*
measurement development, 197
preliminary findings and ongoing investigations, 197–198
in preschool children, 196–198
Marital status, 65–66. *See also* Domestic violence
conflict, 67
distressed marital couples, 66–67
evaluation of gender differences, 74
Masculinity, 68
Masters and Johnson diagnostic criteria, 134
Maternal deprivation. *See* Feeding disorders
MDD. *See* Major depressive disorder
MDI. *See* Mental Developmental Index
Mediator, 283–284
Memory, **158**
Men
andropause, 105
male erectile disorder, **27**
natural killer cell activity in, 11
premature ejaculation, **27**
with schizophrenia, 16
suicide rates, 69
use of services for mental and addictive problems by disorder and sex, **118–120**
vs. women seeking treatment, 117, 118–120
Menopause, 89, 104–105
Menstruation, menstrual-cycle timing, 109
Mental Developmental Index (MDI), 234
Mental disorders
as causes of medical morbidity, 312–313
in childhood, xvii
definition, 305
in the elderly, xvii, 311–312
impact and role of gender on diagnosis of, 134–135
use of services for treatment by sex, 119
Mental retardation, sex/gender ratio, **23**
Mixed language disorder, sex/gender ratio, **23**
Moderator, 283
Mood disorders
in the elderly, 276–278
lifetime prevalence by sex, compared, **37**
nosology in preschool children, 191–200
sex/gender ratio, **25**
use of services for treatment by sex, 118
MRI. *See* Magnetic resonance imaging
Mutism, sex/gender ratio, **23**

Narcissistic personality disorder, sex/gender ratio, **27**
Narcolepsy, sex/gender disorder, **26**
National Comorbidity Survey (NCS), 33, **32**
lifetime prevalence of psychiatric disorders by sex, compared, **37**
sex differences in psychiatric disorders assessment, 34, 36, 38, **37**
National Epidemiologic Survey on Alcohol and Related Conditions (NESARC), 33, 32
lifetime prevalence of psychiatric disorders by sex, compared, **37**
prevalence of DSM-IV personality disorders by sex, **38**
sex differences in psychiatric disorders assessment, 34, 36, 37, 38
National Institute of Mental Health (NIMH), xv
National Institute on Alcohol Abuse and Alcoholism (NIAAA), xv

National Institute on Drug Abuse (NIDA), xv
National Institutes of Health, xv
National Institutes of Health Roadmap, 105, 110
National Violence Against Women Survey, 92
NCS. *See* National Comorbidity Survey
NEO Personality Inventory—Revised (NEO PI-R), 71
NEO PI-R. *See* NEO Personality Inventory—Revised
NESARC. *See* National Epidemiologic Survey on Alcohol and Related Conditions
Neurobiology
 of autism, 264
 comparison studies of behavior and, 57
 importance of neurobiological/environmental interactions, 73–74
 literature gaps and proposed research agenda, 55–59
 neuroanatomic sex differences, 57
 sex differences
  in brain neurochemistry, 50–51
  in the effects of drugs and alcohol, 55
  in genetic vulnerability, 51–52
  in the neurobiological response to childhood adversity, 92–93
  in physiology and vulnerability to medical illness and pain, 54–55
  in stress responses, 52–54
 sex/gender and, 47–63
  mechanisms of sexual differentiation, 48–49
  sex differences in brain anatomy, 49–50
Neuroimaging, as biomarkers, 320–321
Neuroplasticity, 173
New Zealand
 diagnoses of psychiatric disorders assessment, **35**
 lifetime prevalence of major depression and bipolar disorder, by sex, compared, **39**
 lifetime prevalence of panic disorder, social phobia, and obsessive-compulsive disorder by sex, compared, 40
See National Institute on Alcohol Abuse and Alcoholism
Nicotine use, sex/gender ratio, **24**
NIDA. *See* National Institute on Drug Abuse
Nightmare disorder, sex/gender ratio, **26**
NIMH. *See* National Institute of Mental Health
Nursing home care, 310

Obsessive-compulsive disorder (OCD), 36
 lifetime prevalence by sex, compared, **40**
 prevalence of DSM-IV by sex, **38**
 sex/gender ratio, **25**
 use of services for treatment by sex, 118
Occupation, gender and, 8
OCD. *See* Obsessive-compulsive disorder
ODD. *See* Oppositional defiant disorder
Opioid use, sex/gender ratio, **24**
Oppositional defiant disorder (ODD). *See also* Attention-deficit/hyperactivity disorder
 validation of age-adjusted criteria, 192
Oppositional defiant disorder (ODD), sex/gender ratio, **23**
Orientation, long-term vs. short-term, 68
Osteoarthritis, **13**

Overanxious disorder, studies in children less than 5 years of age, **203–205**
Oxytocin system, 51

Pain disorder
sex differences in physiology and vulnerability to, 54–55
sex/gender ratio, 25
Palliative care, 309
Panic disorders
lifetime prevalence by sex, compared, **37, 40**
sex/gender ratio, 25
use of services for treatment by sex, 118
PAPA. *See* Preschool Age Psychiatric Assessment
Paranoid personality disorder
prevalence of DSM-IV by sex, **38**
sex/gender ratio, 27
Parent–child relationship, 146. *See also* Sleep disorders
diagnosis of anxiety disorders in infants, toddlers, and preschool children, 206
feeding disorder associated with lack of reciprocity, 232–233
parental role in diagnosing psychopathology in infants, toddlers, and preschool children, 149
Parent-of-origin effects, 52
Parkinson's disease, 296
sex/gender ratio, 24
Pathological gambling, sex/gender ratio, **27**
PDD. *See* Pervasive developmental disorder
Pedophilia, sex/gender ratio, **27**
Personality
assessment of, 72
five-factor model, 70–71
sociocultural factors, gender and, 70–73
Personality disorders, 22
epidemiological research, 43
lifetime prevalence by sex, compared, **37**
prevalence of DSM-IV disorders by sex from NESARC, **38**
sex/gender ratio, **27–28**
sociocultural factors, gender and, 70–73
Pervasive developmental disorder (PDD), 163, 169, 259. *See also* Autism
sex/gender ratio, 23
PET. *See* Positron emission tomography
Phencyclidine use, sex/gender ratio, **24**
Phobias
studies in children less than 5 years of age, **203–205**
use of services for treatment by sex, 118
Phonological disorder, sex/gender ratio, **23**
Physical activity, gender and, 8
Pica, sex/gender disorder, **23**
Pick's disease, sex/gender ratio, **24**
Picky eating. *See* Feeding disorders
Plasticity, 171–172, 173
Polycystic ovarian syndrome, 58
Positron emission tomography (PET), 49–50, 55, 283
as biomarker, 320
Postpartum-onset depression, 103–104, 106–107
DSM definition, 109
Posttraumatic feeding disorder, 236
proposed diagnostic criteria, 236
research findings, 236
Posttraumatic stress disorder (PTSD), 91
advances in developmental neuroscience, 156–159, **158**
DSM-IV symptomatology, 152–153

measurement of symptomatology in young children, 154–155
nosology for, 151–156, **154–156**
phenomenology, 155–156, **156**
rates by DSM-IV criteria compared with alternative criteria of preschool children, **154**
research for validation, 159–160
research in infants, toddlers, and preschool children, 151–162
sex/gender ratio, **25**
symptomatology, **156**
in women, 12–13, 67
Power-distance, 68
Pregnancy
lifelong implications of, 107–108
postpartum-onset depression, 103–104
Premenstrual dysphoric disorder, 22, 103
Preschool Age Psychiatric Assessment (PAPA), 147, 183, 195, 197, 202, 253
Preschool children
bipolar disorder in, 196–198
depression, 191–196
diagnosis of anxiety disorders in, 201–214
diagnosis of psychopathology, 145–150
disruptive behavior disorders in, 243–257
mania in, 196–198
night waking dyssomnia, **222**
nosology of mood disorders in, 191–200
rates of posttraumatic stress disorder by DSM-IV criteria compared with alternative criteria of preschool children, **154**
research for posttraumatic stress disorder, 151–162
sleep onset dyssomnia, 223
Present State Examination, 177
Prevention of Suicide in Primary Care Elderly: Collaborative Trial (PROSPECT), 338
Progesterone, 54
Progressive supranuclear palsy (PSP), 299
PROSPECT. *See* Prevention of Suicide in Primary Care Elderly: Collaborative Trial
PSP. *See* Progressive supranuclear palsy
Psychiatric disorders. *See also* DSM-V
clinical validators of diagnoses, 113–125
course of, 116
coverage in representative samples of the general population, 42–43
determinants of gender differences in psychopathology, 38, 41
diagnosing psychiatric disorders in medically ill elderly patients, 305–315
context-dependent mental disorders, 307–311
limits of parsimony, 306–307
dying and, 308–310
epidemiological surveys of the general population, **32, 35,** 32–34
gender and prevalence of, 31–45
geriatric syndromes and mental disorders, 311–312
lifetime prevalence by sex, compared, **37**
model for late-life, **292**
phenomenology, 114–116
psychiatric health outcomes, 110
research agenda
for clinical validators of diagnoses, 121–122
for DSM-V and beyond, 41–43
for the elderly, 313
risk factors to sex differences, 42
sex differences as assessed in the ECA, NCS, and NESARC, 34, 36, **39, 40**

Psychiatric disorders *(continued)*
sociocultural influences development, 74–75
treatment response, 117, 121
treatment-seeking behavior, 117, 118–120
Psychiatry
classification systems, 140
life span approach to, 105–107
sex and gender disorders by year, 8–10, 9
Psychopathology
according to DSM-IV, 170
determinants of gender differences in, 38, 41
development of sex/gender over the life span and its relation to psychopathology, 85–89
diagnosis in infants, toddlers, and preschool children, 145–150
importance of sex/gender in, 12–13, 14, **13**
measurement in children under the age of 6, 177–189
available measures, 182–183
impairment and, 183–184
lack of a standard out-of-home setting, 178–179
lack of self-reports of symptoms, 178
objections to DSM-style diagnoses in younger children, 179–182
role of gender in childhood trauma and risk for adult psychopathology, 89–92
sex/gender differences in childhood behavior and, 85–86
Psychosocial factors, impact on late-life depression, 329–342
Psychotic depression, 278
Psychotic disorders, sex/gender ratio, 25
PTSD. *See* Posttraumatic stress disorder
Puberty, 87–88. *See also* Adolescents; Childhood
cyclical effects, 88
level effects, 88
studies of psychiatric illnesses and, 109–110
timing effects, 87–88
transition effects, 88
Puerto Rico
diagnoses of psychiatric disorders assessment, **35**
lifetime prevalence of major depression and bipolar disorder, by sex, compared, **39**
lifetime prevalence of panic disorder, social phobia, and obsessive-compulsive disorder by sex, compared, **40**
Pyromania, sex/gender ratio, **27**

Race, 42
RAD. *See* Reactive attachment disorder
RDC. *See* Research Diagnostic Criteria
Reactive attachment disorder (RAD), 163–176. *See also* Feeding disorders
advances in developmental psychopathology of, 164–167
construct validity, 166–167
in school-age children, 167
studies of institutionalized and post-institutionalized children, 165–166
studies of maltreated children, 164–165
case studies, 164
current state of the science, 163–164
DSM-IV definition, 168–170
phenotype for, 167–170
research, 170–172
Reproductive status
gender and, 8

study of effects of, 57–58
in women, 101–112
research opportunities and a research agenda, 108–110
women with psychiatric episodes and reproductive events, 108–109
Research
approach, 15–16
in both genders, 110
on clinical features, 141
for clinical validators of diagnoses, 121–122
developmental perspective on childhood trauma, 93–95
on diagnosis of psychiatric disorders in medically ill elderly patients, 313
on diagnosis of psychopathology in infants, toddlers, and preschool children, 145–150
on gender, 141–142
impact and role of gender on diagnosis of mental disorders, 134–135
for late-life depression, 299–300
life course epidemiology approach, 15–16
for posttraumatic stress disorder in infants, toddlers, and preschool children, 151–162
on psychosocial risk factors of late-life mental illness, 335–339
on reactive attachment disorder, 163–176
sex/gender, 8–10, 9
in sociocultural factors and gender, 74–76
in women's reproductive health, 108–110
A Research Agenda for DSM-V, xvi
Research Diagnostic Criteria—Preschool Age, 206–207
Research diagnostic criteria (RDC), 221
Respiratory sinus arrhythmia (RSA), 157, **158**
Rett's disorder, sex/gender ratio, **23**
Rickets, 51
RSA. *See* Respiratory sinus arrhythmia
Rumination, sex/gender ratio, **23**

SARS. *See* Severe acute respiratory syndrome
Schedule for Affective Disorders and Schizohrenia, Epidemiological Version, 196
Schedule for Affective Disorders and Schizophrenia for School-Age Children, 253
Schizoaffective disorder
in the elderly, 280
sex/gender ratio, **25**
Schizoid personality disorder
prevalence of DSM-IV by sex, **38**
sex/gender ratio, 27
Schizophrenia
course of, 116
diagnostic criteria, 130
in the elderly, 278–280
in men, 16
neurobiological research, 321–323
prevalence in men and women, 114
sex and gender by year, 8–10, **9**
sex/gender ratio, **25**
use of services for treatment by sex, **119**
in women, 15–16, 102, 130
Schizophreniform disorder, sex/gender ratio, **25**
Schizotypal personality disorder, sex/gender ratio, **27**
School-age children, reactive attachment disorder in, 167
Sedative use, sex/gender ratio, **24**
Sensory food aversions, 235–236
proposed diagnostic criteria, 235
research findings, 235–236
Separation anxiety disorder
sex/gender ratio, **23**
studies in children less than 5 years of age, **203–205**

Severe acute respiratory syndrome (SARS), 291
Sex
  assigned, 85
  chromosomal, 83
  definition, 10
  genetic, 83–84
  genital, 84–85
  gonadal, 84
Sex dimorphisms, 54
Sex/gender
  childhood adverse experiences and psychopathological outcome, 94
  childhood adversity, 94
  definition, 10–11
  developmental perspective on childhood trauma, 81–100
  development over the life span and its relation to psychopathology, 85–89
  diagnostic criteria, 127–137
  differences in childhood behavior and psychopathology, 85–86
  dimensions of, 83–85
  DSM-IV-TR focus on gender ratios, 22, 24, 26, 28
  DSM's approach to gender, 19–29
  empirical identification of gender-biased diagnostic criteria, 43
  environment and, 8
  importance in nonpsychiatric illness, 11–12
  importance in psychopathology, 12–13, **13**, **14**
  importance of gender in illness and psychopathology, 7–8
  journals for sex- and gender-specific effects, 10
  mental health research, 8–10, 9
  as a multidimensional childhood developmental construct, 82–83
  multidimensional developmental approach to the role of, 94–95
  neurobiology and, 47–63
  overview, 3–6
  prevalence of psychiatric disorders and, 31–45
  psychiatric disorders by year, **9**
  research approach, 15–16
    in both genders, 110
  role in childhood trauma and risk for adult psychopathology, 89–92
  sex vs. gender in childhood development, 82
  sociocultural factors, 65–79
  use of services for mental and addictive problems by disorder and sex, 117, **118–120**
  variable partitioning, 103
Sex hormones, 54
Sex steroids, stress and, 94
Sexual behavior, definition, 11
Sexual desire, definition, 11
Sexual development
  in adulthood, 89
  in childhood, 86–87
  in puberty, 87–88
Sexual differentiation, 48–49
Sexual dimorphism, 91
Sexual disorders, sex/gender ratio, 27
Sexual identity, definition, 11
Sexual masochism, sex/gender ratio, 27
Sexual orientation, definition, 11
Sexual sadism, sex/gender ratio, 27
Single-photon emission computed tomography (SPECT), 283
SLE. *See* Systemic lupus erythematosus
Sleep disorders. *See also* Parent–child relationship
  classification in infants and toddlers, 215–226
    advances in developmental sciences, 217, 221, **218–220**

developmentally informed genotype, 221–222, **222**, **223**
research agenda and recommendations, 222–225
state of the science, 215–217
night waking dyssomnia in toddlers and preschoolers, 222
research, 224–225
research review, **218–220**
sex/gender ratio, **26**
sleep onset dyssomnia in toddlers and preschoolers, **223**
Sleep terror disorder, sex/gender ratio, **26**
Sleepwalking disorder, sex/gender ratio,**26**
Smoking. *See* Nicotine use
Social isolation, 330
Social phobia
diagnosis in infants, toddlers, and preschool children, 209–210
lifetime prevalence by sex, compared, **37**, **40**
studies in children less than 5 years of age, **203–205**
use of services for treatment by sex, **118**
Socioculture, 65–79
anxiety disorders and, 66–69
cultural aspects of eating disorders, 69–70
depression and, 66–69
etiological models of DSM-defined disorders, 74
gender and, 70–73
literature gaps and recommended research agenda, 74–76
personality and, 70–73
personality disorders and, 70–73
research on effect on personality disorders, 75
suicide and, 66–69
Socioeconomic status, 332, 335
Somatization disorder, 128
gender-neutral diagnostic criteria, 129
gender-specific threshold for diagnosis, 131
sex/gender ratio, **25**
use of services for treatment by sex, **119**
Somatoform disorders, sex/gender ratio, **25**
SPECT. *See* Single-photon emission computed tomography
Spitz, Rene, 191–192
Steroids, 12
sexual differentiation and, 48–49
stress response systems and sex steroids, 94
Stress
gender and, 58
sex differences in response to, 52–54
sex/gender-specific effects of life events and, 94
sex steroids and, 94
vulnerability to, 90–91
Stroke, 296
Stuttering, sex/gender ratio, **23**
Substance-related disorders
in the elderly, 281–282
lifetime prevalence by sex, compared, 37
sex/gender ratio, 24
Suicide. *See also* Death
gender differences in, 67–68
in late-life depression, 339
in men, 69
rates, 69
sociocultural factors and, 66–69
in women, 69
Sympathetic nervous system, 53
Systemic lupus erythematosus (SLE), in women, 11

Taiwan
diagnoses of psychiatric disorders assessment, **35**
lifetime prevalence of major depression and bipolar disorder, by sex, compared, **39**

Taiwan *(continued)*
lifetime prevalence of panic disorder, social phobia, and obsessive-compulsive disorder by sex, compared, **40**
Tanner stage, 88
Taste aversion. *See* Feeding disorders
Temperament, 208, **251–252**
Testotoxicosis, 52
Tic disorders, sex/gender ratio, **23**
Toddlers. *See also* Infancy
classification of sleep disorders in, 215–226
diagnosis of anxiety disorders in, 201–214
diagnosis of psychopathology, 145–150
night waking dyssomnia, **222**
research for posttraumatic stress disorder, 151–162
sleep onset dyssomnia, **223**
Tourette's disorder, sex/gender ratio, **23**
Toxins, exposure to, 7–8
Traffic accidents, **13**
Transvestic fetishism, sex/gender disorder, **27**
Trauma, 331
impact on gender differences in rates of disorders, 42
Trichotillomania, sex/gender ratio, **27**
Turner syndrome, 83

Uncertainty–avoidance, 68
United States
diagnoses of psychiatric disorders assessment, **35**
lifetime prevalence of major depression and bipolar disorder, by sex, compared, **39**
lifetime prevalence of panic disorder, social phobia, and obsessive-compulsive disorder by sex, compared, **40**

Vagal tone, 157
Vaginismus, **27**
Vasopressin-producing neurons, 51
Vineland Adaptive Behavior Scales, 194
Voyeurism, sex/gender disorder, **27**

White papers. *See A Research Agenda for DSM-V*
WHO. *See* World Health Organization
Williams syndrome, 169, 172
Wilms tumor, 84
Women
cardiovascular disease in, 11–12
depression in, 12
female orgasmic disorder, **27**
female sexual arousal, **27**
lifelong implications of pregnancy, 107–108
menopause, 89, 104–105
vs. men seeking treatment, 117, **118–120**
posttraumatic stress disorder in, 12–13, 67, 106–107
with psychiatric episodes and reproductive events, 108–109
reproductive health, 101–112
with schizophrenia, 15–16, 102, 130
suicide rates, 69
symptoms of heart attack, 12
systemic erythematosus lupus in, 11
use of services for mental and addictive problems by disorder and sex, **118–120**
vaginismus, **27**
World Health Organization (WHO), xvii
World Mental Health Study 2000, 34

X-linked traits, 51

Y-linked traits, 52